BINDING PROTEIN

Edited by **Kotb Abdelmohsen**

Binding Protein
http://dx.doi.org/10.5772/2897
Edited by Kotb Abdelmohsen

Contributors
Magda Reyes-López, Jesús Serrano-Luna, Carolina Piña-Vázquez, Mireya de la Garza, Jennifer L. Bath, Amber E. Ferris, Elif Ozkirimli Olmez, Berna Sariyar Akbulut, Kate A. Redgrove, R. John Aitken, Brett Nixon, Kotb Abdelmohsen, Monde Ntwasa, Minoru Takahashi, Daisuke Iwaki, Yuichi Endo, Teizo Fujita, Daniel Beisang, Paul R. Bohjanen, Irina A. Vlasova-St. Louis

Published by InTech
Janeza Trdine 9, 51000 Rijeka, Croatia

Publishing Process Manager Dragana Manestar
Technical Editor InTech Prepress, Novi Sad
Cover InTech Design team

Additional hard copies can be obtained from orders@intechopen.com

Binding Protein, Edited by Kotb Abdelmohsen
p. cm.
ISBN 978-953-51-0758-3

For EU product safety concerns:
IN TECH d.o.o., Prolaz Marije Krucifikse Kozulić 3, 51000 Rijeka, Croatia,
info@intechopen.com or visit our website at intechopen.com.

Meet the editor

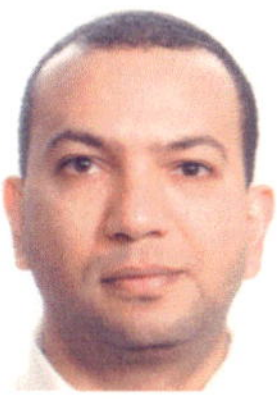

Kotb Abdelmohsen was born in Egypt. He studied at Ain Shams University, Cairo, Egypt, where he received a B.Sc. degree in chemistry and biochemistry in 1995-1996. From 1996 to 2000, he joined the Biochemistry department at Oslo University, Norway, where he received a master degree in biochemistry. From 2000 to 2003, he was a Fellow at Heinrich Heine University (Duesseldorf), Germany, school of medicine, where he received a Ph.D. degree in biochemistry. From 2004 to 2009 he was a post-doc at the National Institutes of Health (NIH), National Institutes on Aging. Currently he is a Staff Scientist at the NIH. For several years his work focused on the mechanisms that regulate gene expression patterns under different conditions including cell damage and diseases such as cancer. He is particularly interested in post-transcriptional processes, mRNA turnover and translation. His studies include global and gene-specific analyses of mRNA stability and translation, the identification of target RNA sequences associated with RNA-binding proteins (RBPs) that modulate mRNA stability and translation, the elucidation of the functions of RBP function in response to stress agents and proliferative signals, the investigation of microRNAs (miRNAs), and long non-coding RNAs (lncRNAs) that modulate gene expression, cell proliferation, replicative senescence, and aging.

Contents

Preface

Proteins are the driving force for all cellular processes. They regulate several cellular events through binding to different partners in the cell. They are capable of binding to other proteins, peptides, DNA, and also RNA. These interactions are essential in the regulation of cell fates and could be important in drugs development. For example RNA interacting proteins regulate gene expression through the binding to different mRNAs. These mRNAs could be involved in important cellular processes such as cell survival or apoptosis. This book contains review articles dealing with protein interactions with the above mentioned factors. The enclosed articles could be informative and stimulating for readers interested in protein binding partners and the consequences of such interactions.

Kotb Abdelmohsen, PhD
Laboratory of Molecular Biology and Immunology National Institute on Aging,
National Institutes of Health Biomedical Research Center
USA

Chapter 1

Transferrin Binding Proteins as a Means to Obtain Iron in Parasitic Protozoa

Magda Reyes-López, Jesús Serrano-Luna,
Carolina Piña-Vázquez and Mireya de la Garza

Additional information is available at the end of the chapter

http://dx.doi.org/10.5772/48288

1. Introduction

Iron is the fourth most abundant element on Earth and is essential for almost all living organisms. However, it is not accessible to cells in every environment. Ferric iron solubility is low at physiological pH, and in aerobic environments, ferrous iron is highly toxic. Thus, iron is not free but bound to proteins [Clarke *et al.*, 2001; Taylor and Kelly, 2010]. In complex organisms, the majority of iron is intracellularly sequestered within heme-compounds or iron-containing proteins or is stored in ferritin.

Extracellular ferric iron is bound to lactoferrin (LF) and transferrin (TF). Lactoferrin is found mainly in secretions such as milk, saliva, mucosal secretions, and other secretory fluids. TF is the iron transporter that allows cellular iron uptake. Additionally, TF and LF maintain Fe^{3+} in a soluble and stable oxidation state, avoiding the generation of toxic free radicals through the Fenton reaction ($Fe^{2+} + H_2O_2 \rightarrow Fe^{3+}$ OH^- + OH), which are deleterious to most macromolecules [Clarke *et al.*, 2001; Wandersman and Delepelaire, 2004; Halliwell and Gutteridge, 2007; Gkouvatsos *et al.*, 2012].

1.1. Transferrin and the transferrin receptor: An overview

TF is mainly found in serum and lymph. It binds two atoms of Fe^{3+} with high affinity (Ka of 10^{-23} M). TF is a single-chain glycoprotein with a molecular mass of approximately 80 kDa and two homologous lobes. Its saturation is indicative of body iron stores; under normal conditions, only 30% of the TF iron-binding sites are saturated. TF and LF maintain the free iron concentration at approximately 10^{-18} M in body fluids, a concentration too low to sustain bacteria and parasite growth [Bullen, 1981]. The relative low TF saturation and high affinity for iron allows TF to maintain a low iron concentration in the serum, thus acting as the first line of defense against infections in that fluid by preventing invading microorganisms from acquiring the iron essential for their growth [Kaplan, 2002; Wandersman and Delepelaire, 2004; Halliwell and Gutteridge, 2007; Gkouvatsos *et al.*, 2012].

Virtually all cells express a transferrin receptor (TFR) on their surface; the quantity of receptor molecules reflects the cellular iron requirement. Human TFR (*Hs*TFR) is a glycoprotein of 180 kDa formed by two disulfide-bonded homodimers. The TFR/TF complex is endocytosed inside clathrin-coated vesicles in practically all cell types. In early endosomes, the content of the vesicle is acidified to approximately pH 5.5. This low pH weakens iron-TF binding; then, the iron is removed, reduced by a ferrireductase (Steap3), and transported out of the vacuole via the divalent metal ion transporter-1 (DMT1) to form the cellular labile iron pool (LIP); this pool consists of a low-molecular-weight pool of weakly chelated iron (ferrous and ferric associated to ligands) that rapidly passes through the cell. Both apoTF (TF without iron) and TFR return to the cell membrane to recycle the TF back to the bloodstream to bind iron in another cycle. At physiological pH, TFR has a much higher affinity for iron-loaded TF (holoTF) than for apoTF [Halliwell and Gutteridge, 2007; Sutak *et al.*, 2008; Gkouvatsos *et al.*, 2012]. There are two different TF receptors, TFR1 and TFR2. TFR1-mediated endocytosis is the usual pathway of iron uptake by body cells. TFR2 participates in low-affinity binding of TF, supporting growth in a few cell types, but the true role of TFR2 is unknown [Halliwell and Gutteridge, 2007; Gkouvatsos *et al.*, 2012].

2. Transferrin and pathogens

The effective acquisition of iron is indispensable for the survival of all organisms. To survive, bacteria, fungi and parasitic protozoa in particular require iron to colonize multicellular organisms. In counterpart, their hosts have to satisfy their own iron requirements and simultaneously avoid iron capture by pathogens. It is very important to the host iron-control strategy to keep this element away from invading pathogens: intracellular and extracellular iron stores are meticulously maintained so that they are unavailable for invaders. As a consequence, pathogens have evolutionarily developed several strategies to obtain iron from the host, e.g., specialized iron uptake mechanisms from host iron-binding proteins, such as TF, through the use of specific TF binding proteins or receptors [Wilson and Britigan, 1998; Wandersman and Delepelaire, 2004; Halliwell and Gutteridge, 2007; Sutak *et al.*, 2008; Weinberg 2009].

2.1. Prokaryotic pathogens

Although it is out of the scope of this chapter, it is important to briefly mention as a reference what has been found in other pathogens such as prokaryotes. Bacteria have evolved specific and efficient mechanisms to obtain iron from various sources that they may contact in their diverse habitats and to compete for this element with other organisms sharing the same space. Some pathogenic bacteria can produce and secrete siderophores, which are low molecular-weight compounds with more affinity than the host proteins for Fe^{3+}; iron-charged siderophores are recognized by bacterial-specific receptors that deliver iron into the cell. Other bacteria directly bind iron from host iron compounds and proteins such as heme, hemoglobin, LF, TF and ferritin [Wooldridge and Williams, 1993; Wilson and Britigan, 1998; Wandersman and Delepelaire, 2004]. Studies in Gram negative bacteria describe their interactions with host iron-containing proteins through outer membrane (OM) receptors; the iron goes through the inner membrane (IM) and is subsequently stored. Iron regulates genes encoding receptor biosynthesis and the uptake of iron proteins [Wandersman and Delepelaire, 2004; Halliwell and Gutteridge, 2007].

Species of the *Neisseriaceae* and *Pasteurellaceae* families are the most studied. They acquire iron directly from host TF, through a receptor on the OM that contacts holo-TF and extracts its iron and transports it across this membrane. The receptor is formed by two proteins: TF-binding protein A (TbpA) and TF-binding protein B (TbpB). TbpA is similar to a classical receptor; it is an integral membrane protein that depends on TonB for energy transduction between the OM and IM. TbpA transports ferric ions across the OM [Cornelissen *et al.*, 1992]. TbpB is a surface-exposed lipoprotein that binds TF independently [Gray-Owen and Schryvers, 1995]. Participation of TbpB is essential for colonizing the host and acquiring iron from TF and displays specificity by binding only TF from the infected animal species [Calmettes *et al.*, 2011]. Once the Fe^{3+} is in the periplasm, it is transported to the cytosol through the FbpABC transporter, which is composed of FbpA, a periplasmic iron-binding protein, and an ABC transporter, formed by the permease FbpB and the ATP-binding protein FbpC [Khun *et al.*, 1998; Nikaido, 2003; Wandersman and Delepelaire, 2004].

TbpB-deficient mutants of *Actinobacillus pleuropneumoniae*, a pathogen of the pig respiratory tract, are neither virulent nor able to colonize its host; thus TbpB is required for iron acquisition *in vivo* [Baltes *et al.*, 2002; Wandersman and Delepelaire, 2004]. Surface lipoproteins such as TbpB have been targeted for vaccine development because they elicit a strong immune response, and antibodies (Abs) to this specific surface lipoprotein are bactericidal. Nevertheless, there is an insufficient cross-protective response induced by an individual receptor protein to be considered as a suitable vaccine antigen [Calmettes *et al.*, 2011]. The abundance of iron acquisition systems present in most pathogenic species undoubtedly reflects the diversity of the potential iron sources in the various niches. Some studies have shown that the iron acquisition systems are important determinants of virulence and that the inactivation of only one system decreases virulence. Bacterial OM receptors can show variability, enabling the pathogen to escape from the host immune system [Wandersman and Delepelaire, 2004].

2.2. Unicellular eukaryotic pathogens

Binding proteins to host iron-containing proteins are also important determinants of virulence in protozoa, as has been deduced from the diversity of iron acquisition systems that have been identified in these protists. In this review, we discuss the current knowledge of transferrin binding proteins (Tbps) in some important parasites. These pathogens possess elaborate control systems for iron uptake from the mammalian hosts that they invade, and these systems ensure their success as parasites. Intracellular parasites are able to live inside of a number of body cells and obtain iron from these sites; for example, in erythrocytes, parasites have free access to hemoglobin as an iron source, debilitating the host by causing anemia and other major problems. Parasites that are phagocytosed by macrophages need to avoid the oxidative stress response of these cells; one of these responses is the production of toxic radicals derived from the oxygen metabolism, and ferrous iron is responsible for their production by Fenton's reaction. However, some parasites not only evade oxidative stress but are also able to survive and multiply inside macrophages; these parasites need to acquire iron for their own growth and to produce the enzyme superoxide-dismutase (SOD), which protects the parasites against toxic radicals. One macrophage's strategy to prevent iron availability to parasites is to sequester this metal through different cleavage mechanisms, such as by reducing the expression of TFR1, the main cellular iron-uptake protein [Mulero and Brock, 1999]. Other mechanisms include increasing the synthesis of ferritin, the main iron-storage protein of the cell, and increasing the expression of ferroportin, the main protein that releases iron from the cell [Das *et al.*, 2009]. Nevertheless, as we will see next, pathogenic parasites have evolved several counterstrategies to stay inside macrophages and acquire cellular iron.

2.2.1. *Trypanosomatids*

Trypanosomatid parasites face different challenges in their fight for iron in the diverse niches that they inhabit inside a host. In extra- and intracellular parasitic forms, iron plays roles in infection as well as in metabolism. Studies of parasite iron acquisition have led to extraordinary therapeutic possibilities of interfering with parasite survival inside the host.

2.2.1.1. *Trypanosoma brucei*

T. brucei is most likely the most-studied parasitic protozoan with respect to iron acquisition from host TF. This parasite is responsible for producing sleeping sickness or human African trypanosomiasis, a disease widespread throughout the African continent. It causes at least 50,000–70,000 cases every year, which can be fatal if not treated correctly [Kinoshita, 2008]. The transmission vector is the tsetse fly, which inoculates *T. brucei* parasites in the blood of its mammalian host during feeding. Trypanosomiasis presents two stages: first, trypanosomes are observed in the hemolymphatic system, producing fever, splenomegaly, adenopathies, endocrine disarrays, and cardiac, neurological and psychological disorders. In this stage, trypanosomes multiply rapidly, infecting the spleen, liver, lymph nodes, skin, heart, eyes and the endocrine system. In the second stage, trypanosomes are distributed in the central nervous system (CNS) leading to several sensory, motor and psychic disorders and ending in death [Kennedy, 2005; de Sousa *et al.*, 2010].

Use of host transferrin by *T. brucei*

In mammals, *T. brucei* lives as a trypomastigote in the bloodstream and tissue fluids [Bitter *et al.*, 1998; Subramanya, 2009; Taylor and Kelly, 2010; Johnson and Wessling-Resnick, 2012]. As an extracellular parasite, it depends on endocytosis to take up nutrients from the host blood [Subramanya, 2009]. This organism uses host TF as the main iron source for growth and has the ability to bind TF from several origins, thus increasing its capacity to colonize a large range of mammals [Salmon *et al.*, 2005]. This ability is important because by taking up different TFs, the parasite favors its own growth without being affected by the host immune system due its variability, leading to chronic infection; in this way, the ability to switch between different TFR genes allows *T. brucei* to cope with the large sequence diversity in the TFs of its hosts [Bitter *et al.*, 1998; Van Luenen *et al.*, 2005]. In contrast, *T. equiperdum* presents a restricted host range, infecting only horses [Isobe *et al.*, 2003; Witola *et al.*, 2005].

T. brucei **transferrin receptor (TbTFR)**

T. brucei binds TF through a transferrin receptor, *Tb*TFR. Although *Tb*TFR and human transferrin receptor (*Hs*TFR) bind the same iron transport protein (TF), they have no detectable amino acid homology [Borst, 1991; Schell *et al.*, 1991; Taylor and Kelly, 2010]. *Tb*TFR is present in only bloodstream forms and not in insect forms of the *T. brucei* life cycle. In fact, *T. evansi*, a derivative of *T. brucei*, does not appear to have a life cycle stage in an insect vector; it presents similar TFR to *T. brucei* [Kabiri and Steverding, 2001]. *Tb*TFR is encoded by two of the expression-site associated genes (*ESAGs)*, *ESAG6* and *ESAG7*, of the variant surface glycoprotein (VSG), the major surface antigen of the bloodstream form of *T. brucei*. ESAG6 and ESAG7 proteins evolved to bind TF [Salmon *et al.*, 1994; Salmon *et al.*, 1997]. The *VSG* gene is at a telomeric expression site (ES) that contains at least seven expression-site associated genes. Each strain of *T. brucei* contains 20 different copies of *ESAG* with a corresponding 20 copies of *Tb*TFR, but only a single ES is active at a time. The receptor expression occurs independently of the ES employed for antigenic variation [Borst, 1991; Schell *et al.*, 1991; Salmon *et al.*, 1994; Salmon *et al.*, 1997; Salmon *et al.*, 2005; Van Luenen *et al.*, 2005]. Antigenic variation prevents receptors from being recognized by the immune system and allows parasites to use TF from different mammalian hosts [Borst, 1991; Bitter *et al.*, 1998]. The surface of the parasite bloodstream form is covered with VSG protein, which is required for nutrient uptake; its variability provides protection from the mammalian immune system [Schell *et al.*, 1991; Taylor and Kelly, 2010]. When some parasites in the population switch VSG gene expression, they produce resistant phenotypes. VSG are powerful antigens, and the initial set of Abs is no longer useful for controlling trypanosomiasis. A proliferation of survivors is produced with posterior infection of the CNS, when parasites move across the blood-brain barrier [Kinoshita, 2008].

*Tb*TFR is a heterodimer consisting of ESAG7, a 42 kDa soluble protein attached to the membrane by the 50-60 kDa ESAG6 protein through a glycosyl-phosphatidylinositol (GPI) residue in the C-terminal tail [Borst, 1991; Schell *et al.*, 1991; Ligtenberg *et al.*, 1994; Salmon *et al.*, 1994; Steverding *et al.*, 1995; Salmon *et al.*, 1997; Steverding, 2000; Maier and Steverding, 2008; Taylor and Kelly, 2010]. ESAG6 and ESAG7 can homodimerize, but only heterodimers bind TF; thus, each subunit provides a necessary component for the specific ligand-binding site [Salmon *et al.*, 1994; Salmon *et al.*, 1997]. The two subunits show differences in their C-terminal region in the four blocks of 5-16 amino acids that generate the ligand binding site. The sequence of the N-terminal half is highly conserved [Salmon *et al.*, 1997]. Near the middle part of the gene is a hypervariable region of approximately 32 nucleotides [Pays, 2006].

Affinity binding of *Tb*TFR for TF is important when the host begins to make a significant Ab response against invariant regions of the receptor that could interfere with TF uptake [Borst, 1991; Salmon *et al.*, 1994; Steverding *et al.*, 1995; Steverding, 2003; Steverding, 2006; Stijlemans *et al.*, 2008]. In some cases, these Abs compete with TF for the receptor binding site, and only a high-affinity receptor could maintain the required iron level for trypanosome replication [Bitter *et al.*, 1998]. Nevertheless, during the course of trypanosomiasis, Abs produced against the *Tb*TFR are too low to deprive the parasite of iron [Steverding, 2006]. This factor could be important for the characteristic anemia observed in chronic illness, in which TF levels are decreased. Because iron is sequestered by macrophages and bloodstream pathogens can obtain iron, the "anemia of chronic infection" results, and erythropoiesis diminishes because there is no available iron to produce hemoglobin. Then, parasites produce a high affinity receptor to TF, which is present in very low quantities [Taylor and Kelly, 2010].

There is a controversy surrounding the purpose of the TFR variability. Some authors report that each TFR encoded by trypanosomatids is slightly different and that these differences affect the binding affinity to TF from different hosts [Van Luenen *et al.*, 2005; Pays, 2006]. Other researchers propose that each receptor with low or high affinity allows trypanosome growth independent of the *in vitro* or *in vivo* TF levels [Salmon *et al.*, 2005]. After the synthesis and heterodimer formation of *Tb*TFR, this receptor is transported to the flagellar pocket by the conventional route of glycoproteins. The flagellar pocket is the site for exocytosis and endocytosis in bloodstream trypanosomes, and it is formed by an invagination of the plasma membrane at the arising flagellum. This pocket protects the parasite from Abs and cell-mediated cytotoxic mechanisms directed against important functionally conserved proteins such as the TFR (Fig. 1) [Balber, 1990; Borst, 1991; Schell *et al.*, 1991; Van Luenen *et al.*, 2005].

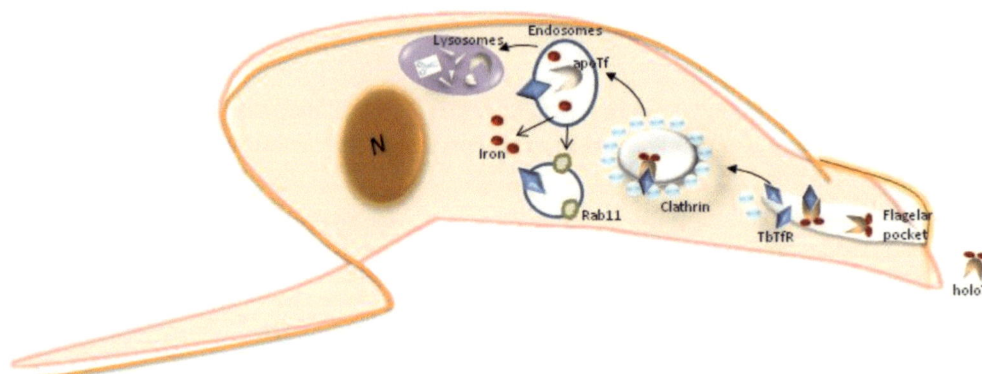

Figure 1. Transferrin endocytosis and iron acquisition in *Trypanosoma brucei*. Transferrin is bound by the *Tb*TFR localized at the flagellar pocket; the complex is then internalized in clathrin-coated pits. The pH is acidified in the endosomes, and the iron is released and transported to the cytoplasm. Apotransferrin is degraded in lysosomes, and the TFR is recycled to the membrane by Rab11-positive vesicles.

VSG proteins leave the flagellar pocket and spread from there to cover the surface, but receptors such as *Tb*TFR are prevented from spreading [Borst, 1991; Mussmann *et al.*, 2004].

Apparently, TFR is retained in the flagellar pocket by the single GPI anchor, while those that present two GPI anchors are targeted to the cell surface [Schwartz *et al.*, 2005; Taylor and Kelly, 2010]. Then, GPI is essential for the correct formation of the VSG coat, for the expression of *Tb*TFRs on the flagellar pocket, and to signal for clathrin-coated endocytosis [Allen *et al.*, 2003]. The lack of TFR leads to lethality; for this reason, some authors have proposed the GPI biosynthetic pathway as a target for the development of anti-trypanosome drugs [Kinoshita, 2008].

Retention of the receptor in the flagellar pocket is a very regulated and saturable process. *Tb*TFR expression depends on the host in which the trypanosome finds itself and on the quantity of iron present. Upregulation of TFR gene expression produces a mislocalization of the receptor onto the cytoplasmic membrane, most likely resulting in binding to more TF molecules. The upregulation of the receptor expression implies that the parasite can sense the reduction in TF availability by sensing cytosolic iron [Van Luenen *et al.*, 2005].

Signal transduction and endocytosis of transferrin by clathrin-coated vesicles

On the flagellar pocket membrane, *Tb*TFR captures TF, and the complex is endocytosed in clathrin-coated pits in a saturable way [Borst, 1991; Schell *et al.*, 1991; Salmon *et al.*, 1994; Taylor and Kelly, 2010] . TF endocytosis is a temperature- and energy-dependent process (Fig. 1) [Ligtenberg *et al.*, 1994; Steverding *et al.*, 1995]. Other proteins that participate in the endocytosis of TF are dynamin, epsin, the adaptor AP-2 [Allen *et al.*, 2003], and small GTPases such as *Tb*Rab5A, β-adaptin [Morgan *et al.*, 2001; Pal *et al.*, 2003], and phosphatidylinositol-3 kinase (PI-3K), *Tb*VPS34 [Hall *et al.*, 2005]. Interestingly, *Tb*TFR does not discriminate between apoTF and holo-TF [Steverding *et al.*, 1995; Steverding, 2003]. TF endocytosis is activated by diacylglycerol (DAG), a diffusible second messenger produced in GPI digestion by the GPI-phospholipase C (GPI-PLC) expressed in bloodstream *T. brucei*. GPI-PLC can cleave intracellular GPIs, producing DAG and inositolphosphoglycan. DAG receptors in trypanosomatids contain a divergent C1_5 domain and DAG signaling pathway that depends on protein tyrosine kinase (PTK) for the activation of proteins in the endocytic system by the phosphorylation of clathrin, actin, adaptins, and other components of this machinery. TF uptake depends on PTK because TF endocytosis diminishes when Tyrphostin A47, an inhibitor of PTK, is used in *T. brucei* and *Leishmania mayor,* another member of the trypanosomatid family [Subramanya and Mensa-Wilmot, 2010].

When the ligand-receptor complex is delivered into the endosomes, the acidic pH triggers the release of iron from TF and the formed apo-TF dissociates from the receptor [Steverding, 2000]. The TFR is recycled into the flagellar pocket via *Tb*Rab11 vesicles [Steverding *et al.*, 1995; Jeffries *et al.*, 2001]. TF is delivered into the lysosomes, where it is degraded by the cathepsin-like protein, *Tb*catB. A small reduction in *Tb*catB produces the accumulation of TFR within the flagellar pocket and the upregulation of TFR levels as a response to iron starvation [Maier and Steverding, 1996; O'Brien *et al.*, 2008]. Later, degraded fragments are exocytosed by the same Rab11 vesicles (Fig. 1) [Steverding *et al.*, 1995; Pal *et al.*, 2003; Hall *et al.*, 2005]. *Tb*TFR has a long half-life, so the receptor is not degraded with TF but is recycled back to the flagellar pocket in approximately 11 min [Kabiri and Steverding, 2000; Kabiri and Steverding, 2001].

The mechanism by which iron crosses to the cytoplasm from the endolysosomal system has not yet been determined; it could be through a ferric reductase. In the *T. brucei* genome, two putative ferric reductases have been found, a cytochrome b561-type (*Tb*927.6.3320) and an NADPH-dependent flavoprotein (*Tb*11.02.1990). These enzymes could act in cooperation with some divalent putative cation transporters, but none of them have been related with iron transport [Taylor and Kelly, 2010].

Iron storage

Depending on the growth conditions, *Tb*TFR can be found at very low concentrations of approximately 1.0 – 2.3 x 10^3 molecules per cell [Borst, 1991; Steverding *et al.*, 1995] or 1.88 – 2.71 x 10^4 molecules per cell [Salmon *et al.*, 1994]; thus, the parasite is very efficient at taking iron from TF. TF is taken up at rates 100–1000 times higher than those for phase fluid endocytosis [Borst, 1991]. The iron necessity is approximately 85,000 Fe^{3+} ions/parasite/generation [Steverding *et al.*, 1995] to 1.4 x 10^6 atoms/trypanosome [Schell *et al.*, 1991], but its requirements are approximately 40,000 Fe^{3+} per generation [Steverding, 2003]. For this reason, it is possible that *T. brucei* accumulates iron in some way [Steverding *et al.*, 1995]. When iron provisions are depleted due to TF starvation, a rapid increase in *Tb*TFR takes place, and the capacity to capture TF increases [Mussmann *et al.*, 2004]. During chronic trypanosomiasis in cattle, anemia occurs, in which the host TF level is decreased and the bloodstream pathogens develop the ability to grow at very low iron concentrations [Steverding *et al.*, 1995]. It is in this stage of iron deprivation and chronic infection when a TFR other than *Tb*TFR, with higher affinity for its ligand, is produced; this occurs because *Tb*TFR is not able to discriminate between holo- and apo-TF [Taylor and Kelly, 2010].

Iron chelation and therapeutic improvement

In the absence of iron, the parasite DNA synthesis rate decreases, oxidative stress levels increase, electron transfer stops, and other functions are affected, all of them leading to death. Iron chelation affects *T. brucei* growth; thus, it could be a therapeutic method for combating the infection. The iron chelator deferoxamine (DFO) prevents iron incorporation in newly synthesized enzymes, decreasing the growth rate and oxygen consumption [Taylor and Kelly, 2010]. Acute iron starvation leads to a rapid increase in *Tb*TFR, allowing an increased capacity to uptake TF [Mussmann *et al.*, 2004].

*Tb*TFR is immunologically important, and it has been studied for its antigenic potential in the production of vaccines. Using the complete collection of TFRs as a vaccine, the proliferation of trypanosomes was blocked; however, some authors are not convinced and suggest that antigenic variation makes the production of a vaccine against sleeping sickness improbable [Kinoshita, 2008]. *ESAG*s could also be targets for immune attack. Flagellar pocket proteins were used for immunization of mice and were able to confer protection against superinfection with trypanosomes [Olenick *et al.*, 1988]. A functional *Tb*TFR was expressed in insect cells and could be helpful in crystallographic studies to determine the structure and characterize the interface between TF and its receptor, which could lead to a new approach to combat infection [Maier and Steverding, 2008]. TF uptake is very important in trypanosomes for obtaining iron, so endocytic uptake systems were developed earlier in evolution compared with TF endocytosis in mammalian cells. Nevertheless, this process has numerous similarities between the two groups.

2.2.1.2. *Trypanosoma cruzi*

This parasite causes human Chagas disease, a chronic and debilitating condition affecting 40 million people in Africa, South America, Europe, and Asia, according to data of the World Health Organization (WHO). *T. cruzi* is transmitted either by an insect vector that has access to the host via breaches in the skin or through mucosal membranes, mainly the conjunctiva or the gastric mucosa. It is an obligate intracellular parasite that disseminates from the initial infection site to the heart and smooth muscle, with several rounds of invasion, growth and egression from infected cells during acute infection. Very little is known regarding the early interaction between the parasite and its host that facilitates the establishment of infection [Mott *et al.*, 2011].

***T. cruzi* transferrin receptor (TcTFR) and endocytosis**

It has been suggested that the internalization of TF is mediated by a receptor in *T. cruzi*. However, until now, there is no biochemical evidence of the presence of a TFR. Epimastigote forms of *T. cruzi* could use a TFR to obtain iron and transport TF through uncoated vesicles formed in the most posterior portion of the cytostome/cytopharynx system, a plasma membrane invagination that penetrates deeply into the cytoplasm towards the nucleus. All the endocytic vesicles formed in the cytostome are uncoated and are associated with lipid raft markers in detergent membrane-resistant (DMR) domains [Correa *et al.*, 2007]. Endocytic vesicles originate either from the cytostome or from the flagellar pocket, and they fuse with early endosomes and then with reservosomes (prelysosomal compartments); endocytosed TF is taken into the reservosomes, which are structures that present numerous proteases [Correa *et al.*, 2008; Cunha-e-Silva *et al.*, 2010; Rocha *et al.*, 2010]. Other proteins that participate in endocytosis have been identified, such as *Tc*Rab7, an indicator of high traffic between the Golgi apparatus and reservosomes, and *Tc*Rab11, which is involved in the recycling process [Cunha-e-Silva *et al.*, 2010; Rocha *et al.*, 2010]. Amastigote forms replicate in the host cell cytoplasm, where TF is almost absent, so the relevance of these forms during infection is not clear. The importance of the receptor is observed in trypomastigotes in the bloodstream and epimastigotes in bloodmeal, where TF was observed in the reservosome [Soares and de Souza, 1991; Soares *et al.*, 1992].

Iron chelation

There is not enough information about how cytoplasmic iron is taken up by *T. cruzi* parasites. They replicate in macrophage cytoplasm; therefore, the macrophage iron-withholding response would benefit the parasite, allowing access to iron [Taylor and Kelly, 2010]. An increase of parasitemia and mortality associated with high levels of iron were observed, as was a reduction in parasitemia with the use of chelants such as DFO or benznidazole [Lalonde and Holbein, 1984; Taylor and Kelly, 2010; Johnson and Wessling-Resnick, 2012]. The obtained iron is stored in specialized electron-dense organelles; these organelles are different from lysosomes and reservosomes [Scott *et al.*, 1997]. The infection in mouse models involves the production of anemia. This anemia is due to interference with the stimulation of the IFN-induced GTPase LRG-47, which produces severe effects in the hematopoietic system [Taylor and Kelly, 2010]. When the parasite is extracellular, it must obtain nutrients from host proteins. The possibility of infecting several organisms makes it possible that this parasite could use different iron sources, including TF. Because TF accumulation reported an organelle in which TF could be accumulated could exist. Very little is known about the *T. cruzi* iron uptake mechanisms either in its different extracellular or intracellular forms of its life cycle.

2.2.2. *Entamoeba histolytica*

E. histolytica is the causal protozoan agent of amoebiasis in humans, a disease characterized by dysentery and intestinal ulcers. The parasite is able to invade and destroy tissues, affecting not only the large intestine but also other extra-intestinal organs such as the liver; these infections can be fatal. Amoebiasis shows high level of morbidity and mortality worldwide, particularly in developing countries. Worldwide, 500 million people are infected with *E. histolytica,* causing disease in 50 million and 100,000 deaths each year [Ali *et al.*, 2008; Anaya-Velázquez and Padilla-Vaca, 2011].

Iron and *E. histolytica*

Iron is essential for *E. histolytica* trophozoites living inside the human host because these parasites require a high quantity of iron (approximately 100 μM) for growing *in vitro* and are able to use iron from several iron-binding proteins [López-Soto *et al.*, 2009b]. High amoebic damage was caused in the liver of hamsters that were fed with ferrous gluconate. In addition, there is a significant relationship between amoebic growth and the mechanisms of iron acquisition modulated by determinants of virulence [Diamond *et al.*, 1978; Smith and Meerovitch, 1982]. Within the host, amoebae face the hostility of nonspecific defense systems such as oxidative stress and the lack of nutrients. Several protective mechanisms have been developed by *E. histolytica,* such as the induction of the superoxide dismutase (SOD) gene under iron-limited conditions; this enzyme defends amoeba from the toxicity and damage caused by oxygen metabolites. Thus, SOD is useful during tissue invasion, when amoebae are exposed to great amounts of superoxide radicals [Bruchhaus and Tannich, 1994a].

If iron is reduced in the culture medium to < 20 μM, amoebae do not survive. Several studies have shown responses of the parasite to the absence or excess of iron and to the presence of iron-containing proteins [Serrano-Luna *et al.*, 1998; Reyes-López *et al.*, 2001; León-Sicairos *et al.*, 2005; López-Soto *et al.*, 2009a]. The concerted use of strategies to bind and use iron from different sources provides the parasite with the ability to use various host proteins for its benefit. In the absence of iron, *E. histolytica* expresses several genes that encode for cysteine proteases CP1, CP2 and CP3; these proteases are virulence factors, as they degrade the mucus barrier in the intestinal epithelium. However, there is no information concerning the mechanisms for iron regulation in this parasite. Genes involved in translation were identified to be expressed in the absence of iron [Park *et al.*, 2001], as occurs with the ferric uptake regulator (Fur) in bacteria and in iron responsive element (IRE) and IRE-binding proteins of mammalian cells [Wang *et al.*, 2007].

Use of host iron-containing proteins

E. histolytica has developed specific mechanisms to obtain iron from host iron-containing proteins. This assertion is based on the parasite growth *in vitro* in media depleted of iron and to which different iron proteins have been added. Trophozoites have been tested in cultures with hemoglobin, LF, TF, ferritin, and as the sole iron sources, and all of them have been utilized by the parasite for growth [Serrano-Luna *et al.*, 1998; Reyes-López *et al.*, 2001; León-Sicairos *et al.*, 2005; López-Soto *et al.*, 2009b]. In this way, amoebae could ensure the presence of iron for the colonization of the different organs and tissues involved in amoebic infection.

***E. histolytica* transferrin binding proteins, EhTFbps**

Iron-loaded TF (holoTF) but not apoTF binds to the *E. histolytica* trophozoite surface. Interestingly, this parasite has two methods of obtaining iron from TF: one is mediated by receptor-independent internalization [Welter *et al.*, 2006] and the other is through three specific TF-binding proteins (*Eh*TFbps) of 70, 96 and 140 kDa of molecular mass, identified by overlay assays with holoTF. The 140 kDa protein is recognized by an anti-*Hs*TFR mAb B3/25 (Boehringerheim cat. No. 1118-048), and the 96 kDa protein is recognized by the anti-*Hs*TFR mAb H68.4 (Zymed cat. No. 13-6800). Apparently, the *Eh*TFR forms a complex with TF to be endocytosed (Fig. 2). Using pharmacological and immunofluorescence microscopy studies, the participation of clathrin protein in the endocytic process was demonstrated. Once inside the vacuoles, TF is transported into the endolysosomal system [Reyes-López *et al.*, 2001; Reyes-López *et al.*, 2011]. However, when the endocytic process was followed using high TF concentrations, the TF was internalized independently of the binding protein [Reyes-López *et al.*, 2011]. This result is in agreement with the observation that TF internalization is unsaturable [Welter *et al.*, 2006]. The presence of clathrin has been demonstrated in some protozoa [Morgan *et al.*, 2001] and in *E. histolytica* [León-Sicairos *et al.*, 2005; López-Soto *et al.*, 2009a; Reyes-López *et al.*, 2011]; clathrin may be important in parasites for the acquisition of nutrients. The gene encoding the clathrin protein has been identified in the *E. histolytica* genome [Loftus *et al.*, 2005]. Once inside the lysosomes, TF could be degraded by specific cysteine proteases (Fig. 2) (our unpublished data), as was observed in *T. brucei.*

In addition to the phagocytosis of erythrocytes to use hemoglobin, the direct binding of host TF to specific proteins on the amoeba surface may be another strategy used to capture iron in the blood and liver, which is important in the human host invasion process of this parasite. The 96 kDa protein was identified as the enzyme acetaldehyde/alcohol dehydrogenase-2 (*Eh*ADH2) by mass spectrometry after its isolation by immunoprecipitation with the mAb H68.4 [Reyes-López *et al.*, 2011]; to our knowledge, this report is the first in which an enzyme was shown to bind TF in parasitic protozoa. Internalization of TF through a receptor is a fast, saturable, and temperature-, time-, and concentration-dependent process. It is possible that the *Eh*ADH2 protein, which requires iron for its activity, participates in the regulation of iron-Tf uptake and utilization. *Eh*ADH2 enzyme is essential for amoeba survival and is able to discriminate between iron-loaded TF and apoTF, possibly because iron is the enzyme cofactor of the protein [Espinosa *et al.*, 2009].

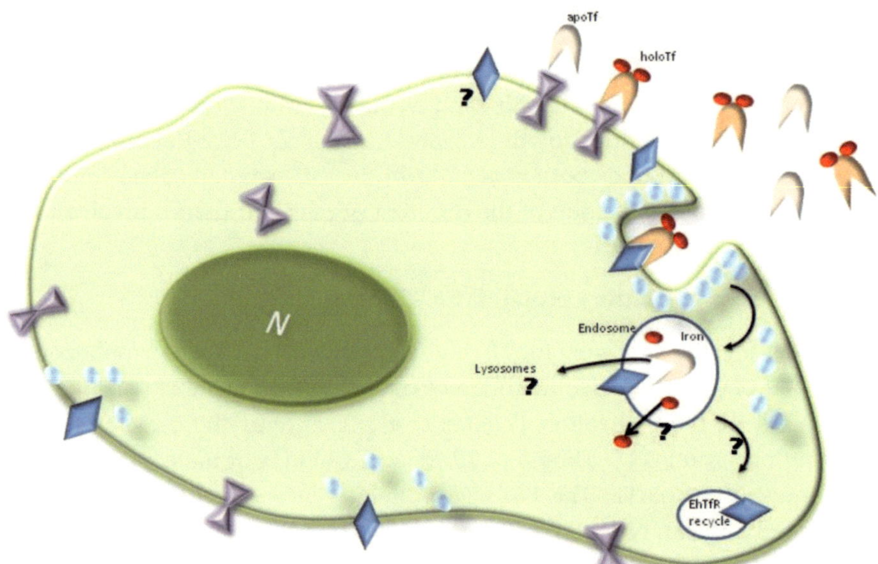

Figure 2. Transferrin endocytosis in *Entamoeba histolytica*. HoloTF is detected by the *Eh*Tbp and the TFR and internalized in clathrin-coated pits.

It has been reported that bacteria such as *Staphylococcus aureus* and *Staphylococcus epidermidis* use the enzyme glyceraldehyde-3-phosphate dehydrogenase (GAPDH) to bind TF [Modun and Williams, 1999], and the parasite *Trypanosoma brucei* uses an organelle in which TF could be accumulated could exist.GAPDH for binding LF rather than TF [Tanaka *et al.*, 2004]. Apparently, glycolytic enzymes have several functions; an example is enolase, which also regulates the activity of cytosine 5-methyltransferase 2 (Dnmt2), an enzyme that catalyses DNA and tRNA methylation in amoeba [Tovy *et al.*, 2010]. The *Eh*ADH2 amino acid sequence and that predicted for the *Hs*TFR are not similar, so the recognition of both proteins by the mAb could be explained by a structural connection. *Eh*ADH2 is an essential enzyme used for obtaining energy by glucose fermentation [Bruchhaus and Tannich, 1994b; Yang *et al.*, 1994; Flores *et al.*, 1996; Espinosa *et al.*, 2001; Avila *et al.*, 2002; Chen *et al.*, 2004; Espinosa *et al.*, 2004; Espinosa *et al.*, 2009]. Due to the properties of *Eh*ADH2, such as its ability to bind to host extracellular matrix proteins, its presence on the cell membrane, and its requirement for iron, the blocking of this enzyme with iron chelators as a therapeutic strategy against *E. histolytica* is an interesting future perspective [Espinosa *et al.*, 2009].

*Eh*TFbp is able to bind TF with either high or with low affinity (1.81 and 1.1-5.7 x 10^{-9} M). This observation could be due to the presence of two binding proteins or only one protein with two different affinities [Reyes-López *et al.*, 2011]. Comparing the affinity for TF in bacteria (0.7 a 4 x 10^{-7} M) [Pintor *et al.*, 1993] and *Trypanosoma cruzi* (2.8 X 10^{-6} M) [Testa, 2002], the amoebic receptor presents the higher affinity. The fact that *E. histolytica* trophozoites possess a variety of mechanisms to obtain iron from TF is advantageous to the parasite. However, in amoebiasis, the host usually has lower iron levels and TF saturation than that showed in uninfected people; this defense is a normal response to limit iron from pathogens during infection, a phenomenon known as hypoferremia of infection [Van Snick *et al.*, 1974; Otto *et al.*, 1992; Jurado, 1997; Griffiths *et al.*, 1999; Weinberg, 1999; Weinberg 2009]. Further studies are necessary to comprehend the role of all the proteins that participate in the iron acquisition system of TF and in the iron metabolism of this important parasite.

2.2.3. *Tritrichomonas foetus*

T. foetus is a venereal protozoan pathogen of cattle that infects the female genital tract, resulting in abortion, endometritis, and infertility [Manning, 2010; Pereira-Neves *et al.*, 2011]. This parasite has a worldwide distribution and causes significant economic losses to cattle producers. Strains of *T. foetus* have also been recognized that cause diarrhea in cats [Gookin *et al.*, 1999] and mild rhinitis in swine [Lun *et al.*, 2005]. As an obligate parasite, *T. foetus* depends on endogenous bacteria and host secretions for nutrients such as iron. This organism has high iron requirements for *in vitro* cultivation (50–100 μM) [Tachezy *et al.*, 1996], surpassing those of eukaryotic cells, although comparable to other anaerobic amitochondriate protists. *T. foetus* inhabits the vagina, cervix, and the lumen of the bovine uterus, with the last one being characterized as rich in TF [Roberts and Parker, 1974]. Therefore, TF could be an important source of iron for *T. foetus.*

The involvement of iron and holo-TF in *T. foetus* virulence has been examined in experimental infection of mice with the moderately virulent KV-1 strain (~5% mortality rate). Administration of ferric ammonium citrate to infected mice increased the mortality rate to the level associated with the highly virulent LUB-1MIP strain (~80% mortality rate) [Kulda *et al.*, 1999]. When examined *in vitro*, the KV-1 strain showed significantly lower iron acquisition from holo-TF and low molecular mass complexes than the highly virulent strain. These data indicate a correlation between strain virulence and iron acquisition from holo-TF [Kulda *et al.*, 1999]. Growth of parasites using holoTF as a sole iron source has been reported *in vitro* [Tachezy *et al.*, 1996]. Accordingly, iron from ^{59}Fe-TF was efficiently accumulated into *T. foetus*, specifically in the labile iron pool (LIP). Interestingly, the concentration of protein-bound iron that restored 50% cell growth (5 μM for Fe-TF) was approximately 5-fold lower than that of low molecular weight iron complexes [Tachezy *et al.*, 1996; Suchan *et al.*, 2003], indicating that *T. foetus* uses TF iron more efficiently. This finding agrees with results in studies of other pathogens that require higher iron concentrations from these complexes than those from host proteins (holoLF and HG) [Wilson *et al.*, 1994; Jarosik *et al.*, 1998].

Retrieval of iron from TF may depend on the extracellular release of iron from this ligand caused by the acidification of the microenvironment by *T. foetus* [Tachezy *et al.*, 1996]. This hypothesis is based on the observation that the pH of the conditional media decreased from pH 7.4 to 5.6 after incubation with *T. foetus*. As predicted at this pH, there was a marked release of iron from holoTF (up to 47%) measured in the cell-free medium (Fig. 3) [Tachezy *et al.*, 1996]. Iron uptake from TF was almost exponential, which possibly reflected the accelerated release of iron from the protein by the acidification of the cellular microenvironment [Tachezy *et al.*, 1996]. Nevertheless, further studies are needed to demonstrate the actual role of microenvironmental acidification in iron uptake, for example, by measuring the iron uptake by *T. foetus* using a stronger buffered medium to prevent acidification.

Iron uptake from transferrin in *T. foetus*

Iron uptake from TF is a process dependent on the energy produced by glycolysis, as sodium fluoride affected the uptake [Tachezy *et al.*, 1998]. The mechanism also involves extracellular iron reduction from holo-TF. This idea is supported by the inhibitory effect of BPSA (a membrane impermeable, ferrous-iron specific chelator) on iron uptake from holo-TF, as iron is originally in the ferric state in this molecule. Additionally, the presence of ascorbic acid, a strong reducing agent, stimulated iron accumulation by *T. foetus* from holo-TF [Tachezy *et al.*, 1998]. Which mechanism is actually used by *T. foetus* to reduce holo-TF iron is unknown. Iron released from holo-TF could be acquired by a mechanism related or identical to that used for acquisition from the low molecular weight iron chelator nitrilotriacetic acid (Fe-NTA) because these processes displayed similar kinetics and susceptibility to various agents [Tachezy *et al.*, 1998]. Iron uptake from Fe-NTA by this microorganism also depends on iron reduction and is better characterized. Extracellular iron reduction from Fe-NTA seems to be non-enzymatic, as the reduction activity is thermo-labile and unaffected by proteases, and the majority is filterable through a membrane with a cut-off of 3 kDa. Additionally, iron acquisition is not enhanced by the presence of NADH, a nucleotide reported to provide electrons to ferrireductases [Low *et al.*, 1986; Berczi and Faulk, 1992; Riedel *et al.*, 1995]. In fact, trichomonads are able to produce reducing volatile agents such as H_2S [Thong and Coombs, 1987] or methanethiol [Thong *et al.*, 1987], which have been suggested to participate in oxygen detoxification [Thong *et al.*, 1986]. It could be that trichomonads are able to take advantage of their reducing environment to take up iron from holo-TF (Fig. 3). This hypothesis needs to be tested and does not completely rule out the possibility that a ferrireductase may also participate.

The extracellular release of iron from holo-TF could be independent of proteolysis because less than 40% of the parent molecule was digested even after 24 h of contact with extracellular *T. foetus* proteases [Talbot *et al.*, 1991]. Iron acquisition from TF seems to be independent of endocytosis because lysosomotropic bases such as ammonium chloride and chloroquine acting as inhibitors of endosome acidification did not decrease iron accumulation from TF [Tachezy *et al.*, 1998]. However, work from Affonso shows that endocytosis of TF by *T. foetus* actually takes place [Affonso *et al.*, 1994]. It was shown that TF binds to the parasite surface, and because unlabeled TF does not compete with labeled TF, this binding does not seem to be through specific surface receptors. In agreement with this result, holo-TF binding does not display saturable kinetics [Tachezy *et al.*, 1996]. The initial binding of gold-labeled human TF may be due to low-affinity interactions, as occurs with *T. vaginalis* [Peterson and Alderete, 1984]. Gold-labeled TF is internalized by the parasite through endocytic vesicles and concentrated into vacuoles of variable dimension, peripheral tubular and tubulovesicular structures all without a typical clathrin coat. The absence of a specific receptor suggests a principal role for fluid phase endocytosis [Tachezy *et al.*, 1996].

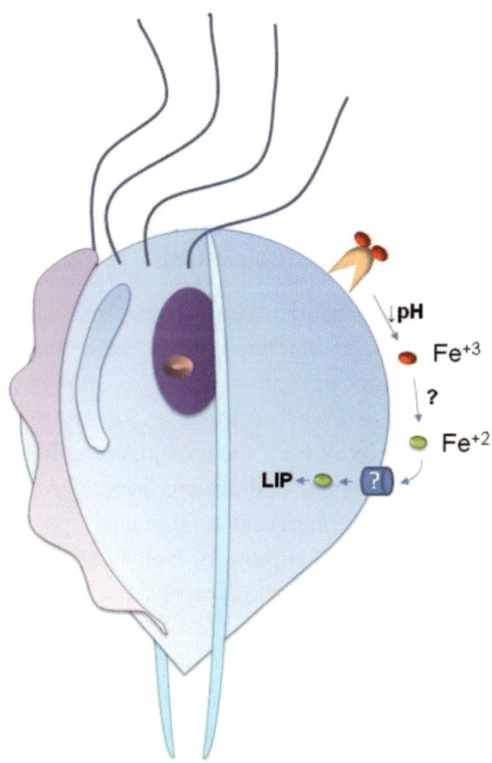

Figure 3. Transferrin acquisition in *Plasmodium falciparum*. The parasite produces its receptor by an unknown mechanism. The receptor is transported to the erythrocyte membrane, where it is able to bind TF . Then the iron from TF is transported back to the parasite by an unknown mechanism.

Further studies are necessary to fully understand the mechanism of iron acquisition from holoTF by *T. foetus*, specifically to characterize the mechanism of iron reduction and of iron transport through the membrane and to clarify the role of holo-TF endocytosis in iron acquisition. Moreover, due to its unusually high nutritional requirement for iron, the inhibition of iron uptake from holo-TF might be an attractive therapeutic strategy against *T. foetus*.

2.2.4. Plasmodium spp.

Malaria is a mosquito-borne infectious disease of humans and other animals caused by parasite protozoa of the genus *Plasmodium*. The disease results from the multiplication of parasites inside red blood cells (erythrocytes), causing fever, headache, splenomegaly, cerebral ischemia, hepatomegaly, hypoglycemia, and hemoglobinuria with renal failure, progressing in severe cases to coma and death [Trampuz *et al.*, 2003]. It is widespread mainly in the tropical and subtropical regions of Sub-Saharan Africa, Asia, and America. Five species of malaria can be transmitted to humans. Severe disease is largely caused by *P. falciparum*, while the diseases caused by *P. vivax*, *P. ovale* [Sutherland *et al.*, 2010] and *P. malariae* are generally milder and rarely fatal. *P. knowlesi* is a zoonosis that causes malaria in macaques but sometimes can infect humans [Fong *et al.*, 1971; Singh *et al.*, 2004]. Malaria has been a widely prevalent disease throughout human history. The World Health Organization has estimated that malaria annually causes 250 million cases [WHO, 2008]. In 2010, it was estimated that 655,000 people died from the disease [WHO, 2010]. However, a 2012 meta-study published in *The Lancet* reported 1,238,000 people dying from malaria in 2010 [Murray *et al.*, 2012]. The majority of cases occur in children under 5 years old [Greenwood *et al.*, 2005]; pregnant women are also especially vulnerable. *P. falciparum* is responsible for the vast majority of deaths associated with the disease [Snow *et al.*, 2005].

The life cycle of malaria parasites in the human body begins when a mosquito infects a person by taking a blood meal. Malaria develops via two phases: an extra-erythrocytic and an intra-erythrocytic phase. The extra-erythrocytic phase involves infection of the hepatic system, whereas the intra-erythrocytic phase involves infection of erythrocytes. When an infected mosquito pierces a person's skin, sporozoites in the mosquito's saliva enter the bloodstream and migrate to the liver, infecting hepatocytes, multiplying asexually and asymptomatically for a period of 8–30 days. After this dormant period in the liver, parasites differentiate to yield thousands of merozoites, which, following rupture of their host cells, escape into the blood and infect red blood cells [Bledsoe, 2005]. The parasite escapes from the liver undetected by wrapping itself with the host cellular membrane. Within the red blood cells, the parasites multiply further, again asexually, periodically breaking out of these cells to invade fresh red blood cells. Several such amplification cycles occur [Sturm *et al.*, 2006]. The parasites are relatively protected from attack by the body's immune system because they reside within the liver and blood cells and are relatively invisible to immune surveillance for most of their life cycle in humans. However, circulating infected blood cells are destroyed in the spleen [Chen *et al.*, 2000].

P. falciparum parasites need iron to support their growth

Treatment with iron supplementation in *Plasmodium*-infected patients increases malaria morbidity [Oppenheimer, 1989]. Interestingly, despite the fact that the intra-erythrocytic parasite is surrounded by hemoglobin, it is unable to utilize this ferrous molecule, and therefore, heme accumulates in hemozoins (crystalline particles) within the parasites [Roth *et al.*, 1986; Goldberg *et al.*, 1990]. The delivery of extracellular iron from serum TF to infected erythrocytes has been postulated [Pollack and Fleming, 1984; Haldar *et al.*, 1986; Rodriguez and Jungery, 1986]. The uptake of ^{125}I- or ^{55}Fe-labeled human TF has been detected in parasitized cells during several days of culture [Pollack and Fleming, 1984]. Furthermore, two independent studies have reported the identification of proteins on the surface of *P. falciparum*-infected erythrocytes that have an affinity for ferric TF [Haldar *et al.*, 1986; Rodriguez and Jungery, 1986]. Rodriguez and Jungery [Rodriguez and Jungery, 1986] described the presence of a 93 kDa protein that bound to a TF affinity-column. These authors claim that this protein could be a parasite-derived TFR, synthesized by *P. falciparum* (*Pf*TFR), because the vast majority of mature erythrocytes lack the expression of TFR (CD71) [Marsee *et al.*, 2010]. Almost at the same time, Haldar et al. [1986] identified another probable *Pf*TFR of 102 kDa synthesized by the intracellular parasite and inserted in the erythrocyte membrane of mature infected cells. This protein recognizes only holoTF. Biochemical analysis indicated that this protein is acylated via 1,2-diacyl-sn-glycerol, which may be important for its association with the membrane. Fry [1989] described a diferric reductase activity in *P. falciparum*-infected erythrocytes. This activity was absent in uninfected mature erythrocytes, suggesting its synthesis and incorporation by *P. falciparum*. The author suggests that the presence of the diferric TF reductase together with the parasite–derived TFR in the erythrocyte membrane could form a TFR –mediated uptake mechanism.

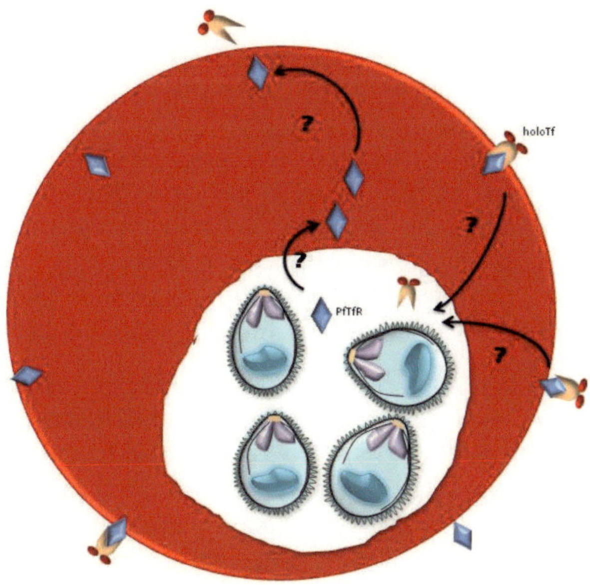

Figure 4. *Tritrichomonas foetus* uptake of iron from Transferrin by a reducing mechanism. HoloTF binds *Tritrichomonas* surface most likely through low-affinity interactions, and then iron is released due to the microenvironment acidification. Ferric iron is reduced to the ferrous form by an unknown mechanism, most likely non-enzymatic, and is then internalized by the parasite to become part of the labile iron pool (LIP).

In contrast, a controversial study performed by Pollack and Vera Schnelle in [1988] was unable to detect a TFR in *P. falciparum*-infected erythrocytes. This study concluded that the binding of TF to the erythrocyte surface was not specific because it was neither saturable nor limited to TF, as LF and albumin were also bound to the parasitized cells. These authors suggested that TF was non-specifically bound and in this way endocytosed and degraded inside the parasite. Furthermore, in [1992], Sánchez-López and Haldar described a TFR-independent iron uptake activity in *P. falciparum*, and this activity was also apparent in uninfected erythrocytes. These authors demonstrated that normal levels of TF in human serum were not required for intra-erythrocytic *P. falciparum* growth. However, although the iron uptake activity was not parasite specific in parasitized erythrocytes, apparently radiolabeled iron (^{55}Fe) was found in association with parasites mechanically released from the infected erythrocyte, indicating that it was delivered to the intracellular organism.

In view of the controversial state of the research regarding to *Plasmodium* TF iron uptake, we think that more careful studies have to be performed to determine whether there is a complete *Pf*TFR in parasitized erythrocytes, in which state the iron travels through the erythrocyte cytoplasm until reaching the parasitic surface, and lastly, how iron is internalized by the parasite (Fig. 4). Another interesting question is that if *P. falciparum* can obtain iron from different sources, which of these sources are important in parasitic iron uptake

2.2.5. Leishmania spp.

Leishmania species are dimorphic-protozoa that cause leishmaniases, a range of diseases displaying a large spectrum of clinical symptoms in mammals. Approximately 2 million new cases occur every year, with an estimate of 150 million people infected around the world [Kaye and Scott, 2011]. Five main species of *Leishmania* can infect human beings: *L. tropica, L. major, L. donovani, L. braziliensis* and *L. mexicana*. There are mainly three clinical forms of infection: the self-healing cutaneous leishmaniasis (CL), the mucocutaneous leishmaniasis (MCL), and the often fatal visceral leishmaniasis (VL) that affects people of the South American continent. The severity of symptoms depends on the parasite species and strain; exposure dose; and genetic, health and immune status of the host [Anstead *et al.*, 2001; Marquis and Gros, 2007; Kaye and Scott, 2011].

Leishmanias can live in two stages: flagellated promastigotes and non-flagellated amastigotes. When promastigotes are inoculated in the host human dermis by the vector insect (sandfly), they are phagocytosed by macrophages, and then transform into amastigotes within a membrane-rounded organelle named the parasitophorous vacuole (PV) that belongs to the endocytic route, and progressively acquires characteristics of a late endosome/lysosome [Courret *et al.*, 2001; Courret *et al.*, 2002]. Inside the PV, the parasites replicate leading to cell lysis, and free parasites infect the surrounding cells. Leishmanias surviving intracellularly produce multiple effects in phagocytes: inhibition of the respiratory burst, prevention of apoptosis, chemotaxis inhibition in both macrophages and neutrophils, and suppression of the Th1 type protective response [Olivier *et al.*, 2005].

Some species of *Leishmania* possess specific transferrin binding proteins

More than 20 years ago, a putative TF binding protein in *L. infantum* promastigotes was reported [Voyiatzaki and Soteriadou, 1990]. The binding of human iron-free ^{125}I-TF to *Leishmania*-purified membrane preparation was found of high affinity (K_d 2.2×10^{-8} M); in addition, this binding was saturable and specific for TF. The affinity of the *Li*Tbp for TF is comparable with that reported in mammalian cells. Interestingly, the anti-human TFR mAb B3/25, which recognizes a Tbp of 140 kDa in *E. histolytica*, did not recognize the *Li*Tbp, suggesting that the *Hs*TFR and *Li*Tbp do not share epitopes. Binding of human apo-TF was also tested on living avirulent *L. infantum* promastigotes, and on *L. mexicana* amastigotes obtained from infected mice with promastigotes. In both cases the binding was specific and saturable, suggesting that the *Li*Tbp is functionally similar to the human TFR. Although the experiments were performed with iron-free TF, these data suggest that both stages of *Leishmania* are able to bind human TF, an important iron protein for the parasite iron requirement; indeed, TF-mediated uptake of iron was observed in these parasites. Later, the same authors isolated and identified the *Li*Tbp as an integral membrane monomeric glycoprotein of 70 kDa [Voyiatzaki and Soteriadou, 1992]. The purification of this receptor was carried out through the use of affinity chromatography with human TF from membrane preparations of *L. infantum* and *L. major* promastigotes.

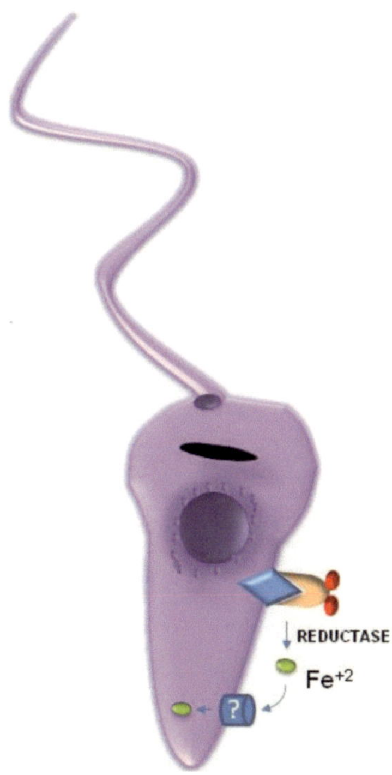

Figure 5. Iron uptake from Transferrin by *Leishmania chagasi* promastigotes. A non-specific receptor, *Lc*Tbp, binds TF, allowing a parasite-associated or secreted reductase to reduce the ferric iron from holoTF, and in this way, the TF affinity for iron diminishes, allowing ferrous iron to be internalized by the parasite.

L. chagasi also showed a 70 kDa protein that binds TF (*Lc*Tbp); however, this protein is not specific for TF because LF and albumin were also bound. Apparently, a parasite-associated or secreted reductase is needed to reduce the ferric iron from holoTF, and in this way, the affinity of TF for iron diminishes allowing iron be internalized by the parasite (Fig. 5)

[Wilson *et al.*, 2002]. *L. chagasi* promastigotes require a lower iron concentration than other parasites (8 μM hemin). Lactoferrin, as an extracellular protein, interacts with promastigotes, and it can be used by them as an iron source *in vitro* [Wilson *et al.*, 1994]. Promastigotes were able to take up ^{59}Fe-LF more rapidly than that from hemin or holoTF, suggesting that iron uptake from holoTF and holoLF occurs via a non-specific receptor because apoLF, apoTF and holoTF competed with holoLF for the uptake. In other experiments [Britigan *et al.*, 1998], it was demonstrated that the binding to TF is markedly greater if this protein is iron-charged; also, if *L. chagasi* does not excrete proteases that cleave TF, then the proteolytic cleavage is not a mechanism to obtain iron in this parasite.

***Leishmania* can live inside macrophages**

The access of iron inside the macrophage's phagosome plays a central role in *Leishmania* infection. Nramp1 protein is located in macrophage lysosomes and in tertiary granules of neutrophils, and it is rapidly recruited towards the membrane of leishmania-containing phagosomes. In that membrane, the iron transporter protein Nramp1 chelates Fe^{2+} in the intraphagosomal environment and in this way, Nramp1 avoids the parasite multiplication and activation of macrophages. However, *L. amazonensis* upregulates the expression of its own ferrous iron transporter LIT1 after being endocytosed by the macrophage. Mutations in *Nramp1* (*Slc11a1*) gene are responsible of mouse propensity to be infected with *Leishmania* because macrophages permit its replication [Forbes and Gros, 2001; Marquis and Gros, 2007; Huynh and Andrews, 2008; Jacques *et al.*, 2010].

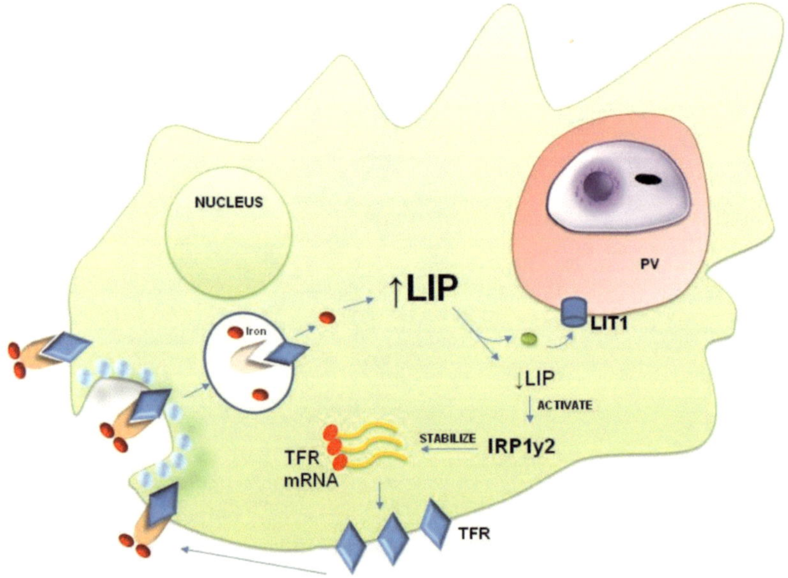

Figure 6. Iron uptake by intracellular *Leishmania donovani* amastigotes. From its parasitophorous vacuole (PV), *Leishmania* expresses its ferrous iron transporter (LIT1) to scavenge iron and deplete the macrophage labile-iron pool (LIP); this activates the host cytosolic iron-responsive element sensor proteins IRP1 and IRP2. These proteins increase the stability of the TFR mRNA , increasing macrophage iron uptake from TF and the intracellular iron parasite needs for survival.

Interestingly, studies with *L. donovani* suggest that there is an intraphagosomal competition for free ferrous-iron between the iron transporters from host and those from the parasite. This competition may, by depleting the macrophage labile-iron pool (LIP) (Fig. 6), activate the host cytosolic iron-responsive element sensor proteins IRP1 and IRP2. These proteins increase the stability of the mRNA of the TFR by binding to iron-responsive elements (IREs) present in the 3′UTR of the TFR1 gene, which in turn leads to increased production of the TFR1 and, thus, to TF-mediated iron uptake [Das *et al.*, 2009]. In this study, the authors clearly demonstrate that instead of macrophages sequester iron, virulent parasites directly scavenge iron from the host LIP (Fig. 6), which activates the interaction IRE-IRP leading to an up-regulation of the macrophage′ TFR1, increasing the intracellular iron needed for parasite survival.

2.2.6. *Toxoplasma gondii*

Toxoplasma gondii is an intracellular obligate protozoan that belongs to the phylum *Apicomplexa* and is unique in invading a large diversity of mammals and birds [Ossorio *et al.*, 1994; Ajioka *et al.*, 1998; Joiner and Roos, 2002]. It is thought that approximately 25% of the world human population is infected by *Toxoplasma* [Tenter *et al.*, 2000]. Toxoplasmosis can produce severe damage in humans with often fatal results, mainly in immunosuppressed patients suffering from AIDS or cancer and in people undergoing immunosuppressive treatments. The most frequent damages include chorioretinitis with consecutive loss of vision and damage to the CNS, lungs, and heart, and when infection occurs during pregnancy, parasites reach the placenta and infect the fetus, causing abortion [Luft and Remington, 1992; Barragan and Sibley, 2002]. However, in immune competent people, infection occurs in a transitory and asymptomatic fashion. The success of *T. gondii* as an intracellular pathogen is based on its high capacity for invasion and dissemination in practically all tissues due to its migration through biological barriers such as intestinal, hematic-encephalic, hematic-ocular, and placental; parasites can be detected in amniotic, cerebrospinal, bronchoalveolar, ocular, pleural and ascitic fluids, as well as in urine and peripheral blood [Derouin and Garin, 1991; Barragan and Hitziger, 2008; Unno *et al.*, 2008]. Due to the high incidence of toxoplasmosis in AIDS patients, in the last few years, much attention has been placed on the pathology caused by this parasite.

The *T. gondii* life cycle involves two types of hosts: definitive hosts, which include members of the *Felidae* family such as the domestic cat in which the sexual reproduction cycle takes place, and intermediate hosts, which include warm-blood animals such as cattle, sheep, pigs, and humans in which asexual reproduction occurs [Dubey, 1998; Tenter *et al.*, 2000]. Parasite replication takes place in the gut, resulting in the production of oocysts, which are shed in the feces. After sporulation, the resultant sporozoites are infective when ingested by humans and other mammals, and tachyzoites multiply and enter into all host nucleated cells, creating the parasitophorous vacuole (PV), a highly specialized non-fusogenic compartment [Martin *et al.*, 2007] delimited by a membrane that allows the passage of small molecules [Gail *et al.*, 2004]. After the parasite undergoes repeated replication rounds, the host cells lyse and tachyzoites are disseminated via the blood and lymph. When the host immune system becomes activated due to the presence of the parasite, immune cells such as macrophages and lymphocytes respond with proliferation, activation, and the release of diverse cytokines including IFN-γ. The presence of IFN-γ induces tachyzoite differentiation in bradyzoites and modification of the infected host cell in tissue cysts, in which this form of the parasite remains in latency for several years, giving rise to chronic infections [Dimier and Bout, 1998].

Role of iron in cell invasion by *T. gondii*

Iron is an essential component in the intracellular survival and multiplication of *T. gondii*. Obtaining iron from the invaded host cell is a key process that *Toxoplasma* has to regulate to secure an adequate provision at the intravacuolar level. As a strategy, the parasite activates the increase of iron regulator proteins (IRPs), which apparently function to stabilize the TFR mRNA of host cells; therefore, a high expression of TFR is induced at the membrane in the invaded cells, leading to TF-iron capture, which is taken up by intracellular tachyzoites to aid in proliferation (Fig. 7). This positive regulation seems to be mediated by soluble factors secreted by *Toxoplasma* that are not yet identified [Gail *et al.*, 2004]. As occurs with other parasites, iron chelating agents such as deferoxamine can limit tachyzoite development. This effect is reverted through the addition of exogenous holo-TF or ferrous sulfate as sources of Fe, conditions that allow successful intracellular replication of the parasite and demonstrate the importance of iron in the intracellular development of this parasite [Dimier and Bout, 1998; Mahmoud, 1999].

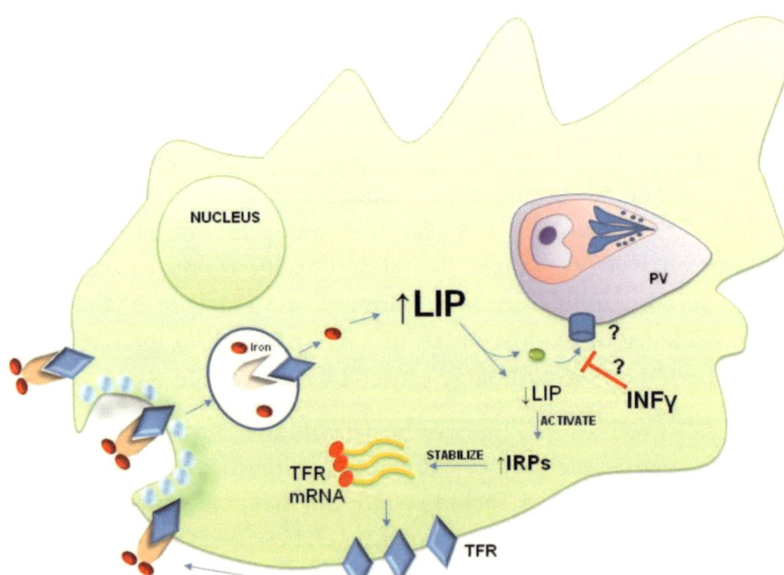

Figure 7. Iron uptake by intracellular *Toxoplasma gondii*. *T. gondii* lives inside a parasitophorous vacuole (PV) within the host cell; from there, it sequesters iron and depletes the macrophage labile-iron pool (LIP), activating the host cytosolic iron-responsive element sensor proteins (IRPs). These proteins increase the stability of the TFR mRNA , increasing host cell iron uptake from TF . This positive regulation system increases the intracellular iron that the parasite requires for survival. Iron uptake by the parasite is limited by TNFγ through an unknown mechanism.

In addition to the participation of macrophages and neutrophils in the immune response to *Toxoplasma,* fibroblasts, endothelia, and intestinal cells might also protect against this pathogen, most likely through a mechanism that involves the incorporation of iron from plasma TF, consequently limiting the availability of Fe resources to the parasite. An alternative strategy is the participation of exogenous IFN-γ in the inhibition of intracellular tachyzoite replication, a phenomenon observed in a dose-dependent manner in primary cultures of rat enterocytes. Interestingly, the exogenous addition of ferrous sulfate or holo-TF neutralizes entirely the effect of IFN-γ on the enterocytes. Although the precise molecular events initiated in enterocytes as a result of IFN-γ exposure are not clear, it has been suggested that IFN-γ inhibits tachyzoite replication by a mechanism that involves the limitation of available intracellular Fe (Fig. 7) [Dimier and Bout, 1998].

Dziadek et al. reported in [2005] that *T. gondii* tachyzoites of the BK strain bind to human holoLF but not holoTF, suggesting the presence of specific membrane receptors of *Toxoplasma* to host mucosal LF. Tanaka studied the expression of Lbps on tachyzoites of the RH-strain maintained through Vero cells incubated with labeled bovine LF and bovine TF. Both iron-carrier proteins were recognized by a single protein of 42 kDa, suggesting a non-specific binding to a common receptor [Tanaka *et al.,* 2003]. In additional studies, it was determined that both the absence and the excess of Fe produce an inhibition of the intracellular proliferation of RH-strain tachyzoites grown in cultured host cells, however, the mechanism of action by which this phenomenon occurs is unknown [Tanaka *et al.,* 1997].

3. Concluding remarks

Our knowledge of iron-uptake mechanisms from host TF by parasitic protozoa has improved in the past few years. These new insights have demonstrated the importance of effective iron uptake for virulence and increased the understanding of several mechanisms. Although substantial progress has been made, there is surprisingly little information available, including information about *T. brucei* and *T. cruzi,* which have been extensively studied, present interesting differences in their iron internalization mechanisms, and have enormous therapeutic potential. In other pathogens with serious medical implications as *Leishmania, P. falciparum* and *E. histolytica,* there is very limited information available, although the importance of iron for their survival is evident.

It is necessary to obtain more knowledge on the iron acquisition mechanisms in unicellular eukaryotic pathogens in order to develop new chemotherapeutic strategies that avoid the utilization of host iron by these parasitic organisms that have intense iron requirements.

Author details

Magda Reyes-López, Jesús Serrano-Luna and Carolina Piña-Vázquez and Mireya de la Garza*
Departamento de Biología Celular, Centro de Investigación y de Estudios Avanzados del IPN, Mexico DF, Mexico

* Corresponding Author

Acknowledgement

This work was supported by CONACyT, Mexico, project 60102.

4. References

Affonso AL, Benchimol M, Ribeiro KC, Lins U, De Souza W. Further studies on the endocytic activity of *Tritrichomonas foetus*. Parasitol Res. 1994;80(5):403-13.

Ajioka JW, Boothroyd JC, Brunk BP, Hehl A, Hillier L, Manger ID, et al. Gene discovery by EST sequencing in Toxoplasma gondii reveals sequences restricted to the Apicomplexa. Genome Res. 1998 Jan;8(1):18-28.

Ali IKM, Clark CG, Petri Jr WA. Molecular epidemiology of amebiasis. Infection, Genetics and Evolution. 2008;8(5):698-707.

Allen CL, Goulding D, Field MC. Clathrin-mediated endocytosis is essential in *Trypanosoma brucei*. EMBO J. [10.1093/emboj/cdg481]. 2003;22(19):4991-5002.

Anaya-Velázquez F, Padilla-Vaca F. Virulence of *Entamoeba histolytica*: a challenge for human health research. Future Microbiology. 2011 2011/03/01;6(3):255-8.

Anstead GM, Chandrasekar B, Zhao W, Yang J, Perez LE, Melby PC. Malnutrition alters the innate immune response and increases early visceralization following Leishmania donovani infection. Infect Immun. 2001 Aug;69(8):4709-18.

Avila EE, Martinez-Alcaraz ER, Barbosa-Sabanero G, Rivera-Baron EI, Arias-Negrete S, Zazueta-Sandoval R. Subcellular localization of the NAD+-dependent alcohol dehydrogenase in *Entamoeba histolytica* trophozoites. J Parasitol. 2002 Apr;88(2):217-22.

Balber AE. The pellicle and the membrane of the flagellum, flagellar adhesion zone, and flagellar pocket: functionally discrete surface domains of the bloodstream form of African trypanosomes. Crit Rev Immunol. 1990;10(3):177-201.

Baltes N, Hennig-Pauka I, Gerlach G-F. Both transferrin binding proteins are virulence factors in *Actinobacillus pleuropneumoniae* serotype 7 infection. FEMS Microbiology Letters. 2002;209(2):283-7.

Barragan A, Hitziger N. Transepithelial migration by Toxoplasma. Subcell Biochem. 2008;47:198-207.

Barragan A, Sibley LD. Transepithelial migration of Toxoplasma gondii is linked to parasite motility and virulence. J Exp Med. 2002 Jun 17;195(12):1625-33.

Berczi A, Faulk WP. Iron-reducing activity of plasma membranes. Biochem Int. 1992 Dec;28(4):577-84.

Bitter W, Gerrits H, Kieft R, Borst P. The role of transferrin-receptor variation in the host range of *Trypanosoma brucei*. Nature. [10.1038/35166]. 1998;391(6666):499-502.

Bledsoe GH. Malaria Primer for Clinicians in the United States. Southern Medical Journal. 2005;98(12):1197-204.

Borst P. Transferrin receptor, antigenic variation and the prospect of a trypanosome vaccine. Trends in Genetics. 1991;7(10):307-9.

Britigan BE, Lewis TS, McCormick ML, Wilson ME. Evidence for the existence of a surface receptor for ferriclactoferrin and ferrictransferrin associated with the plasma membrane of the protozoan parasite Leishmania donovani. Adv Exp Med Biol. 1998;443:135-40.

Bruchhaus I, Tannich E. Induction of the iron-containing superoxide dismutase in *Entamoeba histolytica* by a superoxide anion-generating system or by iron chelation. Molecular and Biochemical Parasitology. 1994a;67(2):281-8.

Bruchhaus I, Tannich E. Purification and molecular characterization of the NAD(+)-dependent acetaldehyde/alcohol dehydrogenase from *Entamoeba histolytica*. Biochem J. 1994b Nov 1;303 (Pt 3):743-8.

Bullen JJ. The significance of iron in infection. Rev Infect Dis. 1981 Nov-Dec;3(6):1127-38.

Calmettes C, Yu R-h, Silva LP, Curran D, Schriemer DC, Schryvers AB, et al. Structural Variations within the Transferrin Binding Site on Transferrin-binding Protein B, TbpB. Journal of Biological Chemistry. 2011 April 8, 2011;286(14):12683-92.

Clarke TE, Tari LW, Vogel HJ. Structural biology of bacterial iron uptake systems. Curr Top Med Chem. 2001 May;1(1):7-30.

Cornelissen CN, Biswas GD, Tsai J, Paruchuri DK, Thompson SA, Sparling PF. Gonococcal transferrin-binding protein 1 is required for transferrin utilization and is homologous to TonB-dependent outer membrane receptors. Journal of Bacteriology. 1992 September 1, 1992;174(18):5788-97.

Correa JR, Atella GC, Batista MM, Soares MJ. Transferrin uptake in *Trypanosoma cruzi* is impaired by interference on cytostome-associated cytoskeleton elements and stability of membrane cholesterol, but not by obstruction of clathrin-dependent endocytosis. Exp Parasitol. 2008 May;119(1):58-66.

Correa JR, Atella GC, Vargas C, Soares MJ. Transferrin uptake may occur through detergent-resistant membrane domains at the cytopharynx of *Trypanosoma cruzi* epimastigote forms. Mem Inst Oswaldo Cruz. 2007 Nov;102(7):871-6.

Courret N, Frehel C, Gouhier N, Pouchelet M, Prina E, Roux P, et al. Biogenesis of Leishmania-harbouring parasitophorous vacuoles following phagocytosis of the metacyclic promastigote or amastigote stages of the parasites. J Cell Sci. 2002 Jun 1;115(Pt 11):2303-16.

Courret N, Frehel C, Prina E, Lang T, Antoine JC. Kinetics of the intracellular differentiation of Leishmania amazonensis and internalization of host MHC molecules by the intermediate parasite stages. Parasitology. 2001 Mar;122(Pt 3):263-79.

Cunha-e-Silva NL, Celso Sant'Anna, Pereira MG, Souza Wd. Endocytosis in *Trypanosoma cruzi*. The Open Parasitology Journal 2010:98-101.

Chen M, Li E, Stanley SL, Jr. Structural analysis of the acetaldehyde dehydrogenase activity of *Entamoeba histolytica* alcohol dehydrogenase 2 (EhADH2), a member of the ADHE enzyme family. Mol Biochem Parasitol. 2004 Oct;137(2):201-5.

Chen Q, Schlichtherle M, Wahlgren M. Molecular aspects of severe malaria. Clin Microbiol Rev. 2000 Jul;13(3):439-50.

Das NK, Biswas S, Solanki S, Mukhopadhyay CK. Leishmania donovani depletes labile iron pool to exploit iron uptake capacity of macrophage for its intracellular growth. Cell Microbiol. 2009 Jan;11(1):83-94.

de Sousa K, Atouguia J, Silva M. Partial Biochemical Characterization of a Metalloproteinase from the Bloodstream Forms of *Trypanosoma brucei brucei* Parasites. The Protein Journal. 2010;29(4):283-9.

Derouin F, Garin YJ. Toxoplasma gondii: blood and tissue kinetics during acute and chronic infections in mice. Exp Parasitol. 1991 Nov;73(4):460-8.

Diamond LS, Harlow DR, Phillips BP, Keister DB. *Entamoeba histolytica*: iron and nutritional immunity. Arch Invest Med (Mex). 1978;9 Suppl 1:329-38.

Dimier IH, Bout DT. Interferon-gamma-activated primary enterocytes inhibit Toxoplasma gondii replication: a role for intracellular iron. Immunology. 1998 Aug;94(4):488-95.

Dubey JP. Advances in the life cycle of Toxoplasma gondii. Int J Parasitol. 1998 Jul;28(7):1019-24.

Dziadek B, Dzitko K, Dlugonska H. Toxoplasma gondii binds human lactoferrin but not transferrin. Exp Parasitol. 2005 Jun;110(2):165-7.

Espinosa A, Clark D, Stanley SL, Jr. *Entamoeba histolytica* alcohol dehydrogenase 2 (EhADH2) as a target for anti-amoebic agents. J Antimicrob Chemother. 2004 Jul;54(1):56-9.

Espinosa A, Perdrizet G, Paz-y-Miño C G, Lanfranchi R, Phay M. Effects of iron depletion on *Entamoeba histolytica* alcohol dehydrogenase 2 (EhADH2) and trophozoite growth: implications for antiamoebic therapy. Journal of Antimicrobial Chemotherapy. 2009 April 1, 2009;63(4):675-8.

Espinosa A, Yan L, Zhang Z, Foster L, Clark D, Li E, et al. The bifunctional *Entamoeba histolytica* alcohol dehydrogenase 2 (EhADH2) protein is necessary for amebic growth and survival and requires an intact C-terminal domain for both alcohol dahydrogenase and acetaldehyde dehydrogenase activity. J Biol Chem. 2001 Jun 8;276(23):20136-43.

Flores BM, Stanley SL, Jr., Yong TS, Ali M, Yang W, Diedrich DL, et al. Surface localization, regulation, and biologic properties of the 96-kDa alcohol/aldehyde dehydrogenase (EhADH2) of pathogenic *Entamoeba histolytica*. J Infect Dis. 1996 Jan;173(1):226-31.

Fong YL, Cadigan FC, Coatney GR. A presumptive case of naturally occurring *Plasmodium knowlesi* malaria in man in Malaysia. Trans R Soc Trop Med Hyg. 1971;65(6):839-40.

Forbes JR, Gros P. Divalent-metal transport by NRAMP proteins at the interface of host-pathogen interactions. Trends Microbiol. 2001 Aug;9(8):397-403.

Fry M. Diferric transferrin reductase in *Plasmodium falciparum*-infected erythrocytes. Biochem Biophys Res Commun. 1989 Jan 31;158(2):469-73.

Gail M, Gross U, Bohne W. Transferrin receptor induction in Toxoplasma gondii-infected HFF is associated with increased iron-responsive protein 1 activity and is mediated by secreted factors. Parasitol Res. 2004 Oct;94(3):233-9.

Gkouvatsos K, Papanikolaou G, Pantopoulos K. Regulation of iron transport and the role of transferrin. Biochimica et Biophysica Acta (BBA) - General Subjects. 2012;1820(3):188-202.

Goldberg DE, Slater AF, Cerami A, Henderson GB. Hemoglobin degradation in the malaria parasite *Plasmodium falciparum*: an ordered process in a unique organelle. Proc Natl Acad Sci U S A. 1990 Apr;87(8):2931-5.

Gookin JL, Breitschwerdt EB, Levy MG, Gager RB, Benrud JG. Diarrhea associated with trichomonosis in cats. J Am Vet Med Assoc. 1999 Nov 15;215(10):1450-4.

Gray-Owen SD, Schryvers AB. Characterization of transferrin binding proteins 1 and 2 in invasive type b and nontypeable strains of *Haemophilus influenzae*. Infection and Immunity. 1995 October 1, 1995;63(10):3809-15.

Greenwood BM, Bojang K, Whitty CJ, Targett GA. Malaria. Lancet. 2005 Apr 23-29;365(9469):1487-98.

Griffiths WJ, Kelly AL, Cox TM. Inherited disorders of iron storage and transport. Mol Med Today. 1999 Oct;5(10):431-8.

Haldar K, Henderson CL, Cross GA. Identification of the parasite transferrin receptor of *Plasmodium falciparum*-infected erythrocytes and its acylation via 1,2-diacyl-sn-glycerol. Proc Natl Acad Sci U S A. 1986 Nov;83(22):8565-9.

Hall BS, Pal A, Goulding D, Acosta-Serrano A, Field MC. *Trypanosoma brucei:* TbRAB4 regulates membrane recycling and expression of surface proteins in procyclic forms. Experimental Parasitology. 2005;111(3):160-71.

Halliwell B, Gutteridge JMC. Free radicals in biology and medicine. Oxford University Press; 2007.

Huynh C, Andrews NW. Iron acquisition within host cells and the pathogenicity of Leishmania. Cell Microbiol. 2008 Feb;10(2):293-300.

Isobe T, Holmes EC, Rudenko G. The Transferrin Receptor Genes of*Trypanosoma equiperdum* Are Less Diverse in Their Transferrin Binding Site than Those of the Broad-Host Range *Trypanosoma brucei*. Journal of Molecular Evolution. 2003;56(4):377-86.

Jacques I, Andrews NW, Huynh C. Functional characterization of LIT1, the Leishmania amazonensis ferrous iron transporter. Mol Biochem Parasitol. 2010 Mar;170(1):28-36.

Jarosik GP, Land CB, Duhon P, Chandler R, Jr., Mercer T. Acquisition of iron by *Gardnerella vaginalis*. Infect Immun. 1998 Oct;66(10):5041-7.

Jeffries TR, Morgan GW, Field MC. A developmentally regulated Rab11 homologue in *Trypanosoma brucei* is involved in recycling processes. Journal of Cell Science. 2001 July 15, 2001;114(14):2617-26.

Johnson EE, Wessling-Resnick M. Iron metabolism and the innate immune response to infection. Microbes and Infection. 2012;14(3):207-16.

Joiner KA, Roos DS. Secretory traffic in the eukaryotic parasite Toxoplasma gondii: less is more. J Cell Biol. 2002 May 13;157(4):557-63.

Jurado RL. Iron, infections, and anemia of inflammation. Clin Infect Dis. 1997 Oct;25(4):888-95.

Kabiri M, Steverding D. Studies on the recycling of the transferrin receptor in *Trypanosoma brucei* using an inducible gene expression system. European Journal of Biochemistry. 2000;267(11):3309-14.

Kabiri M, Steverding D. *Trypanosoma evansi*: Demonstration of a Transferrin Receptor Derived From Expression Site-Associated Genes 6 and 7. Journal of Parasitology. 2001 2001/10/01;87(5):1189-91.

Kaplan J. Mechanisms of Cellular Iron Acquisition: Another Iron in the Fire. Cell. 2002;111(5):603-6.

Kaye P, Scott P. Leishmaniasis: complexity at the host-pathogen interface. Nat Rev Microbiol. 2011 Aug;9(8):604-15.

Kennedy PGE. Sleeping sickness-human African trypanosomiasis. Practical Neurology. 2005 October 1, 2005;5(5):260-7.

Khun HH, Kirby SD, Lee BC. A *Neisseria meningitidis* fbpABC Mutant Is Incapable of Using Nonheme Iron for Growth. Infection and Immunity. 1998 May 1, 1998;66(5):2330-6.

Kinoshita T. Designing Sleeping Sickness Control. ACS Chemical Biology. 2008 2008/10/17;3(10):601-3.

Kulda J, Poislova M, Suchan P, Tachezy J. Iron enhancement of experimental infection of mice by *Tritrichomonas foetus*. Parasitol Res. 1999 Aug;85(8-9):692-9.

Lalonde RG, Holbein BE. Role of iron in *Trypanosoma cruzi* infection of mice. The Journal of Clinical Investigation. 1984;73(2):470-6.

León-Sicairos N, Reyes-López M, Canizalez-Roman A, Bermudez-Cruz RM, Serrano-Luna J, Arroyo R, et al. Human hololactoferrin: endocytosis and use as an iron source by the parasite *Entamoeba histolytica*. Microbiology. 2005 Dec;151(Pt 12):3859-71.

Ligtenberg MJ, Bitter W, Kieft R, Steverding D, Janssen H, Calafat J, et al. Reconstitution of a surface transferrin binding complex in insect form *Trypanosoma brucei*. EMBO J. 1994 Jun 1;13(11):2565-73.

Loftus B, Anderson I, Davies R, Alsmark UC, Samuelson J, Amedeo P, et al. The genome of the protist parasite *Entamoeba histolytica*. Nature. 2005 Feb 24;433(7028):865-8.

López-Soto F, Gonzalez-Robles A, Salazar-Villatoro L, León-Sicairos N, Piña-Vazquez C, Salazar EP, et al. *Entamoeba histolytica* uses ferritin as an iron source and internalises this protein by means of clathrin-coated vesicles. Int J Parasitol. 2009a Mar;39(4):417-26.

López-Soto F, León-Sicairos N, Reyes-López M, Serrano-Luna J, Ordaz-Pichardo C, Piña-Vázquez C, et al. Use and endocytosis of iron-containing proteins by *Entamoeba histolytica* trophozoites. Infection, Genetics and Evolution. 2009b;9(6):1038-50.

Low H, Sun IL, Navas P, Grebing C, Crane FL, Morre DJ. Transplasmalemma electron transport from cells is part of a diferric transferrin reductase system. Biochem Biophys Res Commun. 1986 Sep 30;139(3):1117-23.

Luft BJ, Remington JS. Toxoplasmic encephalitis in AIDS. Clin Infect Dis. 1992 Aug;15(2):211-22.

Lun ZR, Chen XG, Zhu XQ, Li XR, Xie MQ. Are *Tritrichomonas foetus* and *Tritrichomonas suis* synonyms? Trends Parasitol. 2005 Mar;21(3):122-5.

Mahmoud MS. Effect of deferoxamine alone and combined with pyrimethamine on acute toxoplasmosis in mice. J Egypt Soc Parasitol. 1999;29(3):791-803.

Maier A, Steverding D. Low affinity of *Trypanosoma brucei* transferrin receptor to apotransferrin at pH 5 explains the fate of the ligand during endocytosis. FEBS Letters. 1996;396(1):87-9.

Maier A, Steverding D. Expression and purification of non-glycosylated *Trypanosoma brucei* transferrin receptor in insect cells. Experimental Parasitology. 2008;120(2):205-7.

Manning K. Update on the diagnosis and management of *Tritrichomonas foetus* infections in cats. Top Companion Anim Med. 2010 Aug;25(3):145-8.

Marquis JF, Gros P. Intracellular Leishmania: your iron or mine? Trends Microbiol. 2007 Mar;15(3):93-5.

Marsee DK, Pinkus GS, Yu H. CD71 (transferrin receptor): an effective marker for erythroid precursors in bone marrow biopsy specimens. Am J Clin Pathol. 2010 Sep;134(3):429-35.

Martin AM, Liu T, Lynn BC, Sinai AP. The Toxoplasma gondii parasitophorous vacuole membrane: transactions across the border. J Eukaryot Microbiol. 2007 Jan-Feb;54(1):25-8.

Modun B, Williams P. The Staphylococcal Transferrin-Binding Protein Is a Cell Wall Glyceraldehyde-3-Phosphate Dehydrogenase. Infection and Immunity. 1999 March 1, 1999;67(3):1086-92.

Morgan GW, Allen CL, Jeffries TR, Hollinshead M, Field MC. Developmental and morphological regulation of clathrin-mediated endocytosis in *Trypanosoma brucei*. Journal of Cell Science. 2001 July 15, 2001;114(14):2605-15.

Mott GA, Costales JA, Burleigh BA. A Soluble Factor from *Trypanosoma cruzi* inhibits Transforming Growth Factor-Induced MAP Kinase Activation and Gene Expression in Dermal Fibroblasts. PLoS ONE. 2011;6(9):e23482.

Mulero V, Brock JH. Regulation of iron metabolism in murine J774 macrophages: role of nitric oxide-dependent and -independent pathways following activation with gamma interferon and lipopolysaccharide. Blood. 1999 Oct 1;94(7):2383-9.

Murray CJ, Rosenfeld LC, Lim SS, Andrews KG, Foreman KJ, Haring D, et al. Global malaria mortality between 1980 and 2010: a systematic analysis. Lancet. 2012 Feb 4;379(9814):413-31.

Mussmann R, Engstler M, Gerrits H, Kieft R, Toaldo CB, Onderwater J, et al. Factors Affecting the Level and Localization of the Transferrin Receptor in *Trypanosoma brucei*. Journal of Biological Chemistry. 2004 September 24, 2004;279(39):40690-8.

Nikaido H. Molecular Basis of Bacterial Outer Membrane Permeability Revisited. Microbiology and Molecular Biology Reviews. 2003 December 1, 2003;67(4):593-656.

O'Brien TC, Mackey ZB, Fetter RD, Choe Y, O'Donoghue AJ, Zhou M, et al. A Parasite Cysteine Protease Is Key to Host Protein Degradation and Iron Acquisition. Journal of Biological Chemistry. 2008 October 24, 2008;283(43):28934-43.

Olenick JG, Wolff R, Nauman RK, McLaughlin J. A flagellar pocket membrane fraction from *Trypanosoma brucei rhodesiense*: immunogold localization and nonvariant immunoprotection. Infection and Immunity. 1988 January 1, 1988;56(1):92-8.

Olivier M, Gregory DJ, Forget G. Subversion mechanisms by which Leishmania parasites can escape the host immune response: a signaling point of view. Clin Microbiol Rev. 2005 Apr;18(2):293-305.

Oppenheimer SJ. Iron and malaria. Parasitol Today. 1989 Mar;5(3):77-9.

Ossorio PN, Dubremetz JF, Joiner KA. A soluble secretory protein of the intracellular parasite Toxoplasma gondii associates with the parasitophorous vacuole membrane through hydrophobic interactions. J Biol Chem. 1994 May 27;269(21):15350-7.

Otto BR, Verweij-van Vught AM, MacLaren DM. Transferrins and heme-compounds as iron sources for pathogenic bacteria. Crit Rev Microbiol. 1992;18(3):217-33.

Pal A, Hall BS, Jeffries TR, Field MC. Rab5 and Rab11 mediate transferrin and anti-variant surface glycoprotein antibody recycling in *Trypanosoma brucei*. Biochem J. 2003 Sep 1;374(Pt 2):443-51.

Park S-J, Lee S-M, Lee J, Yong T-S. Differential gene expression by iron-limitation in *Entamoeba histolytica*. Molecular and Biochemical Parasitology. 2001;114(2):257-60.

Pays E. The variant surface glycoprotein as a tool for adaptation in African trypanosomes. Microbes and Infection. 2006;8(3):930-7.

Pereira-Neves A, Campero CM, Martinez A, Benchimol M. Identification of *Tritrichomonas foetus* pseudocysts in fresh preputial secretion samples from bulls. Vet Parasitol. 2011 Jan 10;175(1-2):1-8.

Peterson KM, Alderete JF. Iron uptake and increased intracellular enzyme activity follow host lactoferrin binding by *Trichomonas vaginalis* receptors. J Exp Med. 1984 Aug 1;160(2):398-410.

Pintor M, Ferreirós CM, Criado MT. Characterization of the transferrin-iron uptake system in *Neisseria meningitidis*. FEMS Microbiology Letters. 1993;112(2):159-65.

Pollack S, Fleming J. *Plasmodium falciparum* takes up iron from transferrin. Br J Haematol. 1984 Oct;58(2):289-93.

Pollack S, Schnelle V. Inability to detect transferrin receptors on *P. falciparum* parasitized red cells. Br J Haematol. 1988 Jan;68(1):125-9.

Reyes-López M, Bermudez-Cruz RM, Avila EE, de la Garza M. Acetaldehyde/alcohol dehydrogenase-2 (EhADH2) and clathrin are involved in internalization of human transferrin by *Entamoeba histolytica*. Microbiology. 2011 Jan;157(Pt 1):209-19.

Reyes-López M, Serrano-Luna JJ, Negrete-Abascal E, León-Sicairos N, Guerrero-Barrera AL, de la Garza M. *Entamoeba histolytica:* transferrin binding proteins. Exp Parasitol. 2001 Nov;99(3):132-40.

Riedel HD, Remus AJ, Fitscher BA, Stremmel W. Characterization and partial purification of a ferrireductase from human duodenal microvillus membranes. Biochem J. 1995 Aug 1;309 (Pt 3):745-8.

Roberts GP, Parker JM. Macromolecular components of the luminal fluid from the bovine uterus. J Reprod Fertil. 1974 Oct;40(2):291-303.

Rocha GM, Seabra SrH, de Miranda KR, Cunha-e-Silva N, de Carvalho TMU, de Souza W. Attachment of flagellum to the cell body is important to the kinetics of transferrin uptake by *Trypanosoma cruzi*. Parasitology International. 2010;59(4):629-33.

Rodriguez MH, Jungery M. A protein on *Plasmodium falciparum*-infected erythrocytes functions as a transferrin receptor. Nature. 1986 Nov 27-Dec 3;324(6095):388-91.

Roth EF, Jr., Brotman DS, Vanderberg JP, Schulman S. Malarial pigment-dependent error in the estimation of hemoglobin content in *Plasmodium falciparum*-infected red cells: implications for metabolic and biochemical studies of the erythrocytic phases of malaria. Am J Trop Med Hyg. 1986 Sep;35(5):906-11.

Salmon D, Geuskens M, Hanocq Fo, Hanocq-Quertier J, Nolan D, Ruben L, et al. A novel heterodimeric transferrin receptor encoded by a pair of VSG expression site-associated genes in T. brucei. Cell. 1994;78(1):75-86.

Salmon D, Hanocq-Quertier J, Paturiaux-Hanocq F, Pays A, Tebabi P, Nolan DP, et al. Characterization of the ligand-binding site of the transferrin receptor in *Trypanosoma brucei* demonstrates a structural relationship with the N-terminal domain of the variant surface glycoprotein. EMBO J. [10.1093/emboj/16.24.7272]. 1997;16(24):7272-8.

Salmon D, Paturiaux-Hanocq Fo, Poelvoorde P, Vanhamme L, Pays E. *Trypanosoma brucei:* growth differences in different mammalian sera are not due to the species-specificity of transferrin. Experimental Parasitology. 2005;109(3):188-94.

Sanchez-López R, Haldar K. A transferrin-independent iron uptake activity in *Plasmodium falciparum*-infected and uninfected erythrocytes. Mol Biochem Parasitol. 1992 Oct;55(1-2):9-20.

Scott DA, Docampo R, Dvorak JA, Shi S, Leapman RD. In Situ Compositional Analysis of Acidocalcisomes in *Trypanosoma cruzi*. Journal of Biological Chemistry. 1997 October 31, 1997;272(44):28020-9.

Schell D, Evers R, Preis D, Ziegelbauer K, Kiefer H, Lottspeich F, et al. A transferrin-binding protein of *Trypanosoma brucei* is encoded by one of the genes in the variant surface glycoprotein gene expression site. EMBO J. 1991 May;10(5):1061-6.

Schwartz KJ, Peck RF, Tazeh NN, Bangs JD. GPI valence and the fate of secretory membrane proteins in African trypanosomes. Journal of Cell Science. 2005 December 1, 2005;118(23):5499-511.

Serrano-Luna JdJ, Negrete E, Reyes M, de la Garza M. *Entamoeba histolytica* HM1:IMSS: Hemoglobin-Degrading Neutral Cysteine Proteases. Experimental Parasitology. 1998;89(1):71-7.

Singh B, Kim Sung L, Matusop A, Radhakrishnan A, Shamsul SS, Cox-Singh J, et al. A large focus of naturally acquired *Plasmodium knowlesi* infections in human beings. Lancet. 2004 Mar 27;363(9414):1017-24.

Smith JM, Meerovitch E. Specificity of iron requirements of *Entamoeba histolytica* in vitro. Arch Invest Med (Mex). 1982;13 Suppl 3:63-9.

Snow RW, Guerra CA, Noor AM, Myint HY, Hay SI. The global distribution of clinical episodes of *Plasmodium falciparum* malaria. Nature. 2005 Mar 10;434(7030):214-7.

Soares MJ, de Souza W. Endocytosis of gold-labeled proteins and LDL by *Trypanosoma cruzi*. Parasitol Res. 1991;77(6):461-8.

Soares MJ, Souto-Padron T, De Souza W. Identification of a large pre-lysosomal compartment in the pathogenic protozoon *Trypanosoma cruzi*. Journal of Cell Science. 1992 May 1, 1992;102(1):157-67.

Steverding D. The transferrin receptor of *Trypanosoma brucei*. Parasitology International. 2000;48(3):191-8.

Steverding D. The significance of transferrin receptor variation in *Trypanosoma brucei*. Trends in Parasitology. 2003;19(3):125-7.

Steverding D. On the significance of host antibody response to the *Trypanosoma brucei* transferrin receptor during chronic infection. Microbes and Infection. 2006;8(12-13):2777-82.

Steverding D, Stierhof YD, Fuchs H, Tauber R, Overath P. Transferrin-binding protein complex is the receptor for transferrin uptake in *Trypanosoma brucei*. The Journal of Cell Biology. 1995 December 1, 1995;131(5):1173-82.

Stijlemans B, Vankrunkelsven A, Brys L, Magez S, De Baetselier P. Role of iron homeostasis in trypanosomiasis-associated anemia. Immunobiology. 2008;213(9-10):823-35.

Sturm A, Amino R, van de Sand C, Regen T, Retzlaff S, Rennenberg A, et al. Manipulation of host hepatocytes by the malaria parasite for delivery into liver sinusoids. Science. 2006 Sep 1;313(5791):1287-90.

Subramanya S. Glycosylphosphatidylinositol-specific phospholipase C regulates transferrin endocytosis in the African trypanosome. Biochemical journal. 2009;417(3):685.

Subramanya S, Mensa-Wilmot K. Diacylglycerol-Stimulated Endocytosis of Transferrin in Trypanosomatids Is Dependent on Tyrosine Kinase Activity. PLoS ONE. 2010;5(1):e8538.

Suchan P, Vyoral D, Petrak J, Sut'ak R, Rasoloson D, Nohynkova E, et al. Incorporation of iron into *Tritrichomonas foetus* cell compartments reveals ferredoxin as a major iron-binding protein in hydrogenosomes. Microbiology. 2003 Jul;149(Pt 7):1911-21.

Sutak R, Lesuisse E, Tachezy J, Richardson DR. Crusade for iron: iron uptake in unicellular eukaryotes and its significance for virulence. Trends in Microbiology. 2008;16(6):261-8.

Sutherland CJ, Tanomsing N, Nolder D, Oguike M, Jennison C, Pukrittayakamee S, et al. Two nonrecombining sympatric forms of the human malaria parasite *Plasmodium ovale* occur globally. J Infect Dis. 2010 May 15;201(10):1544-50.

Tachezy J, Kulda J, Bahnikova I, Suchan P, Razga J, Schrevel J. *Tritrichomonas foetus*: iron acquisition from lactoferrin and transferrin. Exp Parasitol. 1996 Jul;83(2):216-28.

Tachezy J, Suchan P, Schrevel J, Kulda J. The host-protein-independent iron uptake by *Tritrichomonas foetus*. Exp Parasitol. 1998 Oct;90(2):155-63.

Talbot JA, Nielsen K, Corbeil LB. Cleavage of proteins of reproductive secretions by extracellular proteinases of *Tritrichomonas foetus*. Can J Microbiol. 1991 May;37(5):384-90.

Tanaka T, Abe Y, Inoue N, Kim WS, Kumura H, Nagasawa H, et al. The detection of bovine lactoferrin binding protein on *Trypanosoma brucei*. J Vet Med Sci. 2004 Jun;66(6):619-25.

Tanaka T, Abe Y, Kim WS, Xuan X, Nagasawa H, Igarashi I, et al. The detection of bovine lactoferrin binding protein on Toxoplasma gondii. J Vet Med Sci. 2003 Dec;65(12):1377-80.

Tanaka T, Omata Y, Narisawa M, Saito A, Shimazaki K, Igarashi I, et al. Growth inhibitory effect of bovine lactoferrin on Toxoplasma gondii tachyzoites in murine macrophages: role of radical oxygen and inorganic nitrogen oxide in Toxoplasma growth-inhibitory activity. Vet Parasitol. 1997 Jan;68(1-2):27-33.

Taylor MC, Kelly JM. Iron metabolism in trypanosomatids, and its crucial role in infection. Parasitology. 2010;137(06):899-917.

Tenter AM, Heckeroth AR, Weiss LM. Toxoplasma gondii: from animals to humans. Int J Parasitol. 2000 Nov;30(12-13):1217-58.

Testa U. Proteins of iron metabolism. CRC Press; 2002.

Thong KW, Coombs GH. *Trichomonas* species: homocysteine desulphurase and serine sulphydrase activities. Exp Parasitol. 1987 Apr;63(2):143-51.

Thong KW, Coombs GH, Sanderson BE. S-Adenosylmethionine metabolism and transsulphuration reactions in trichomonads. Acta Universitatis Carolinae-Biologica. 1986;30:293-8.

Thong KW, Coombs GH, Sanderson BE. L-methionine catabolism in trichomonads. Mol Biochem Parasitol. 1987 Apr;23(3):223-31.

Tovy A, Siman Tov R, Gaentzsch R, Helm M, Ankri S. A new nuclear function of the *Entamoeba histolytica* glycolytic enzyme enolase: the metabolic regulation of cytosine-5 methyltransferase 2 (Dnmt2) activity. PLoS Pathog. 2010 Feb;6(2):e1000775.

Trampuz A, Jereb M, Muzlovic I, Prabhu RM. Clinical review: Severe malaria. Crit Care. 2003 Aug;7(4):315-23.

Unno A, Suzuki K, Xuan X, Nishikawa Y, Kitoh K, Takashima Y. Dissemination of extracellular and intracellular Toxoplasma gondii tachyzoites in the blood flow. Parasitol Int. 2008 Dec;57(4):515-8.

Van Luenen HGAM, Kieft R, Mußmann R, Engstler M, Ter Riet B, Borst P. Trypanosomes change their transferrin receptor expression to allow effective uptake of host transferrin. Molecular Microbiology. 2005;58(1):151-65.

Van Snick JL, Masson PL, Heremans JF. The involvement of lactoferrin in the hyposideremia of acute inflammation. J Exp Med. 1974 Oct 1;140(4):1068-84.

Voyiatzaki CS, Soteriadou KP. Evidence of transferrin binding sites on the surface of Leishmania promastigotes. J Biol Chem. 1990 Dec 25;265(36):22380-5.

Voyiatzaki CS, Soteriadou KP. Identification and isolation of the Leishmania transferrin receptor. J Biol Chem. 1992 May 5;267(13):9112-7.

Wandersman Cc, Delepelaire P. BACTERIAL IRON SOURCES: From Siderophores to Hemophores. Annual Review of Microbiology. 2004;58(1):611-47.

Wang W, Di X, D'Agostino RB, Torti SV, Torti FM. Excess Capacity of the Iron Regulatory Protein System. Journal of Biological Chemistry. 2007 August 24, 2007;282(34):24650-9.

Weinberg ED. Iron loading and disease surveillance. Emerg Infect Dis. 1999 May-Jun;5(3):346-52.

Weinberg ED. Iron availability and infection. Biochimica et Biophysica Acta (BBA) - General Subjects. 2009;1790(7):600-5.

Welter BH, Powell RR, Laughlin RC, McGugan GC, Bonner M, King A, et al. *Entamoeba histolytica*: Comparison of the role of receptors and filamentous actin among various endocytic processes. Experimental Parasitology. 2006;113(2):91-9.

WHO. World Malaria Report 2008. Journal [serial on the Internet]. 2008 Date: Available from: http://www.who.int/malaria/publications/atoz/9789241563697/en/index.html.

WHO. World Malaria Report summary. Journal [serial on the Internet]. 2010 Date: Available from:
http://www.who.int/malaria/world_malaria_report_2010/malaria2010_summary_keypoints_en.pdf.

Wilson ME, Britigan BE. Iron Acquisition by Parasitic Protozoa. Parasitology Today. 1998;14(9):348-53.

Wilson ME, Lewis TS, Miller MA, McCormick ML, Britigan BE. Leishmania chagasi: uptake of iron bound to lactoferrin or transferrin requires an iron reductase. Exp Parasitol. 2002 Mar;100(3):196-207.

Wilson ME, Vorhies RW, Andersen KA, Britigan BE. Acquisition of iron from transferrin and lactoferrin by the protozoan *Leishmania chagasi*. Infect Immun. 1994 Aug;62(8):3262-9.

Witola WH, Sarataphan N, Inoue N, Ohashi K, Onuma M. Genetic variability in ESAG6 genes among *Trypanosoma evansi* isolates and in comparison to other Trypanozoon members. Acta Tropica. 2005;93(1):63-73.

Wooldridge KG, Williams PH. Iron uptake mechanisms of pathogenic bacteria. FEMS Microbiology Reviews. 1993;12(4):325-48.

Yang W, Li E, Kairong T, Stanley SL, Jr. *Entamoeba histolytica* has an alcohol dehydrogenase homologous to the multifunctional adhE gene product of *Escherichia coli*. Mol Biochem Parasitol. 1994 Apr;64(2):253-60.

Chapter 2

The Potential Role of Binding Proteins in Human Parasitic Infections: An In-Depth Look at the Novel Family of Nematode-Specific Fatty Acid and Retinol Binding Proteins

Jennifer L. Bath and Amber E. Ferris

Additional information is available at the end of the chapter

http://dx.doi.org/10.5772/50654

1. Introduction

Nematodes (phylum Nematoda) diverged from other animals between 600–1,200 million years ago [1] and have become one of the most diverse animal phyla on earth, second only to arthropods. Many nematodes are parasites of plants, animals, and humans, posing major global ecological and economic challenges. Close to 30,000 species have been identified [1], with an estimated one million species thought to exist [2]. An astounding 16,000+ species are parasites of plants and animals, causing diseases worldwide of major socio-economic importance. In agriculture, the current financial losses caused by parasites to domesticated animals and crops greatly affect farm profitability and exacerbate challenges to global food production and distribution. Root-knot nematodes alone infect more than 3,000 plant species and cause an estimated $100 billion annual loss worldwide [3].

Nematode genomes encode for proteins specific to the phylum Nematoda, and are critically important for understanding nematode biology [4-6]. Proteins specific to the phylum Nematoda are ideal targets for drugs with low toxicity to the host and the environment. Despite the importance of nematode-specific proteins and protein families, few have been identified and very little information regarding them is available on public databases [7].

Recent studies have investigated a novel, nematode-specific family of proteins, the fatty acid and retinol binding (FAR) proteins of the phylum Nematoda. The limited information available regarding this family of proteins, as well as the areas that are poorly understood concerning their *in vivo* function(s), will be described herein. It is likely that advances in the study of this family of proteins may be significant for a broad range of scientists in understanding animal parasitism, nematode evolution and parasite-control methods.

The nematode model organism, *Heligmosomoides polygyrus,* has long been used to study nematode biology, especially as it pertains to chronic nematode infections [8,9]. It is widely believed by parasitologists that the chronicity of nematode parasite infections is directly linked to the parasite's ability to alter its immediate environment, decreasing the effectiveness of the host's responses to the invading organism. There is evidence to suggest that alteration of the parasite's environment is achieved by the release of an excretory/secretory (E/S) molecule from the parasitic nematode [8]. There is also research to support this hypothesis using the model organism *H. polygyrus,* including studies investigating the role of an E/S FAR protein from *H. polygyrus,* termed Hp-FAR-1 [10]. *H. polygyrus* is now also used as a model for studying the role of FAR proteins in nematode biology and development, nutrient acquisition and lipid sequestration [10].

It was recently discovered that parasitic nematodes of plants, animals and humans secrete these structurally novel FAR proteins into the tissues they occupy [11].This family of proteins has been shown to be highly conserved across animal parasitic nematodes. The lipid-binding characteristics of FAR proteins across multiple families of parasitic nematodes, and their presence at the host-parasite interface, lends support to the idea that this nematode-restricted family of proteins may play a crucial role in the life cycle of the roundworms, providing essential lipids they cannot synthesize themselves [12], and possibly directly in the parasitism of their animal hosts. It is speculated by researchers that these proteins may interfere with intercellular lipid signaling to manipulate the defense reactions of the host or acquire essential lipids for the nematodes [10,13,14].

The highly conserved nematode-specific FAR proteins are thought to play a critical role in lipid sequestration and delivery from the host to the nematode of a broad range of essential fatty acids, retinoids and other nutrients. Hydrophobic lipophilic molecules such as fatty acids, eicosanoids, retinoids and steroids have important functions both as energy sources and in metabolic signaling [15]. They affect fundamental processes such as gene transcription, cell development, inflammation and the immune response [16-18].

2. Previous research on parasitic FAR proteins

To support the growing evidence that FAR proteins play an active role in nematode development and survival when in contact with host tissue, researchers have performed RT-PCR to determine the developmental stage specificity of *hp-far-1* mRNA transcription in third stage larvae (L_3), fourth stage larvae (L_4) and adult *H. polygyrus* [10].These data obtained provide further evidence to suggest that FAR proteins may play a crucial role in nematode lifecycle. This research demonstrates the transcription of the *hp-far-1* gene from the L_3 larval stage of *H. polygyrus,* as well as the L_4 and adult stages of the parasite. In addition, these studies analyzed the production of a FAR protein during stages in which the parasite is embedded within the host tissue, potentially in direct contact with mediators of host immunity [10]. These findings provide a context by which FAR proteins could theoretically sequester nutrients and fatty acids, as well as alter tissue environments, based on the sequestration or delivery of small lipid ligands, as previously speculated [11,14,19].

Based on secondary structure analysis, the structure of FAR proteins are clearly unlike that of any family of lipid-binding proteins, and also structurally distinct from proteins known from any organisms- from bacteria to plants to humans, increasing the possibility that they may present useful targets for drug development [20].

Below is an example of an abbreviated, ClustalW alignment demonstrating the conservation of amino acids from human parasitic FAR proteins across the phylum Nematode (Figure 1):

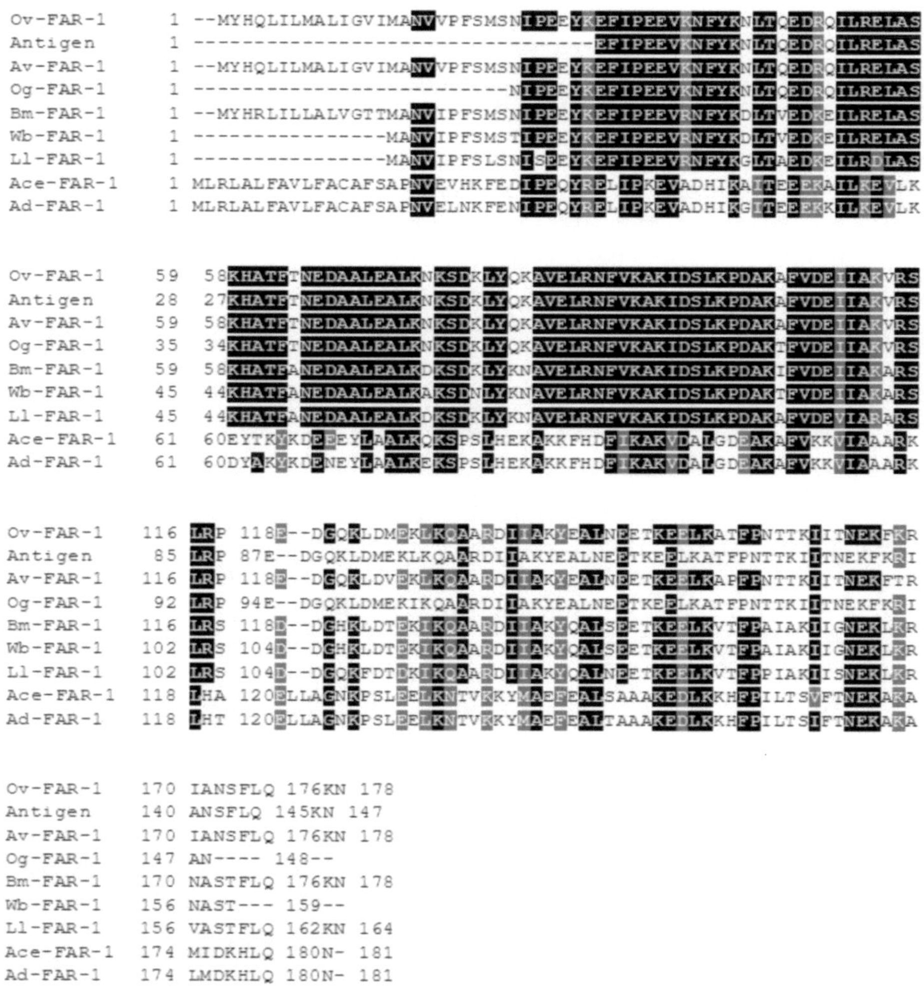

Figure 1. Amino acid sequence alignment of putative homologs of human parasitic FAR proteins from *Onchocerca volvulus* (Ov-FAR-1, AAC32662 and Antigen Maltose Binding Protein "Antigen", AAA65186), *Anthocheilenema vitae* (Av-FAR-1, AAM28244), *Onchocerca gutturosa* (Og-FAR-1, AAL33789) *Brugia malayia* (Bm-FAR-1, U69169), and *Wuchereria bancrofti* (Wb-FAR-1, AAL33794), *Loa loa* (Ll-FAR-1, AAK84218) *Ancyclostoma ceylanicum* (Ace-FAR-1, AAC76809), *Ancylostoma duodenale* (Ad-FAR-1, ABR87004). Sequences were aligned using ClustalW with a filter of 80% identity and prepared for display by BOXSHADE. Identical amino acids are shaded in black, and similar substitutions in gray. Amino acids common to every sequence are marked by an asterisk below the alignment.

There is not three-dimensional structural information available for parasitic FAR proteins and there is little information available regarding key amino acids involved in the function of parasitic FARs. The empirical structural information that exists for FAR proteins is a circular dichroism analysis showing that the Ov-FAR-1 protein from *Onchocerca volvulus*, demonstrating that it is rich in alpha-helices [21].

A study conducted in 2009 reported the X-ray crystallographic structure of Ce-FAR-7 from *C. elegans*, however, this is a non-parasitic nematode belonging to a different evolutionary group [15] Parasitic nematodes possess one or two types of FAR proteins [11,14], but the free-living *C. elegans* produces eight FAR proteins (Ce-FAR-1 to 8) [13]. They belong to three groups, group A (Ce-FAR-1, 2 and 6), group B (Ce-FAR-1, 4 and 5) and group C (Ce-FAR-7 and 8) [13]. Group A has the highest sequence identity to FARs from parasitic nematodes, such as Hp-FAR-1, Ov-FAR-1 (*O. volvulus*, human parasite) and Gp-FAR-1 (*Globodera pallida*, plant parasite) [21]. Although the sequence identity among parasitic FARs is high [14,21], the sequence identity of Ce-FAR-7 (the only FAR protein for which structural information is available) with other FAR proteins is extremely low [15], making data on Ce-FAR-7 more complicated for use in identifying key functional amino acids. In fact, of all of the *C. elegans* FAR proteins, Ce-FAR-7 is the least representative of known FAR proteins [13,14,21]. In contrast to other FAR proteins, Ce-FAR-7 exhibits minimal binding of 11-((5-dimethylaminonaphthalene-1-sulphonyl)amino)undecanoic acid (DAUDA) and, although Ce-FAR-7 induces fluorescence emission enhancements in cis-parinaric acid and retinol, it does so much less so than other FAR proteins [13]. Thus, is has been speculated that Ce-FAR-7 is functionally discrete from others [13].

In addition, a previous study investigating key amino acids in FAR ligand binding was performed on the FAR protein from the plant parasitic nematode *G. pallida*, Gp-FAR-1 [14]. In this study, several amino acids in the protein were altered by site-directed mutagenesis and, although the intrinsic fluorescence analysis of one mutant protein into which a tryptophan residue had been inserted supported computer-based predictions of the position of this residue at the protein's interior, the remaining substitutions produced no marked changes in ligand binding [14]. Therefore, this study concluded that the amino acids they had selected did not have any direct and essential involvement in the binding of ligands [14].

Thus, as it stands, there is a significant dearth of information available detailing amino acids that play a key role in ligand binding and protein function for FARs. Future work is likely to provide information on the key amino acids involved in fatty acid and lipid binding, which is essential to a basic understanding of FAR function and evolution, and the ability to utilize FAR proteins as a target for nematode-control measures.

To date, several FAR proteins, from a multitude of different nematode species, have been identified, recombinantly produced, isolated, and characterized [10,11,13,14].

FAR proteins discovered have been analyzed for fatty acid and retinol binding capabilities using spectrofluorimetry and fluorescence-based ligand-binding assays. Most commonly, fluorescence emission spectra were recorded at 20°C with the fluorescent fatty acid analog DAUDA or retinol diluted in PBS, as well as oleic acid diluted in PBS for competitive binding studies [10,11,13,14].

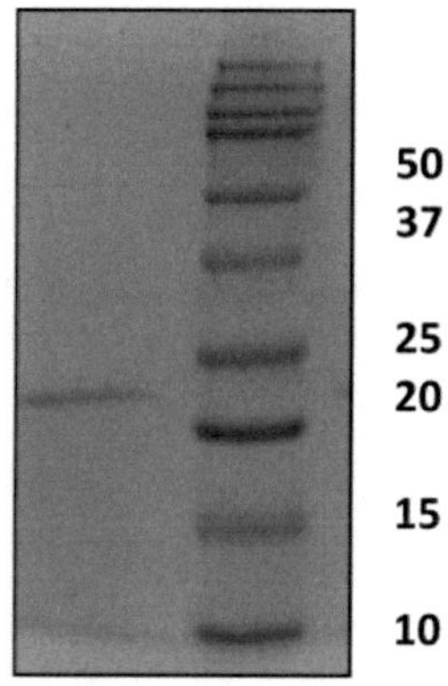

Image from Bath et al. 2009 Identification of an Immunogenic, Secreted Fatty Acid and Retinol-Binding Protein (Hp-FAR-1) from Heligmosomoides polygyrus. J. Nemat. 41(3):228-233.

Figure 2. Example of an SDS-PAGE of recombinant His-tagged FAR protein (in this case, Hp-FAR-1), produced by nickel-affinity chromatography.

Figures 3-5 demonstrate the specific results obtained for the FAR protein from *H. polygyrus*, Hp-FAR-1, which are fairly representative of binding patterns displayed by nematode FAR proteins.

Figure 3 shows Hp-FAR-1 binding characteristics, which are typical for parasitic FAR proteins, demonstrating the FAR protein bound to the fluorophore-tagged fatty acid DAUDA to produce a significant blue shift in its peak emission from 543 nm to 484 nm, which is unusually large for lipid transporter proteins but typical for FAR proteins [11,13,14,21], and indicative of a highly apolar binding site. Figure 4 shows that the addition of oleic acid to Hp-FAR-1:DAUDA complexes displaced DAUDA from the protein's binding site very efficiently, and complete replacement was observed at a ligand:competitor ratio of approximately 1:9. Figure 5 shows binding of retinol by Hp-FAR-1 which is indicated by a substantial increase in fluorescence emission intensity when retinol is added to a solution of Hp-FAR-1 in buffer [10].

Phosphorylation is one of the most common post-translational modifications that occurs on cellular proteins [22]. This process causes changes in the function, activity, localization, and/or stability in about 30 percent of cellular proteins [23]. A preliminary paper investigating the more distantly related Ce-FAR-7 protein presents evidence to suggest that retinol binding is positively regulated by CKII phosphorylation at a conserved site located near the binding pocket associated with retinol binding [15]. Previous research has also demonstrated that this is 100% conserved across all plant, animal and human parasitic nematode FAR proteins known to date [10,14,15,19].

Given this high conservation of the CKII phosphorylation site, and the overall high identity of the orthologs involved, it is reasonable to assume that CKII phosphorylation may also play a role in parasitic FAR:retinol binding. However, such studies have not yet been conducted, and basic questions regarding the role of the phosphorylation in parasitic nematodes, the impact of phosphorylation of K_ds of ligand binding, and possible shifts in preference for ligands have not been analyzed.

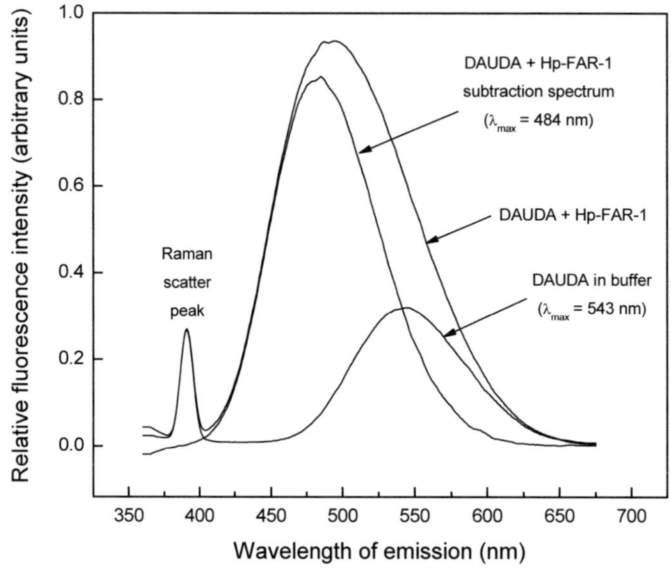

Figure from Bath et al. 2009 Identification of an Immunogenic, Secreted Fatty Acid and Retinol-Binding Protein (Hp-FAR-1) from Heligmosomoides polygyrus. J. Nemat. 41(3):228-233.

Figure 3. Binding of DAUDA by Hp-FAR-1 indicated by a substantial increase in fluorescence emission by DAUDA and the subtraction spectrum showing a significant blue shift in peak emission.

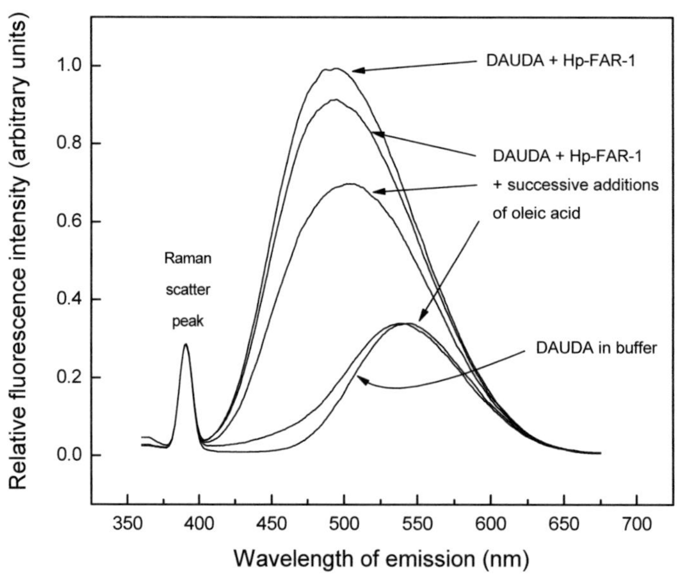

Figure from Bath et al. 2009 Identification of an Immunogenic, Secreted Fatty Acid and Retinol-Binding Protein (Hp-FAR-1) from Heligmosomoides polygyrus. J. Nemat. 41(3):228-233.

Figure 4. Highly efficient displacement of DAUDA from Hp-FAR-1 by successive additions of oleic acid. The concentration of compounds in the cuvette were approximately 1 μM DAUDA, and approximately 0.08 μM, 0.9 μM, and 9 μM oleic acid in the successive additions.

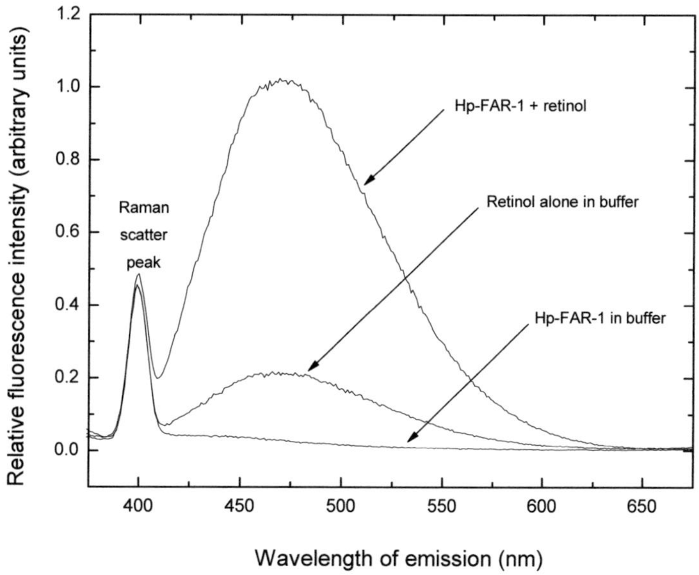

Figure from Bath et al. 2009 Identification of an Immunogenic, Secreted Fatty Acid and Retinol-Binding Protein (Hp-FAR-1) from Heligmosomoides polygyrus. J. Nemat. 41(3):228-233.

Figure 5. Binding of retinol by Hp-FAR-1 indicated by a substantial increase in fluorescence emission intensity when retinol is added to a solution of Hp-FAR-1 in buffer.

Ligand binding by Hp-FAR-1. Protein was mixed with environment-sensitive fluorescent ligands DAUDA (panel A), oleic acid (panel B) or retinol (panel C).

Analysis of the impact of phosphorylation on parasitic FAR proteins is of great interest for future studies because the initial binding capabilities of the analyzed Ce-FAR-7 are distinctly different than those of the distantly human and animal parasitic FARs, and thus one cannot make the assumption that CKII phosphorylation has the same role in parasitic FARs. While the results from Ce-FAR-7 suggest that the retinol binding site (P2) is probably regulated by CKII, the fatty acid binding pocket (P1) was not affected by phosphorylation. However, Ce-FAR-7's affinity for retinol is an order of magnitude lower than that for fatty acids, implying that, in contrast to the other FAR family members, transport of retinoids is not the major function of Ce-FAR-7 [15]. Thus, it is still unknown if the FAR protein affinity for signaling lipids, such as retinoids, is regulated in parasitic FARs, and if it is, how phosphorylation impacts the K_ds of the bound ligands.

Nematode FARs may function in scavenging, transport and metabolism of hydrophobic lipophilic molecules such as fatty acids, eicosanoids, retinoids, and steroids. These molecules have important functions as energy sources and are used in metabolic and developmental processes of embryogenesis, glycoprotein synthesis, growth and cellular differentiation [24,25]. Parasites cannot synthesize all of the lipids required for metabolism, but instead rely on a ready-made supply from their host. FAR proteins might facilitate uptake, transport and distribution of these molecules to specific target tissues [24].

Secretion of FARs into host tissues by parasites may, however, have significance beyond mere resource acquisition, in particular as depletion of these substances can significantly alter the tissue environment. For example, retinol has intrinsic importance in collagen synthesis and tissue repair mechanisms in a variety of tissues including the skin and the gut [26]. Retinol also prevents the decline in IgA and Th2 cytokine levels [27].

Cellular responses to *H. polygyrus* are an active area of research [9,28,29], and more recently there has been a surge of interest in the FAR family of proteins from organisms such as *H. polygyrus*, with respect to their potential role in altering their environment [10,11,21,30]. It is even speculated that the ability of FAR proteins to sequester RA results in cellular and cytokine alterations in the nematode's environment, a phenomenon that historically could have allowed nematodes to take advantage of a new niche, vertebrate parasitism.

3. Future directions and parasitic FARs as targets in drug development

There is an increasing interest by laboratories in investigating FAR proteins [11,14-15,30]. Continued studies will provide invaluable information as to exactly which amino acids are key in the binding of fatty acids and retinol, as well as the possible *in vivo* function(s) of nematode FAR proteins. These data would also enhance our understanding of the basic structural information for understanding the mode of action of FAR proteins and investigation of inhibitors of lipid binding.

A fuller appreciation of the function of FAR protein secretion will require a more detailed analysis and understanding of what parasitic FARs bind. Do they, for example, preferentially bind inflammatory mediators, their metabolic products or other potential pharmacologically active lipid mediators? Interference with such binding activities would likely have significant effects on the survival of nematodes and the impact of FARs on tissue dwelling and disease processes, and would further justify the relevance of targeting these molecules for drug targeting and/or vaccine development.

It is speculated, based on bioinformatic analyses, phylogenic studies, and the high conservation of FAR proteins amongst parasitic nematodes, that the evolution of FAR proteins may have been a precursor to nematode parasitism [13]. As such, it is also of interest to explore naturally occurring sequence variations, to determine which conserved regions or amino acids are imperative for ligand binding. Results from such studies are likely to shed more light on the role of FAR proteins in parasitism, with implications for their possible role(s) in the adaptation of free-living to parasitic lifestyles, by combining our knowledge of protein function with our information about sequence conservation from species to species.

Of particular interest for investigating the potential role of FARs in human parasitic diseases are the FAR affinities for the many vitamin A derivatives and fatty acids that are known to regulate expression of genes through the retinoic acid receptors (RARs) and retinoid X receptors (RXRs). These include RA in both of its stereoisomeric forms, all-trans retinoic acid

(ATRA, binds RARs) and 13-cis-retinoic acid (binds RAR). In addition, 9-cis-retinoic acid, which is converted from 13-cis-retinoic acid (binds RARs and RXRs) [31]. Two other RAR-interacting retinoids have been identified in tissue: all-trans 13,14-dihydroretinoic acid and beta –apoands-14′-carotenal [32,33]. Phytanic acid [34], docosahexaenoic acid [35] and other unsaturated fatty acids [36] have been proposed as additional/alternative ligands for RXRs. Future research may investigate the binding abilities FARs to leukotrienes and prostaglandins, both of which are compounds involved in the inflammatory response [18].

As the screening of potential FAR ligands broadens, it will provide researchers with a much fuller appreciation of the potential function of FAR protein secretion. The information gained with respect to ligands bound would be useful in the design and analysis of FAR studies aiming to target FARs in parasites, by demonstrating the potential pathways that interference with FAR binding activities are likely to effect.

Investigating the potential role(s) of FAR proteins in parasitic nematodes at a range of physiologically relevant temperatures is an area of research that should not be overlooked, in the event that ligand binding dissociation constants (Kds) are temperature sensitive. Such an expansion of the analysis to include additional temperatures may be quite relevant, as previous research has demonstrated significant variation in the binding affinities of various proteins to their ligands with regard to environmental temperature [37], and nematode-specific FAR proteins have been shown to be heat-stable [13,20]. Given that plant-parasitic nematodes are much more prevalent during warmer seasons and in tropical climates [38-40] and that animal parasites would, by their nature, inhabit warmer environments, it seems possible that FAR studies conducted to date, at 20°C, may not accurately reflect the binding properties of this family of protein *in vivo.*

The investigation of the role of phosphorylation by comparing the Kds for the most commonly tested ligands (DAUDA, oleic acid and RA) will likely be expanded by subjecting phosphorylated FAR proteins to a broader panel of ligands, to determine if the binding preferences and Kds for a broader range of ligands are altered upon phosphorylation. This knowledge would shed light on our basic understanding of nematode development and biology, by investigating the role of the conserved CKII phosphorylation site on FAR proteins with respect to ligand binding capabilities and respective Kds. The function of the N-terminal conserved CKII phosphorylation site on FARs may be important for ligand-binding. When phosphorylated, it may increase or decrease the affinity of the binding pockets for the binding of any number of essential fatty acids, retinoids and other nutrients that nematodes are not able to synthesize on their own [12]. Such knowledge sheds light on the possible *in vivo* roles of FARs in small lipid sequestration and delivery. This information directly impacts our understanding of basic nematode biology, development, and parasitism as hydrophobic lipophilic molecules such as fatty acids, eicosanoids, retinoids and steroids have important functions both as energy sources and in metabolic signaling [15] and affect fundamental processes such as gene transcription, cell development, inflammation and the immune response [16-18].

The ability of FAR proteins to bind fatty acids and retinoids is a characteristic of particular interest to parasitologists, due to the proteins potential function in nutrient acquisition, manipulation of the parasite's environment, and countering host defense reactions [24,41,42]. Retinoids, in particular, have the potential to regulate the expression of multiple genes by various mechanisms [43], through the binding of either RARs or RXRs [28]. When bound with ligand, the receptors transactivate specific cis-elements of target genes, known as Retinoic Acid Response Elements (RAREs). It is through this mechanism that retinol acts to positively regulate the T cell-derived cytokine interleukin 4 (IL-4). This is a key finding with respect to animal and human parasitism, in that localized host IL-4 levels are directly correlated to host protection [9,28,29], and thus a parasites' ability to regulate local IL-4 levels through an E/S protein may, in fact, be key to their survival.

Continued research in this area of FAR protein function will likely provide invaluable information regarding the possible *in vivo* function(s) of nematode FAR proteins, specifically with regard to the role they play in nematode survival and their possible use as targets in parasite-control methods. Such specific information about FAR proteins and their role in nematode survival could prove instrumental for nematologists, plant and animal parasitologists, agriculturalists and disease specialists.

Our growing understanding of the nematode-specific family of protein continues to provide invaluable information regarding the possible *in vivo* function(s) of nematode FAR proteins in parasitism and disease. Enhanced understanding of FAR proteins and their role in nematode biology could prove instrumental for plant and animal parasitologists, agriculturalists, cell biologists, evolutionists, and disease specialists. Continued enlightenment will also contribute to our fundamental understanding of how the evolution of FAR proteins may have contributed to the adaptation of free living nematodes, such as *C. elegans* (having eight known FAR proteins), to parasitic lifestyles.

Author details

Jennifer L. Bath*
Biology Department, Concordia College, Moorhead, MN, USA

Amber E. Ferris
Aldevron, LLC, Fargo, ND, USA

Acknowledgement

The authors would like to thank Kelsey Swagger (William Mitchell College of Law, St. Paul, MN) and Tyler Chase (Concordia College, Moorhead, MN) for their production of the ClustalW alignment of the parasitic FAR protein sequences.

* Corresponding Author

4. References

[1] Blaxter, M. *Caenorhabditis elegans* is a nematode. Science 1998; 282(5396) 2041-2046.

[2] Lambshead, P.J., Brown, C.J., Ferrero, T.J., Hawkins, L.E., Smith, C.R., Mitchell, N.J. Biodiversity of nematode assemblages from the region of the Clarion-Clipperton Fracture Zone, an area of commercial mining interest. BMC Ecology 2003, 3:1.

[3] Ibrahim, H.M., Hosseini, P., Alkharouf, N.W., Hussein, E.H., Gamal El-Din, Ael. K., Aly, M.A., Matthews, B.F. Analysis of Gene expression in soybean (Glycine max) roots in response to the root knot nematode *Meloidogyne incognita* using microarrays and KEGG pathways. BMC Genomics 2001; 12(1) 220.

[4] Curtis, R.H. Plant parasitic nematode proteins and the host parasite interaction. Briefings in Functional Genomics & Proteomics 2007; 6(1) 50 -58.

[5] Davis, E.L., Hussey, R.S., Baum, T.J. Getting to the roots of parasitism by nematodes. Trends Parasitol 2004; 20(3) 134-141.

[6] Lilley, C.J., Urwin, P.E., Atkinson, H.J. Characterization of plant nematode genes: identifying targets for a transgenic defence. Parasitology 1999; 118(Suppl) S63-72.

[7] Yin, Y., Martin, J., Abubucker, S., Wang, Z., Wyrwicz, L., Rychlewshi, L., McCarter, J.P., Wilson, R.K., Mitreva, M. Molecular determinants archetypical to phylum Nematoda. BCM Genomics 2009; 10:114.

[8] Behnke, J.M., Barnard, C.J., Wakelin, D. Understanding chronic nematode infections: evolutionary considerations, current hypotheses and the way forward. Int. J. Parasitol. 1999; 22(7) 861-907.

[9] Gustad, T., Robinson, M. Memory TH2 cells induce alternatively activated macrophages to mediate protection against nematode parasites. Paras. Immunol. 1996; 18:87-93.

[10] Bath, J.L, Robinson, M., Kennedy, M.W., Agbasi, C., Linz, L., Maetzold, E., Scheidt, M., Knox, M., Ram, D., Hein, J., Clark, C., Drees, J. Identification of an Immunogenic, Secreted Fatty Acid and Retinol-Binding Protein (Hp-FAR-1) from *Heligmosomoides polygyrus*. J. Nemat. 2009; 41(3) 228-233.

[11] Garofalo, A., Klager, S.L., Rowlinson, M.C., Nirmalan, N., Klion, A., Allen, J.E., Kennedy, M.W., Bradley, J.E. The FAR proteins of filarial nematodes: secretion, glycosylation and lipid binding characteristics. Mol. Biochem. Parasitol. 2002; 122:161-170.

[12] Barrett, J. Biochemistry of parasitic helminths. Baltimore, MD: University Park Press; 1981.

[13] Garofalo, A., Rowlinson, M.C., Amambua, N.A., Hughes, J.M., Kelly, S.M., Price, N.C., Cooper, A., Watson, D.G., Kennedy, M.W., Bradley, J.E. The FAR protein family of the nematode *Caenorhabditis elegans* - Differential lipid binding properties, structural characteristics, and developmental regulation. J. Biol. Chem. 2003; 278:8065-8074.

[14] Prior, A., Jones, J.T., Blok, V.C., Beauchamp, J., McDermott, L., Cooper, A., Kennedy, M.W. A surface-associated retinol- and fatty acid-binding protein (Gp-FAR-1) from the potato cyst nematode *Globodera pallida*: lipid binding activities, structural analysis and expression pattern. Biochem. J. 2001; 356:387-394.

[15] Jordanova, R., Groves, M. R., Kostova, E., Woltersdorf, C., Liebau, E., Tucker, P.A. Fatty acid- and retinoid-binding proteins have distinct binding pockets for the two types of cargo. JBC 2009; 284(51) 35818-26.

[16] Hotasmisligil, G. S. Inflammation and Metabolic Disorders. Nature 2006; 444(1721) 860-867.

[17] Cao, H., Gerhold, K., Mayrs, J.R., Wiest, M.M., Watkins, S.M., Hotasmisligil, G.S. Identification of a lipokine, a lipid hormone linking adipose tissue to systemic metabolism. Cell 2008; 134(6) 933-944.

[18] Funk, C.D. Prostaglandins and leukotrienes: advances in eicosanoid biology. Science 2001; 294(5548) 1871-1875.

[19] Basavaraju, S., Zhan, B., Kennedy, M.W., Liu, Y., Hawdon, J., Hotez, P.M. Ac-FAR-1, a 20 kDa fatty acid- and retinol-binding protein secreted by adult *Ancylostoma caninum* hookworms: gene transcription pattern, ligand binding properties and structural characterization. Mol Biochem Parasitol. 2003; 126(1) 63-71.

[20] Fairfax, K. C., Vermeire, J. J., Harrison, L. M., Bungiro, R. D., Grant, W., Husain, S. Z., Cappello, M. Characterisation of a fatty acid and retinol binding protein orthologue from the hookworm *Ancylostoma ceylanicum*. Int. J. Parasit. 2009; 39:1561-1571.

[21] Kennedy, M.W., Garside, L.H., Goodrick, L.E., McDermott, L., Brass, A., Price, N.C., Kelly, S.M., Cooper, A., Bradley, J.E. The Ov20 protein of the parasitic nematode *Onchocerca volvulus* – A structurally novel class of small helix-rich retinol-binding proteins. JBC 1997; 272(47) 29443-48.

[22] Stein A, Pache RA, Bernad P, Pons M, Aloy P. Dynamic interactions of proteins in complex networks: A more structured view. FEBS Journal 2009; 276(19) 5390-405.

[23] Ptacek, J., Snyder, M. Charging it up: Global analysis of protein phosphorylation. Trends in Genetics 2006; 22(10) 545-54.

[24] Kennedy, M.W. The polyprotein lipid binding proteins of nematodes. Biochem Biophys Acta 2000; 1476:149-164.

[25] McDermott, L., Cooper, A., Kennedy, M.W. Novel classes of fatty acid and retinol binding protein from nematodes. Molecular and Cellular Biochemistry 1999; 192(1-2) 69-75.

[26] Bulger, E.M., Helton, W.S. Nutrient antioxidants in gastrointestinal diseases. Gastroenterol Clin North AM. 1998; 27(2) 403-19.

[27] Nikawa T., Odahara K., Koizumi H., Kido Y., Teshima S., Rokutan K., Kishi K. Vitamin A prevents the decline in immunoglobin A and Th2 cytokine levels in small intestinal mucosa of protein-malnourished mice. J. Nutr. 1999; 129(5) 934–941.

[28] Liu, Z., Liu, Q., Pesce, J., Anthony, R.M., Lamb, E., Whitmire, J., Hamed, H., Morimoto, M., Urban Jr., J.F., Gause, W.C., and Anthony, R. Requirements for the development of

IL-4-producing T cells during intestinal nematode Infections: what it takes to make a Th2 cell in vivo. Immunol. Rev. 2004; 201:57-74.

[29] Anthony, R. M., Urban Jr., J. F., Alem, F., Hamed, H. A., Rozo, C. T., Boucher, J., Van Rooijen, N., Gause, W. C. Memory TH2 cells induce alternatively activated macrophages to mediate protection against nematode parasites. Nature Medicine 2006; 12:955-960.

[30] McDermott, L., Kennedy, M.W., McManus, D.P., Bradley, J.E., Cooper, A. How helminth lipid-binding proteins offload their ligands to membranes: differential mechanisms of fatty acid transfer by the ABA-1 polyprotein allergen and Ov-FAR-1 proteins of nematodes and Sj-FABPc of schistosomes. J. Biochem. 2002; 41(21) 6706-6713.

[31] Chambon, P. A decade of molecular biology of retinoic acid receptors. Faseb J. 1996; 10(9) 940-954.

[32] Moise, A.R., Kuksa, V., Blaner, W.S., Baehr, W., Palczewski, K. Metabolism and transactivation activity of 13,14-dihydroretinoic acid. J. Biol. Chem. 2005; 280:27815–27825.

[33] Ziouzenkova, O., Orashanu, G., Sukhova, G., Lau, E., Berger, J.P., Tang, G., Krinsky, N.I., Dolnikowski, G.G., Plutzky, J. Asymmetric cleavage of {beta}-carotene yields a transcriptional repressor of RXR and PPAR responses. Mol. Endocrinol. 2007; 21(1) 77-88.

[34] Lemotte P.K., Keidel S., Apfel C.M. Phytanic acid is a retinoid X receptor ligand. Eur. J. Biochem. 1996; 236:328–333.

[35] de Urquiza, A.M., Liu S., Sjoberg M., Zetterstrom R.H., Griffiths W., Sjovall J., Perlmann T. Docosahexaenoic acid, a ligand for the retinoid X receptor in mouse brain. Science 2000; 290:2140–2144.

[36] Goldstein J.T., Dobrzyn A., Clagett-Dame M., Pike J.W., DeLuca, H.F. Isolation and characterization of unsaturated fatty acids as natural ligands for the retinoid-X receptor. Arch. Biochem. Biophys. 2003; 420:185–193.

[37] Mattingly Jr., J.R., Iriarte, A., Martinez-Carrion, M. Homologous proteins with different affinities for groEL – The refolding of the aspartate aminotransferase isozymes at varying temperatures. JBC 1995; 270(3) 1138-48.

[38] Castagnone-Sereno, P., Bongiovanni, M., Dalmassto, A. Stable virulence against the tomato resistance Mi gene in the parthenogenetic root-knot nematode *Meloidogyne incognita*. Phytopathology 1993; 83(8) 803-805.

[39] Ammiraju, J., Veremis, J., Huang, X., Roberts, P., Kaloshian, I. The heat-stable root-knot nematode resistance gene Mi-9 from *Lycopersicon peruvianum* is localized on the short arm of chromosome 6. Theor. Appl. Genet. 2003; 106(3) 478-84.

[40] Claverie, M., Dirlewanger, E., Cosson, P., Bosselut, N., Lecouls, A.C., Voisin, R., Kleinhentz, M., Lafargue, B., Caboche, M., Calhoub, B., Esmenjaud, D. High-resolution mapping and chromosome landing at the root-knot nematode resistance locus Ma from

Myrobalan plum using a large-insert BAC DNA library. Theor. Appl. Genet. 2004; 109(6) 1318-27.

[41] Kennedy, M.W. Molecular Biology, Biochemistry, and Immunology. In: Kennedy, M.W. and Harnett W (eds.) Parasitic Nematodes. Wallingford and New York: CABI publishing; 2001. p 309-330.

[42] Bradley, J.E., Nirmalan N., Klager S.L., Faulkner H., Kennedy M.W. Trends Parasitol. 2001; 17: 471-475.

[43] Balmer, J.E., Blomhoff, R. Gene expression regulation by retinol acid. J. Lipid Res. 2002; 43(11) 1773-1808.

Chapter 3

Protein-Peptide Interactions Revolutionize Drug Development

Elif Ozkirimli Olmez and Berna Sariyar Akbulut

Additional information is available at the end of the chapter

http://dx.doi.org/10.5772/48418

1. Introduction

Protein-protein interactions form the basis of many cellular processes. Disruption or deregulation of these complex interactions is the main cause of a significant number of human ailments. Consequently, there is intense research effort to design inhibitors that target specific protein-protein interactions. This places intricate protein-protein interactions in the heart of the development for novel drug leads. The emergence of 'omic' technologies, namely genomics, transcriptomics and proteomics, has greatly accelerated our understanding of the protein-protein interaction networks leading to the discovery of a number of proteins and their interaction interface as potential drug targets.

The "druggable proteins" are targeted by commercially viable, and preferably orally bioavailable, therapeutics [1]. These drugs are usually small organic molecules that function as competitive or noncompetitive proteins inhibitors [2]. On the other hand, many "undruggable" proteins are important targets in various disease states. These proteins are considered undruggable because they lack a cavity for the small organic inhibitors to bind and they interact with their protein partners through extensive and flat surfaces. The use of protein based therapeutics expands the repertoire of "druggable proteins" by targeting those proteins that cannot be inhibited by the available small molecules [3]. Besides their improved specificity offered by their high compatibility with the target proteins, the major advantage of peptide therapeutics is their reduced immunogenicity and improved safety. On the other hand, low oral bioavailability, low protease/peptidase resistance, low cellular uptake, high rate of hepatic and renal clearance, high biodegradability and high flexibility are some limitations of peptides as therapeutics [4].

Peptide drugs take advantage of the highly specific and selective interaction between proteins. The peptide is usually based on the sequence of the binding region between the two proteins. The linear sequences might originate from a loop within a structured domain, or from a disordered region in protein termini or between defined domains. In order to achieve desired efficacy, following delivery to the correct cellular compartment, the designed peptide needs to target the appropriate site and bind it. A perfect therapeutic agent is then a short protein sequence that will reach, bind and modulate the function of a target protein for the required amount of time and efficacy. These linear sequences are difficult to discover due to their short length and a tendency to reside in disordered regions in proteins. Increase in the available structural information on the protein – protein interactions has spurred the design of novel peptide therapeuticals. Furthermore, it is now possible to screen and select high affinity peptides for these targets with the advent of peptide libraries and array techniques.

Peptide drugs may function by interacting with different targets such as proteins, lipids, nucleotides or metabolites. Particularly, there is significant research focused on antimicrobial peptides that target lipid cell membranes. This review focuses on the challenges and opportunities in the design and development of peptide based drugs that bind and inhibit some important protein targets.

2. Protein–peptide interactions

Diverse cellular events such as protein and vesicle trafficking, gene expression, DNA repair, control of the cytoskeleton and targeted protein degradation as well as signaling cascades are regulated through dynamic protein interactions [5-7]. Enhancing the efficacy of a peptide therapeutic addressing one of these processes is tightly bound to basic principles governing protein-peptide interactions. Despite their significance and estimated abundance, a large fraction of protein-peptide interactions lack detailed characterization and some questions of scientific and commercial interest remain: How does a peptide overcome the energetic cost involved in switching from an unstructured, flexible peptide to a rigid, well-defined bound structure? What is the recognition process for the binding event? What stabilizes these interactions? If a peptide binds to a protein, what is the spatial configuration and what is the strength of this interaction? If they don't bind each other, can they be made to bind by modifications? The increasing number of resolved protein-peptide structures sheds light into the mechanistic details of binding.

2.1. Protein – Peptide structures in the PDB

The rational design of peptide drugs is stimulated by the availability of structural information on protein – protein complexes. Peptides derived from the binding region of an inhibitor protein usually serve as a starting point in the design of peptide inhibitors against the protein – protein interaction. Coordinate and distance information about the binding interface can be based on X-ray crystallography or NMR methods. Other experimental methods that identify interface residues include alanine scanning mutagenesis [8], chemical modification, mass spectrometry and phage display [9].

We have filtered the Protein Data Bank [10] for the keyword "peptide" in the structure description and with chain length between 5 to 35 amino acids and found a total of 1816 crystal structures and 307 structures determined by solution NMR in March 2012. Additionally, two electron microscopy structures of the *Escherichia coli* 70S ribosome in the presence of the leader peptide were also reported. A 2010 study clustered the complex structures determined by crystallography in the Pep-X database (http://pepx.switchlab.org) [11]. This database contains 505 nonredundant protein-peptide interface complexes. 14% of these complexes are with the Major Histocompatibility Complex, 12% of them are with thrombin and 8% are with alpha-ligand binding domain. Another nonredundant protein – peptide database of 103 structures was reported in 2010 by the Schueler-Furman group [12].

The peptide binding site is usually a large and shallow pocket on the protein surface and it does not change its conformation upon peptide binding. In addition, hydrogen bonds with the peptide backbone and interactions with hot spot residues provide the enthalpic contribution to protein – peptide recognition. The protein – peptide interface is enriched in Leu and Ile as well as aromatic residues. The protein – peptide interface was shown to resemble the core of the protein, with more hydrophobic residues than the protein surface and with the structural motifs found in protein folds [12, 13].

2.2. Protein interaction domains in peptide recognition

It has become apparent that a significant number of protein interactions are commonly formed between conserved protein recognition domains and short linear peptide motifs, often less than 10 amino acids in length [14-17]. Members of a given protein domain family usually recognize a consensus motif but they may recognize different variations of this motif and they may possess unique binding specificities [17-24].

Peptides can interact with globular protein domains in very diverse ways. These include binding of a peptide onto a protein domain by forming an additional beta-sheet, binding to clefts in extended beta or proline type II helical conformations or adoption of a helical conformation. For example, SH2 and phosphotyrosine-binding (PTB) domains recognize phosphotyrosine motifs [6, 25-27], while polyProline helices are recognized by SH3, WW and EVH1 domains [14, 28, 29] (**Figure 1**). 14-3-3 proteins, FHA and WD40 domains recognize phosphothreonine/serine-containing elements [30]; bromo and chromo domains recognize acetylated or methylated lysine [31, 32]; VHL proteins recognize hydroxyproline motifs [33]. On the other hand, short amino acid motifs at the carboxyl termini of target proteins, such as ion channels, are important for recognition by PDZ domains [34].

Design of peptide based inhibitors against proteins with such modules is hampered by the similarity between the recognized peptide sequences. However the structural information available clarifies many ambiguities regarding protein-peptide interactions. The specificity and selectivity of the protein modules in the cell suggest the presence of a mechanism whereby a selective peptide drug can be designed that interferes with the binding of protein domains to their respective partners.

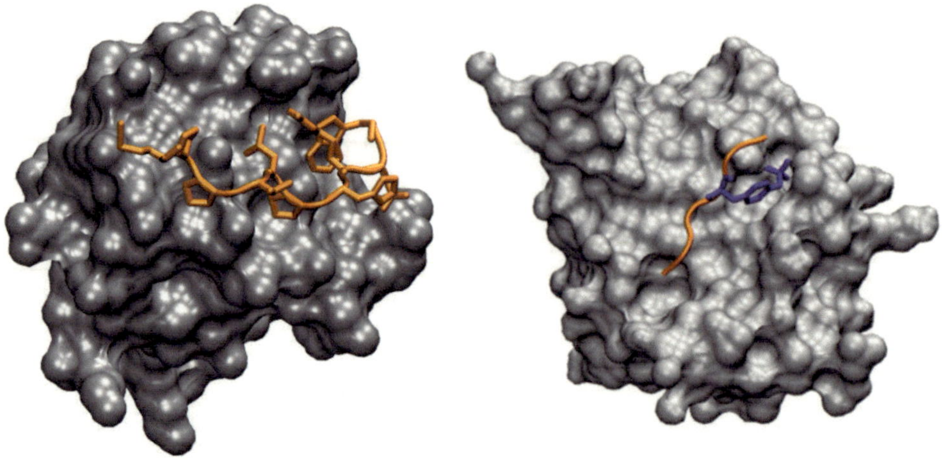

Figure 1. SH3 domain (gray) in complex with a polyproline peptide (PDB code: 1n5z), SH2 domain (gray) in complex with a phosphotyrosine peptide (PDB code: 1sps)

3. Identification/development of peptide ligand drugs

Figure 2 illustrates the primary steps involved in the design and development of peptide ligand drugs. The initial step in peptide drug design is the identification of the protein target. This is usually a protein that is implicated in a disease state. If possible (and/or available), the interaction partners of the target protein are also determined. Information from structure-activity relationship studies is then used for rational design. Structural information of the protein – protein interface is fundamental for rational drug design. If there is no information about the interacting partner, combinatorial approaches, such as phage display, peptide arrays or peptide aptamers, should be used to screen tight binding peptide sequences. Rational design may follow combinatorial approaches to design a peptide sequence with improved specificity and higher affinity. Once a tight binding potential peptide sequence is identified, the peptide is usually modified to enhance stability, uptake and delivery. These may include alteration of amino acids to nonnatural amino acids, cyclization of the peptide or constraining the peptide so that it forms an alpha helix. This modified peptide is a peptidomimetic, which has the properties of the peptide with respect to binding mechanism but also has higher stability and uptake potential than a natural peptide ligand. After *in vitro* tests of the modified peptide, *in vivo* tests and clinical trials are performed. Peptide may undergo further modifications during these tests. The ones that pass clinical trials are then marketed.

3.1. Rational design

Increase in the availability of crystallographic structures of protein complexes has conveyed valuable information for rational drug design efforts [36, 37]. Given a known (or predicted) protein – protein complex structure, inhibitors that target the interface between the two proteins can interfere with this interaction. Design of peptides based on the interface has also been an area of intense research [38, 39].

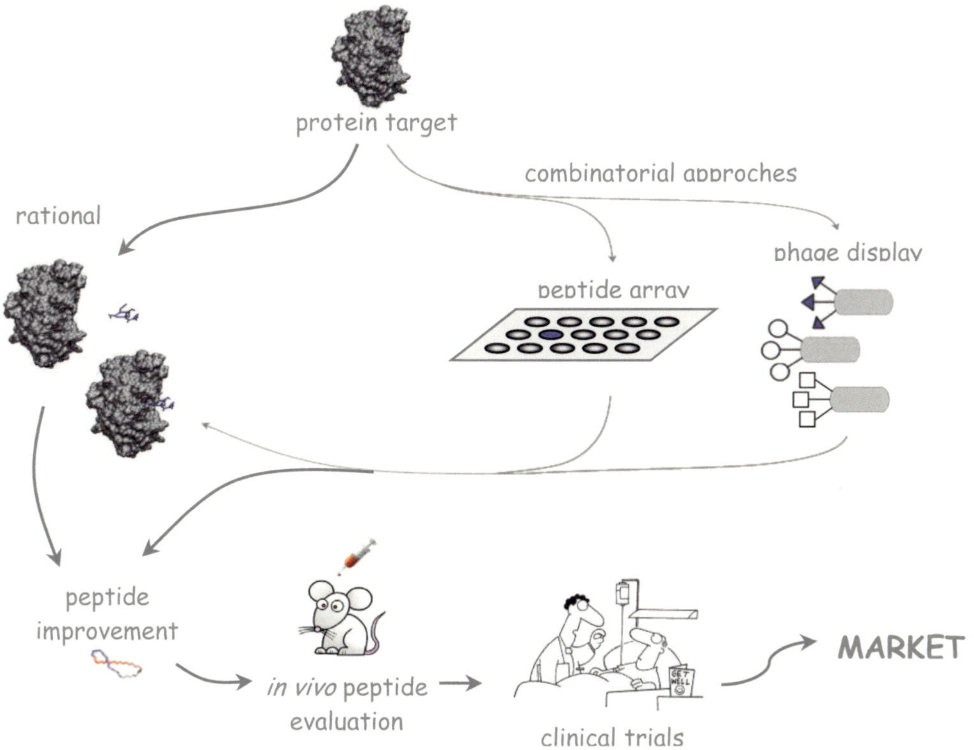

Figure 2. Schematic diagram of drug design (Target protein is beta-lactamase (PDB code: 1zg4, [35]) , photo of the patient in hospital by Randy Glasbergen (www.glasbergen.com, Copyright 2002).

Docking of small organic molecules to protein targets has shown good progress with the advent of docking, virtual screening and pharmacophore building algorithms [40]. However, the prediction of the complex structure between a peptide ligand and its protein partner is not easy due to the flexible nature of peptides. The solution structure and the bound structure of peptides are usually different, with the peptide adopting its bound conformation only in the presence of the protein [41]. In addition, protein – peptide docking studies are further complicated by the absence of a cavity for peptide binding, because protein – peptide interaction sites are usually shallow pockets on the surface [12]. Several algorithms have been proposed for protein – flexible peptide docking. Three recent algorithms are the molecular dynamics based Dynadock [42], the Monte Carlo based FlexPepDock [43] and PepCrawler, which uses the protein – protein interaction interface structure and the Rapidly-exploring Random Trees approach [39].

With the advent of high-throughput technologies, rational drug design led to the development of combinatorial chemistry to provide diverse libraries and arrays for drug discovery [44]. Combined with the screening of libraries and arrays against target proteins, rational drug design is a powerful tool for discovering novel pharmacologically active small peptide leads. These drug leads can further be engineered for the development of future generations of novel therapeuticals.

3.2. Peptide phage display

There are a number of display technologies (phage, ribosome, mRNA, bacterial, etc.) to select peptides for defined proteins targets. In this review, the discussion of display technologies will be restricted to phage display, the most widely utilized display method.

Phage display technique is based on displaying peptides on the surface of a bacteriophage by expressing the peptides as fusions to capsid proteins [45]. Using either lytic or filamentous phage or phagemid vectors, various phage-displayed libraries have been designed but the most common systems are based on filamentous phages in which peptides are fused to coat proteins. The choice of the coat protein is an important factor in modulating the display valency of the fusion protein on the phage particle which can vary between less than one and several thousand copies per virion on average [44]. The fact that a large number of virions occupy a small volume makes it possible to express billions of peptides on phage particles for constructing libraries of the required diversity. In such libraries, each phage displays a unique random peptide. In cases where the peptides are critically big to disrupt the integrity of the capsid at high copies, they can be constrained by cyclization through incorporating pairs of cysteine residues forming intramolecular disulfide bonds [44, 45]. Affinity purification is often used to screen phage displaying peptides of interest. Several rounds of screening might be necessary in order to isolate target specific binders. Finally, the tight binding peptides are identified by rapid sequence analysis [37, 45]. Unlike rational design, screening phage displayed libraries for bioactive ligands requires no prior knowledge of the target structure [44].

Mirror image phage display is an elegant approach to obtain peptide ligands in the D-conformation which are resistant to gut and serum proteases. In principle, the selection is carried out against a target protein synthesized in the D-amino acid configuration (the mirror image of the original target) using a phage library of peptides in the naturally occurring L-conformation. For reasons of symmetry, the mirror images of these phage-displayed peptides interact with the target protein of the natural handedness [46].

3.3. Peptide arrays

Systematically arranged peptides on a solid support, peptide arrays, show great promise in screening lead drugs [47]. Peptide arrays synthesized on cellulose membranes are very versatile and their preparation is very rapid and cost-effective [48]. Peptide arrays are primarily classilified based on the method used for assembly of peptides on the surface of the solid support. The *in situ* peptide array has peptides directly synthesized on the solid surface. In contrast, spotting peptide array relies on immobilization of presynthesized peptides onto a suitably derivatized solid surface [47, 49].

The two techniques used *in situ* peptide synthesis are the photolithographic synthesis (light-directed parallel chemical synthesis) and the SPOT synthesis. The former approach, first reported by Fodor et al [50], uses photolabile protecting groups to simultaneously synthesize thousands of spots, each with a unique peptide sequence. Improvements to this work have been reported by McGall et al [51], Pellois et al [52] and Li et al [53, 54]. In the SPOT technique, first reported by Frank [55, 56], peptides are synthesized by sequential spotting of small volumes of activated amino acids to a porous membrane. Advances have made rapid synthesis of a large number of peptides possible [57]. The advantage of *in situ* technique is that it avoids conventional synthesis of each peptide sequence found on the array.

The spotting array technique is preferable when small numbers of peptides are needed in the array or when the peptides will be used to prepare large numbers of identical arrays. There are currently a variety of methods for slide derivatization and immobilization of peptides to the surface [49]. In any application, chemical surfaces should allow efficient immobilization using the appropriately chosen functional groups present in a peptide. Additionally, the protocol to introduce the functional group, the tag, to the peptide should not be tedious.

3.4. Peptide aptamers

Peptide aptamers are most commonly used as disrupters of protein–protein interactions *in vivo*. They are combinatorial protein molecules (Figure 3), which consist of a variable peptide loop attached at both ends to an inert, constant scaffold protein [58-60]. The scaffold should preferable be small, composed of a single chain, and with a highly stable structure [61]. The choice between different scaffolds such as thioredoxin A (TrxA) [62], staphylococcus nuclease [63], human stefin A [64], and green fluorescent protein [65] is made by taking into account the intended use of the peptide [59]. Scaffold structures restrict the conformation of the peptide such that the loop can only adopt a discrete shape from the conformational space available to it. The variable loop of the aptamer, as constrained on both ends, offers greater specificity and higher affinity for their target surfaces as compared to the free peptide [66]. The higher affinity is a result of lower entropic cost due to binding of a constrained peptide compared with the entropic cost of constraining the peptide upon binding.

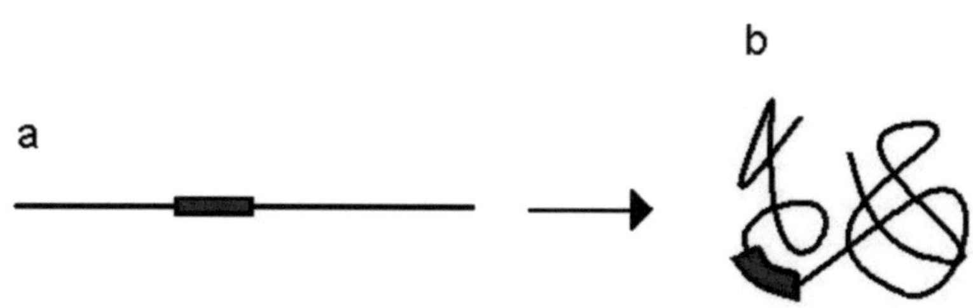

Figure 3. Peptide aptamer, a) unfolded form, b) folded form. Black region shows the scaffold protein and red loop shows the variable peptide.

Once the scaffold has been chosen, the three basic principles followed in aptamer design are (i) generation of a pool of peptides commonly using combinatorial approaches, (ii) selection to find best candidates, and (iii) amplification by expression in bacterial cells, such as *Escherichia coli* [59].

4. Toward a peptide drug with better bioavailability and stability

Peptides are gaining increasing attention as drug leads over small molecule drugs featured by their high affinity and specificity to interact with their targets together with their low toxicity profiles [67]. Unfortunately, the major limitations encountered in stability and delivery, overshadow their remarkable success. To be competitive and profitable, the lead peptide, which is usually designed based on the protein – protein interface, needs to be improved for better cell membrane permeability and stability and ADME (Absorption, Distribution, Metabolism, Excretion) properties [4, 68, 69]. Initial attempts were mainly focused on the improvement of existing peptide leads but the need for peptides with better physicochemical properties and pharmacokinetic profiles eventually has given rise to the field of peptidomimetics, the development of small peptide like compounds with the ability to mimic the structure or action of the raw peptide. The engineering of the desired property carries the new small molecule beyond the capabilities of the raw peptide lead [70].

4.1. Improvement of half life and stability

Peptides can display half lives as short as a few minutes, which is usually too short deliver sufficient drug amounts to target tissues. Consequently, many peptide drugs with exciting pharmacological activities prove to be ineffective *in vivo*. The short half life, which renders the peptide ineffective, is primarily due to its *fast renal clearance*, connected to its hydrophilic property and small size, and its *poor metabolic stability* and *biodegradability* as a result of enzymatic degradation by proteolytic enzymes (proteases and peptidases) of the blood, liver, and kidney. Hence different strategies for targeted modifications of peptide drugs in order to prolong their plasma half lives are highly demanded to improve drugs' pharmacokinetic profiles. [67, 71].

In performing a modification to a peptide drug to protect it from proteolytic cleavage, each peptide drug should be considered as a separate entity since, based on the sequence, each is a target for a different group of enzymes. This makes the detailed knowledge of proteases, their tissue localization and cleavage specificity very essential [71]. Only then can modifications on a particular drug be imposed to improve its susceptibility towards proteolytic enzymes targeting it. Protease resistance can be conferred by substituting the natural amino acids by unnatural amino acids (D-), an N-methyl-alpha-amino acid, or a beta-amino acid. The amide bond between two amino acids may be replaced. The N- or C-termini may be blocked or carbohydrate chains can be added. N-terminus may be esterified or pegylated. In addition, controlled release parenteral delivery, mucosal delivery and transdermal delivery have emerged as alternative strategies to oral delivery which exposes the peptide to stomach acid [4].

Constraining a peptide from an unstructured ensemble of many configurations to a fixed conformation serves two purposes; the conformational heterogeneity of the peptide in the unbound form is reduced, hence reducing the entropic cost associated with binding and more importantly the protease resistance of the peptide is enhanced [72]. Some example strategies of constraining the peptide are to "staple" or crosslink the peptide to assume an alpha helical shape [72] (Figure 4A), to cyclize the beta hairpin form [73] (Figure 4B), or to change the backbone such that it is nonrotatable [74]. Another similar modification mimics the structure of plant derived cyclotides, which contain a cyclic cysteine knot [75] (Figure 4C).

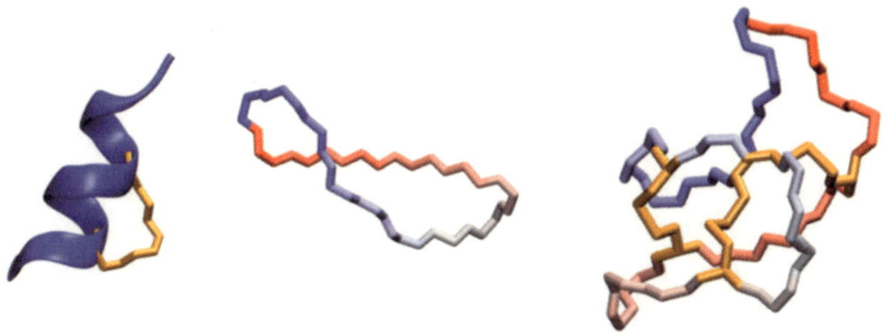

Figure 4. Examples of constrained peptides A) Cyclotide with three disulfide bridges shown in gold [76] 2k7g B) Cyclic beta-hairpin 2ns4 [77] C) Stapled peptide with the so-called staple, or hydrocarbon link shown in gold [78] 2yja

In many cases, modification of the peptide drug significantly increases enzymatic stability, but activity loss is always an issue. Therefore it is important that improved stability counterbalances activity loss. For this reason, co-administration of peptides with inhibitors of enzymes that target the peptide might be offered as an attractive alternative tool to chemical modifications to increase peptide stability [79-81].

4.2. Enhancing uptake and delivery

An important challenge in the design and development of peptide based drugs is their size and hydrophilic character, preventing their spontaneous uptake by the cell. For peptides which target membrane receptors, delivery to the target sites may be made possible with the application of liposomes or nano- and microparticles. On the other hand, in case of peptide drugs that target intracellular proteins, intracellular delivery through the biological membrane is crucial for their efficacy. Since poor uptake and limited delivery has been an important drawback hampering the acceptance of peptide drugs in the pharmaceutical market, different approaches have been proposed to address this problem.

Sustained delivery systems based on biodegradable polymers from renewable resourses such as chitosan and its derivatives, from petroleum resources such as PLGA (poly-lactic-co-glycolic acid) or PGA (polyglycolide) or blends of these have been receiving increasing attention following the nanotechnological advances applicable to peptide delivery [82-84]. As an example, progress made in the use of chitosan in peptide delivery is detailed below.

The polysaccharide based chitosan is a nontoxic linear polymer composed of β-1,4 linked D-glucosamine derived from the deacetylation of the naturally occurring polymer chitin. The biodegradable, biocompatible, bioadhesive, and permeation enhancing properties have made chitosan and its derivatives, such as N-trimethyl chitosan, outstanding polymers for delivery [85]. In addition to nasal, pulmonary, transdermal, and parenteral delivery routes using chitosan-based nano- and microparticle carriers, chitosan coated particles or pegylated chitosan particles receive particular interest for the delivery of peptides [83, 86]. Use of chitosan-based nano- and microparticles for peptide antigens based on luteinizing hormone-releasing hormone [87], peptide hormone insulin [88], glutathione [89, 90], heparin [91], and calcitonin [92] are just a few examples on the application of chitosan in peptide delivery.

Liposomes, regarded as drug delivery vehicles, are also widely used as carriers of peptides. They also enhance the local availability of peptides, protecting them from proteolytic action. Liposomes are artificially prepared microscopic vesicles composed of a lipid bilayer. The therapeutic peptide is encapsulated inside the aqueous compartment surrounded by the lipid membrane. Various types of liposome formulations have been prepared with different dimensions, composition, surface charge and structure to induce specificity and cell targeting [93, 94]. Different liposome formulations were tested for the administration of peptides such as insulin [95], calcitonin [96] and vasoactive intestinal peptide (VIP) [97].

There is significant discussion regarding the use of cell-penetrating peptides (CPPs) as tools to carry peptides to desired targets [37]. CPPs are usually 10-30 amino acids long and harbor a hydrophobic and a basic region. The major advantage of CPPs over antimicrobial peptides, which simply target the lipid membrane, is that CPPs help carry cargo into the cell in an energy independent manner without disrupting the cell membrane, hence can target intracellular enzymes and machinery [98, 99]. Two CPPs that have been studied in detail are the TAT peptide (GRKKRRQRRRPPQ) [100, 101] and penetratin (RQIKIWFQNRRMKWKK) [102, 103] . The mechanism of uptake has been proposed to be by endosomes at low concentrations [98]. Transient pore formation, and resulting direct penetration, was also proposed as a mechanism of uptake for Tat peptide at high concentrations [104]. In direct penetration, the membrane is transiently destabilized by the interaction of the basic residues (Arg) and the negatively charged components of the cell membrane. Another CPP, TP10 (also known as transportan, AGYLLGKINLKALAALAKKIL), lacks arginine residues and has been suggested to be delivered by the endocytotic pathway or by the interaction of the positively charged Lysine residues with the membrane [105, 106]. Structure activity relationship studies on another CPP, pVEC (LLIILRRRIRKQAHAHSK) showed that mutation of arginines to alanine did not abolish uptake, but scrambling the sequence of the peptide or mutating the first five hydrophobic residues to alanine did [107]. Conjugation of peptide drugs to CPPs is particularly relevant in the treatment of diseases which require the relevant peptide to traverse the blood-brain barrier.

5. Therapeutical peptides, present and future

5.1. Current status of peptide drugs

Although the synthesis and clinical use of the first synthetic peptide, insulin, dates back to 1920s [108, 109], it had not been possible to consider peptides as potential drugs before the introduction in 1960s by the 1984 Nobel Chemistry Prize Laureate Bruce Merrifield, of solid phase peptide synthesis, which lowered the production costs and time [110, 111]. Currently, the pharmaceutical industry and its contract manufacturers express their willingness to go into larger scale production using both solid- and solution-phase strategies. Today, there are more than 50 peptide drugs that have been approved for clinical use and the increasing number of peptides entering clinical trials now supports the notion that peptide drugs have a long and secure future. The targeted therapeutic areas of the present peptides include but are not limited to oncology, metabolic, cardiovascular and infectious diseases, all of which represent important markets. Table 1 includes a list of some of the peptide drugs that have reached high global sales (Pechon et al. development trends for peptide therapeutics, peptide therapeutics foundation, 2010 report).

Currently, most of the peptide drugs are peptide hormones (such as insulin) or peptides that mimic hormones [4]. However, the number of peptide drugs that act as enzyme inhibitors [112] or as antimicrobial peptides [113] is increasing.

5.2. Protein targets for potential peptide drugs

New peptide drugs are currently under development for a variety of protein targets. Here we focus on three major disease states, namely HIV infection, cancer and Alzheimer's disease and discuss some of the ongoing research toward the design and development of peptide drugs against these diseases.

Primary HIV infection starts through recognition of its envolope glycoproteins (gp120 and gp41) by the CD4 receptors and CCR5 (macrophage) or CXCR4 (T cell) co-receptors on its target. Upon entry, the envelope protein undergoes a major conformational change and juxtaposes the viral and host membranes. Finally, the viral genome integrates into the host genome. The envelope proteins is the site of primary infection, therefore fusion inhibitor peptides blocking their interaction with the protein targets in the host might be regarded as potential drugs [121]. With this motive, initial efforts of the early 1990s have eventually lead to the development of the first approved anti HIV-agent originally designated DP-178, later T-20 now FUZEON or Enfuviritide, which is a synthetic peptide based on the C-terminal heptad repeat region (C-HR) sequence of HIV-1 gp41 (Table 1) [120]. Although it is highly effective *in vitro*, its limited use due to difficulties encountered in its administration has shown that this drug in this from is not the ultimate solution for HIV treatment. Continued research, supported with structural studies, has shown C34, also derived from the C-HR sequence of gp41, can compete with gp41 [122, 123]. T21 and N36, derived from the N-terminal heptad repeat region (N-HR) were also reported to be potent inhibitors [124, 125]. Based on the fact that peptides derived from C-HR and N-HR regions of gp41 may serve as potent intibitors of HIV entry, intense research effort has been made for the rational design of different inhibitors based on these sequences. This also includes modifications such as incorporation of nonnatural and D-form amino acids (C34M3, [126]), synthesis of chimeric peptides (T1249, [123]) and even construction of fatty acid C-HR based conjugates (DP, [127]). For a detailed list, refer to the review by Naider and Anglister [121]. There is also continued research that focus on the sequences of CCR5 or CXCR4 receptors to design HIV-inhibitor peptides [128].

Peptide	**Brand name**	**Target disease**	**Target protein/ biological action**	**Sequence**	**Reference**
glatiramer acetate	Copaxone, copolymer1	Multiple sclerosis	Unknown	Random mixture of Glu, Ala, Lys, Tyr	[114]
leuprolide acetate	lupron	Prostate cancer, breast cancer	Binds gonadotropin-releasing hormone receptor	Pyr-HWSY-D-LLRP-NHEt	[115]
goserelin acetate	Zoladex	Prostate cancer, breast cancer	luteinising-hormone releasing hormone analog	p-EHWSY-D-S(tBu)-LRP-AzaGly-NH2,	[116]
octreotide acetate	Sandostatin	Acromegaly, carcinoid syndrome		H-D-F-c[CFD-WKTC]-tholacetate	[117]
exenatide	Byetta	Type 2 diabetes mellitus	glucagon-like peptide 1 analog	HGEGTFTSDLSK QMEEEAVRLFIE WLKNGGPSSGA PPPS	[118]
teriparatide	Forteo	osteoporosis		SVSEIQLMHNL GKHLNSMERVE WLRKKLQDVH NF	[119]
enfuvirtide	Fuzeon	HIV	Targets HIV-1 fusion machinery	Ac-YTSLIHSLIEESQ QQELNEQELLE LD KWASLWNW F-NH_2	[120]

Table 1. Some peptide drugs that have reached high global sales

Despite current progress, there is continued challenge in developing anti-HIV peptides due to their rapid renal clearance, poor distribution, and susceptibility to peptidase degradation. Hence search for HIV fusion inhibitors has been extended to screening a wide range of different sources such as red algae Griffithsia. From the algal lectin Griffithsin, a small HIV-1 entry inhibitor of 18-residues, Grifonin-1, was derived and this peptide was found to bind the HIV surface glycoprotein gp120 and block its binding with host surface receptors [129].

Envelope glycoproteins and cell surface receptors do not constitute the only target to prevent HIV infections. The cell-surface expressed nucleolin, which is one of the major RNA binding proteins of the nucleolus and serves as a binding protein for different ligands including HIV, might be another possible target in HIV treatment. The pentameric pseudopeptide HB-19 was found to inhibit HIV infection by binding to the nucleolin and to block the attachment of virus particles to cells. Hence HB-19 represents a potential anti-HIV drug [130, 131]. Since nucleoin at the cell surface is also a binding site for a variety of ligands implicated in tumorigenesis and angiogenesis, its potential as an anticancer drug has also been evaluated [131].

Loss of apoptotic control has been implicated in many disease states ranging from cancer [132] to autoimmune diseases . Caspases, a group of proteases implicated in apoptosis and inflammatory response, are therefore an important drug target. The WEHD tetrapeptide was found to be an optimal peptide sequence for caspase inhibitors using positional scanning synthetic combinatorial library [133] and many variants of this sequence have been designed. These peptidomimetic lead compounds for caspase inhibition, such as Pralnacasan, VX-765, emricasan and NCX-1000, have been recently reviewed by MacKenzie et al. [134]. The structure of caspase-2 in complex with a pentapeptide [135] is shown in Figure 5.

Estrogen receptors have been a drug target in breast and endometrial cancers since they regulate reproduction, maintain bone density and are important for central nervous system function. Peptide inhibitors that mimic and compete with the leucine-rich pentapeptide motif (LXXLL, where X is any residue) of the ER coactivator are promising lead compounds in the design of selective peptide inhibitors [136]. One modification to these lead compounds is using a hydrocarbon link to stabilize them in the alpha-helix form, also known as a stapled peptide [78]. The structure of the estrogen receptor in complex with a staple peptide is shown in Figure 5.

Bcl-2 is another protein involved in apoptosis and it has been the target of many drug design efforts [3]. However, the shallow groove which interacts with its binding partners renders it "undruggable" and therefore peptide based drug design against Bcl-2 has emerged as a promising approach [137]. The structure of Bcl-xL in complex with a Bad peptide is shown in Figure 5.

The phosphotyrosine recognition domain, SH2, is a subunit of many kinases, which are the key players in important signal transduction events. In Src kinases, SH2 – kinase domain intramolecular interaction keeps the kinase in its downregulated form [138], while in Stat3 (signal transducer and activator of transcription 3), the SH2 domain serves as a binding site for downstream signaling [68]. Loss of kinase regulation or constitutive kinase activation has been implicated in cancer and autoimmune diseases. As such, SH2 is an important drug target and SH2 inhibitor design is an area of intense research. The Stat3 SH2 recognition sequence pYXXQ (where pY is the phosphotyrosine and X is any residue) was modified into a lead peptidomimetic, nanomolar affinity was attained [68]. The structure of Grb2 SH2 domain in complex with a pYXN-derivative [139] is shown in Figure 5.

The proline rich AMAP-1 protein interacts with the SH3 domain of cortactin and this complex formation is implicated in tumor invasion [140]. This interface is therefore a drug target in breast cancer invasion and metastasis. The proline rich domain of AMAP-1 was used to design a proline rich peptide [141], which was then made cell-permeable by the addition of the HIV Tat sequence [142].

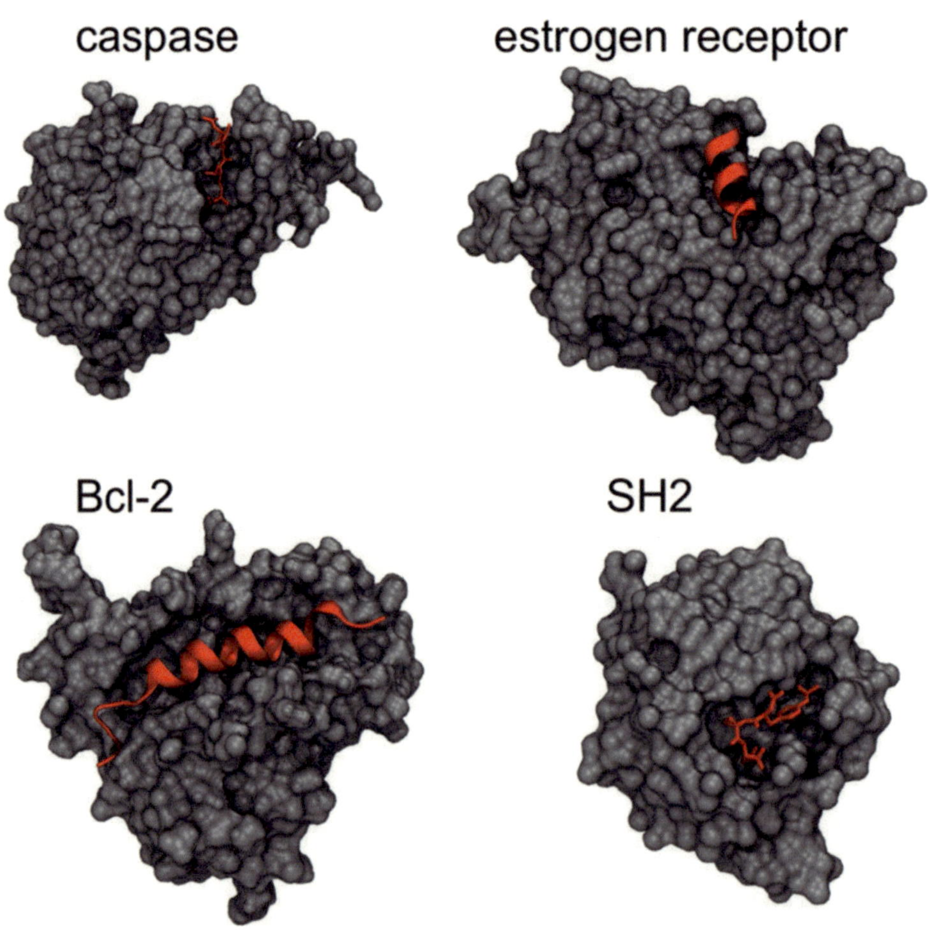

Figure 5. Some of the protein targets discussed in this review and their interaction with their designed peptide ligands. Caspase (PDB code: 3r6l), estrogen receptor (2yja), Bcl-2 (1g5j) and Grb2 SH2 domain (3ov1) are shown in silver surface representation and the peptide ligand is red.

The molecular origins of a number of neurodegenerative disorders such as Alzheimer's, Huntington's, Parkinson's and Creutzfeldt-Jakob diseases have been associated with the aggregation of proteins [143, 144]. In particular, the pathological event in Alzheimer's disease (AD) is the progressive accumulation of 42 residue β-amyloid peptides and resulting formation of insoluble β-amyloid fibrils [145]. Presently there is no cure for the treatment of AD but novel peptides that can inhibit and or reverse this abnormal conformational change are the subject of many recent reports. β-amyloid fibrillogenesis involves the conversion of α-helix/random coil to β-sheet motifs and proceeds via oligomeric and protofibrillar intermediates therefore it can be inhibited by destabilizing the β-sheet-rich β-amyloid intermediates, using β-sheet breaker peptides [146-149]. One example of a β-sheet breaker peptide, which comprises a short fragment of β-amyloid peptide (KLVFF; residues 16-20), can bind full-length β-amyloid peptide and prevent its assembly into amyloid fibrils [150]. The peptide LPFFD derived from another fragment of the β-amyloid peptide (LVFFA; residues 17-21) is another β-sheet breaker that abolishes fibril formation [146, 147] . Permanne et al further modified this peptide to extend the serum half-life and increase the blood-brain barrier permeability [151] . Rationally designed hybrid molecules composed of β-breaker elements combined with aromatic moieties (e.g. D-Trp-α-aminoisobutyric acid) have also emerged as promising leads [152]. Development of beta-sheet breaker peptides have also been reported toward diabetes 2, which is another amyloidogenic disease state [153].

6. Conclusion

As our understanding of complex biological networks increases, different proteins emerge as potential targets for peptide based drug development. Peptides are gaining increasing importance as drug leads over small molecule drugs featured by their high affinity and specificity to interact with the protein targets together with their low toxicity profiles. Many peptides that are currently administered do not meet the required criteria in cost, stability, long serum half-life and delivery. Nevertheless they serve as a source of inspiration for the development future generation peptide drugs. Evaluating the overall success, the increasing number of peptide leads going into clinical trials is a significant triumph for structural biology.

Author details

Elif Ozkirimli Olmez
Bogazici University, Chemical Engineering Department, Istanbul, Turkey

Berna Sariyar Akbulut
Marmara University, Bioengineering Department, Goztepe Campus, Istanbul, Turkey

Acknowledgement

We gratefully acknowledge funding Marmara University Nihad Sayar Foundation for Education, the Bogazici University Research Fund (09HA504P) and Tubitak Research Grant (109M229).

7. References

[1] Hopkins, A.L. and C.R. Groom, *The druggable genome.* Nat Rev Drug Discov, 2002. 1(9): p. 727-30.

[2] Boran, A.D.W. and R. Iyengar, *Systems Pharmacology.* Mt Sinai J Med, 2010. 77(4): p. 333-344.

[3] Verdine, G.L. and L.D. Walensky, *The Challenge of Drugging Undruggable Targets in Cancer: Lessons Learned from Targeting BCL-2 Family Members.* Clinical Cancer Research, 2007. 13(24): p. 7264-7270.

[4] Vlieghe, P., et al., *Synthetic therapeutic peptides: science and market.* Drug Discov Today, 2010. 15(1-2): p. 40-56.

[5] Pawson, T., *Protein modules and signalling networks.* Nature, 1995. 373(6515): p. 573-80.

[6] Pawson, T., M. Raina, and P. Nash, *Interaction domains: from simple binding events to complex cellular behavior.* FEBS Letters, 2002. 513(1): p. 2-10.

[7] Pawson, T., *Assembly of Cell Regulatory Systems Through Protein Interaction Domains.* Science, 2003. 300(5618): p. 445-452.

[8] DeLano, W.L., *Unraveling hot spots in binding interfaces: progress and challenges.* Curr Opin Struct Biol, 2002. 12(1): p. 14-20.

[9] Shoemaker, B.A. and A.R. Panchenko, *Deciphering protein-protein interactions. Part I. Experimental techniques and databases.* PLoS Comput Biol, 2007. 3(3): p. e42.

[10] Berman, H.M., et al., *The Protein Data Bank.* Nucleic Acids Research, 2000. 28(1): p. 235-42.

[11] Vanhee, P., et al., *PepX: a structural database of non-redundant protein-peptide complexes.* Nucleic Acids Research, 2010. 38(Database): p. D545-D551.

[12] London, N., D. Movshovitz-Attias, and O. Schueler-Furman, *The structural basis of peptide-protein binding strategies.* Structure, 2010. 18(2): p. 188-99.

[13] Vanhee, P., et al., *Protein-peptide interactions adopt the same structural motifs as monomeric protein folds.* Structure, 2009. 17(8): p. 1128-36.

[14] Ren, R., et al., *Identification of a ten-amino acid proline-rich SH3 binding site.* Science, 1993. 259(5098): p. 1157-61.

[15] Castagnoli, L., et al., *Selectivity and promiscuity in the interaction network mediated by protein recognition modules.* FEBS Letters, 2004. 567(1): p. 74-9.

[16] Encinar, J.A., et al., *ADAN: a database for prediction of protein-protein interaction of modular domains mediated by linear motifs.* Bioinformatics, 2009. 25(18): p. 2418-24.

[17] Gorelik, M. and A.R. Davidson, *Distinct Peptide Binding Specificities of Src Homology 3 (SH3) Protein Domains Can Be Determined by Modulation of Local Energetics across the Binding Interface.* J Biol Chem, 2012. 287(12): p. 9168-77.

[18] Zarrinpar, A., R.P. Bhattacharyya, and W.A. Lim, *The structure and function of proline recognition domains.* Sci STKE, 2003. 2003(179): p. RE8.

[19] Zarrinpar, A., S.-H. Park, and W.A. Lim, *Optimization of specificity in a cellular protein interaction network by negative selection.* Nature, 2003. 426(6967): p. 676-80.

[20] Stollar, E.J., et al., *Structural, Functional, and Bioinformatic Studies Demonstrate the Crucial Role of an Extended Peptide Binding Site for the SH3 Domain of Yeast Abp1p.* Journal of Biological Chemistry, 2009. 284(39): p. 26918-26927.

[21] Lim, W.A., F.M. Richards, and R.O. Fox, *Structural determinants of peptide-binding orientation and of sequence specificity in SH3 domains.* Nature, 1994. 372(6504): p. 375-9.

[22] Dalgarno, D.C., M.C. Botfield, and R.J. Rickles, *SH3 domains and drug design: ligands, structure, and biological function.* Biopolymers, 1997. 43(5): p. 383-400.

[23] Mayer, B.J., *SH3 domains: complexity in moderation.* J Cell Sci, 2001. 114(Pt 7): p. 1253-63.

[24] Gfeller, D., et al., *The multiple-specificity landscape of modular peptide recognition domains.* Mol Syst Biol, 2011. 7: p. 484.

[25] Kavanaugh, W.M. and L.T. Williams, *An alternative to SH2 domains for binding tyrosine-phosphorylated proteins.* Science, 1994. 266(5192): p. 1862-5.

[26] Blaikie, P., et al., *A region in Shc distinct from the SH2 domain can bind tyrosine-phosphorylated growth factor receptors.* J Biol Chem, 1994. 269(51): p. 32031-4.

[27] Liu, B.A., et al., *The human and mouse complement of SH2 domain proteins-establishing the boundaries of phosphotyrosine signaling.* Mol Cell, 2006. 22(6): p. 851-68.

[28] Chen, H.I. and M. Sudol, *The WW domain of Yes-associated protein binds a proline-rich ligand that differs from the consensus established for Src homology 3-binding modules.* Proc Natl Acad Sci USA, 1995. 92(17): p. 7819-23.

[29] Tonikian, R., et al., *Bayesian modeling of the yeast SH3 domain interactome predicts spatiotemporal dynamics of endocytosis proteins.* PLoS Biol, 2009. 7(10): p. e1000218.

[30] Yaffe, M.B. and A.E. Elia, *Phosphoserine/threonine-binding domains.* Curr Opin Cell Biol, 2001. 13(2): p. 131-8.

[31] Owen, D.J., et al., *The structural basis for the recognition of acetylated histone H4 by the bromodomain of histone acetyltransferase gcn5p.* EMBO J, 2000. 19(22): p. 6141-9.

[32] Bannister, A.J., et al., *Selective recognition of methylated lysine 9 on histone H3 by the HP1 chromo domain.* Nature, 2001. 410(6824): p. 120-4.

[33] Jaakkola, P., et al., *Targeting of HIF-alpha to the von Hippel-Lindau ubiquitylation complex by O2-regulated prolyl hydroxylation.* Science, 2001. 292(5516): p. 468-72.

[34] Doyle, D.A., et al., *Crystal structures of a complexed and peptide-free membrane protein-binding domain: molecular basis of peptide recognition by PDZ.* Cell, 1996. 85(7): p. 1067-76.

[35] Stec, B., et al., *Structure of the wild-type TEM-1 beta-lactamase at 1.55 angstrom and the mutant enzyme Ser70Ala at 2.1 angstrom suggest the mode of noncovalent catalysis for the mutant enzyme.* Acta Crystallographica Section D-Biological Crystallography, 2005. 61: p. 1072-1079.

[36] Sinskey, A., S. Finkelstein, and S. Cooper, *Getting to Rational Drug Design - at Last.* Pharmagenomics, 2002: p. 18-22.

[37] Mason, J.M., *Design and development of peptides and peptide mimetics as antagonists for therapeutic intervention.* Future Med Chem, 2010. 2(12): p. 1813-22.

[38] London, N., et al., *Can self-inhibitory peptides be derived from the interfaces of globular protein-protein interactions?* Proteins, 2010. 78(15): p. 3140-9.

[39] Donsky, E. and H.J. Wolfson, *PepCrawler: a fast RRT-based algorithm for high-resolution refinement and binding affinity estimation of peptide inhibitors.* Bioinformatics, 2011. 27(20): p. 2836-42.

[40] Plewczynski, D., et al., *Can we trust docking results? Evaluation of seven commonly used programs on PDBbind database.* J. Comput. Chem., 2011. 32(4): p. 742-55.

[41] Post, C.B., *Exchange-transferred NOE spectroscopy and bound ligand structure determination.* Curr Opin Str Biol, 2003. 13: p. 581-588.

[42] Antes, I., *DynaDock: A new molecular dynamics-based algorithm for protein-peptide docking including receptor flexibility.* Proteins, 2010. 78(5): p. 1084-104.

[43] Raveh, B., N. London, and O. Schueler-Furman, *Sub-angstrom modeling of complexes between flexible peptides and globular proteins.* Proteins, 2010. 78(9): p. 2029-40.

[44] Molek, P., B. Strukelj, and T. Bratkovic, *Peptide Phage Display as a Tool for Drug Discovery: Targeting Membrane Receptors.* Molecules, 2011. 16(1): p. 857-887.

[45] Smith, G.P. and V.A. Petrenko, *Phage Display.* Chem. Rev., 1997. 97(2): p. 391-410.

[46] Schumacher, T.N., et al., *Identification of D-peptide ligands through mirror-image phage display.* Science, 1996. 271(5257): p. 1854-7.

[47] Panicker, R.C., X. Huang, and S.Q. Yao, *Recent advances in peptide-based microarray technologies.* Comb Chem High Throughput Screen, 2004. 7(6): p. 547-56.

[48] Briant, D.J., et al., *Rapid identification of linear protein domain binding motifs using peptide SPOT arrays.* Methods Mol Biol, 2009. 570: p. 175-85.

[49] Min, D.-H. and M. Mrksich, *Peptide arrays: towards routine implementation.* Curr Opin Chem Biol, 2004. 8(5): p. 554-8.

[50] Fodor, S.P., et al., *Light-directed, spatially addressable parallel chemical synthesis.* Science, 1991. 251(4995): p. 767-73.

[51] McGall, G., et al., *Light-directed synthesis of high-density oligonucleotide arrays using semiconductor photoresists.* Proc Natl Acad Sci USA, 1996. 93(24): p. 13555-60.

[52] Pellois, J.P., et al., *Individually addressable parallel peptide synthesis on microchips.* Nat Biotechnol, 2002. 20(9): p. 922-6.

[53] Li, S., et al., *Photolithographic synthesis of peptoids.* J Am Chem Soc, 2004. 126(13): p. 4088-9.

[54] Li, S., et al., *Photolithographic synthesis of cyclic peptide arrays using a differential deprotection strategy.* Chem Commun (Camb), 2005(5): p. 581-3.

[55] Frank, R., *Spot synthesis – an easy technique for the positionally addressable, parallel chemical synthesis on a membrane support.* Tetrahedron, 1992. 48: p. 9217-9232.

[56] Frank, R., *The SPOT-synthesis technique. Synthetic peptide arrays on membrane supports--principles and applications.* J Immunol Methods, 2002. 267(1): p. 13-26.

[57] Winkler, D.F.H., H. Andresen, and K. Hilpert, *SPOT synthesis as a tool to study protein-protein interactions.* Methods Mol Biol, 2011. 723: p. 105-27.

[58] Colas, P., et al., *Genetic selection of peptide aptamers that recognize and inhibit cyclin-dependent kinase 2.* Nature, 1996. 380(6574): p. 548-50.

[59] Mascini, M., I. Palchetti, and S. Tombelli, *Nucleic acid and peptide aptamers: fundamentals and bioanalytical aspects.* Angew Chem Int Ed Engl, 2012. 51(6): p. 1316-32.

[60] Hoppe-Seyler, F., et al., *Peptide aptamers: specific inhibitors of protein function.* Curr Mol Med, 2004. 4(5): p. 529-38.

[61] Nygren, P.-A. and A. Skerra, *Binding proteins from alternative scaffolds.* J Immunol Methods, 2004. 290(1-2): p. 3-28.

[62] Borghouts, C., C. Kunz, and B. Groner, *Peptide aptamers: recent developments for cancer therapy.* Expert Opin Biol Ther, 2005. 5(6): p. 783-97.

[63] Norman, T.C., et al., *Genetic selection of peptide inhibitors of biological pathways.* Science, 1999. 285(5427): p. 591-5.

[64] Woodman, R., et al., *Design and validation of a neutral protein scaffold for the presentation of peptide aptamers.* Journal of Molecular Biology, 2005. 352(5): p. 1118-33.

[65] Abedi, M.R., G. Caponigro, and A. Kamb, *Green fluorescent protein as a scaffold for intracellular presentation of peptides.* Nucleic Acids Research, 1998. 26(2): p. 623-30.

[66] Crawford, M., R. Woodman, and P. Ko Ferrigno, *Peptide aptamers: tools for biology and drug discovery.* Brief Funct Genomic Proteomic, 2003. 2(1): p. 72-9.

[67] Jenssen, H. and S.I. Aspmo, *Serum stability of peptides.* Methods Mol Biol, 2008. 494: p. 177-86.

[68] Mandal, P.K., et al., *Structure-affinity relationships of glutamine mimics incorporated into phosphopeptides targeted to the SH2 domain of signal transducer and activator of transcription 3.* J. Med. Chem., 2009. 52(19): p. 6126-41.

[69] Mandal, P.K., W.S.-L. Liao, and J.S. McMurray, *Synthesis of phosphatase-stable, cell-permeable peptidomimetic prodrugs that target the SH2 domain of Stat3.* Org Lett, 2009. 11(15): p. 3394-7.

[70] Liskamp, R.M.J., et al., *Peptides and proteins as a continuing exciting source of inspiration for peptidomimetics.* Chembiochem, 2011. 12(11): p. 1626-53.

[71] Werle, M. and A. Bernkop-Schnürch, *Strategies to improve plasma half life time of peptide and protein drugs.* Amino Acids, 2006. 30(4): p. 351-67.

[72] Henchey, L.K., A.L. Jochim, and P.S. Arora, *Contemporary strategies for the stabilization of peptides in the α-helical conformation.* Curr Opin Chem Biol, 2008. 12(6): p. 692-697.

[73] Phichith, D., et al., *Novel peptide inhibiting both TEM-1 β-lactamase and penicillin-binding proteins.* FEBS J, 2010. 277(23): p. 4965-72.

[74] Ward, J.M., et al., *Constraining binding hot spots: NMR and molecular dynamics simulations provide a structural explanation for enthalpy-entropy compensation in SH2-ligand binding.* J Am Chem Soc, 2010. 132(32): p. 11058-70.

[75] Poth, A.G., et al., *Discovery of cyclotides in the fabaceae plant family provides new insights into the cyclization, evolution, and distribution of circular proteins.* ACS Chem Biol, 2011. 6(4): p. 345-55.

[76] Wang, C.K., et al., *Combined X-ray and NMR Analysis of the Stability of the Cyclotide Cystine Knot Fold That Underpins Its Insecticidal Activity and Potential Use as a Drug Scaffold.* Journal of Biological Chemistry, 2009. 284(16): p. 10672-10683.

[77] Athanassiou, Z., et al., *Structure-guided peptidomimetic design leads to nanomolar beta-hairpin inhibitors of the Tat-TAR interaction of bovine immunodeficiency virus.* Biochemistry, 2007. 46(3): p. 741-51.

[78] Phillips, C., et al., *Design and structure of stapled peptides binding to estrogen receptors.* J Am Chem Soc, 2011. 133(25): p. 9696-9.

[79] Pauly, R.P., et al., *Improved glucose tolerance in rats treated with the dipeptidyl peptidase IV (CD26) inhibitor Ile-thiazolidide.* Metab Clin Exp, 1999. 48(3): p. 385-9.

[80] Deacon, C.F., T.E. Hughes, and J.J. Holst, *Dipeptidyl peptidase IV inhibition potentiates the insulinotropic effect of glucagon-like peptide 1 in the anesthetized pig.* Diabetes, 1998. 47(5): p. 764-9.

[81] Ahrén, B., et al., *Inhibition of dipeptidyl peptidase IV improves metabolic control over a 4-week study period in type 2 diabetes.* Diabetes Care, 2002. 25(5): p. 869-75.

[82] Keijzer, C., et al., *PLGA, PLGA-TMC and TMC-TPP nanoparticles differentially modulate the outcome of nasal vaccination by inducing tolerance or enhancing humoral immunity.* PLoS ONE, 2011. 6(11): p. e26684.

[83] Fonte, P., et al., *Chitosan-coated solid lipid nanoparticles for insulin delivery.* Meth Enzymol, 2012. 508: p. 295-314.

[84] Morishita, M. and N.A. Peppas, *Is the oral route possible for peptide and protein drug delivery?* Drug Discov Today, 2006. 11(19-20): p. 905-10.

[85] Garcia-Fuentes, M., N. Csaba, and M.J. Alonso, *Nanostructured Chitosan Carriers for Oral Protein and Peptide Delivery.* TOUCH BRIEFINGS, 2007: p. 16-19.

[86] Amidi, M., et al., *Chitosan-based delivery systems for protein therapeutics and antigens.* Adv Drug Deliv Rev, 2010. 62(1): p. 59-82.

[87] Chua, B.Y., et al., *Chitosan microparticles and nanoparticles as biocompatible delivery vehicles for peptide and protein-based immunocontraceptive vaccines.* Mol Pharm, 2012. 9(1): p. 81-90.

[88] Mahjub, R., et al., *Preparation, statistical optimization, and in vitro characterization of insulin nanoparticles composed of quaternized aromatic derivatives of chitosan.* AAPS PharmSciTech, 2011. 12(4): p. 1407-19.

[89] Ieva, E., et al., *Analytical characterization of chitosan nanoparticles for peptide drug delivery applications.* Anal Bioanal Chem, 2009. 393(1): p. 207-15.

[90] Trapani, A., et al., *A comparative study of chitosan and chitosan/cyclodextrin nanoparticles as potential carriers for the oral delivery of small peptides.* Eur J Pharm Biopharm, 2010. 75(1): p. 26-32.

[91] Krauland, A.H. and M.J. Alonso, *Chitosan/cyclodextrin nanoparticles as macromolecular drug delivery system.* Int J Pharm, 2007. 340(1-2): p. 134-42.

[92] Prego, C., et al., *Chitosan-PEG nanocapsules as new carriers for oral peptide delivery. Effect of chitosan pegylation degree.* J Control Release, 2006. 111(3): p. 299-308.

[93] Ali, M. and N. Manolios, *Peptide Delivery Systems.* Letters in Peptide Science, 2002. 8: p. 289-294.

[94] Tan, M.L., P.F.M. Choong, and C.R. Dass, *Recent developments in liposomes, microparticles and nanoparticles for protein and peptide drug delivery.* Peptides, 2010. 31(1): p. 184-93.

[95] Jain, A.K., et al., *Muco-adhesive multivesicular liposomes as an effective carrier for transmucosal insulin delivery.* J Drug Target, 2007. 15(6): p. 417-27.

[96] Werle, M. and H. Takeuchi, *Chitosan-aprotinin coated liposomes for oral peptide delivery: Development, characterisation and in vivo evaluation.* Int J Pharm, 2009. 370(1-2): p. 26-32.

[97] Hajos, F., et al., *Inhalable liposomal formulation for vasoactive intestinal peptide.* Int J Pharm, 2008. 357(1-2): p. 286-94.

[98] Madani, F., et al., *Mechanisms of Cellular Uptake of Cell-Penetrating Peptides.* Journal of Biophysics, 2011. 2011: p. 1-10.

[99] Guterstam, P., et al., *Elucidating cell-penetrating peptide mechanisms of action for membrane interaction, cellular uptake, and translocation utilizing the hydrophobic counter-anion pyrenebutyrate.* Biochimica Et Biophysica Acta-Biomembranes, 2009. 1788(12): p. 2509-2517.

[100] Vivès, E., P. Brodin, and B. Lebleu, *A truncated HIV-1 Tat protein basic domain rapidly translocates through the plasma membrane and accumulates in the cell nucleus.* J Biol Chem, 1997. 272(25): p. 16010-7.

[101] Futaki, S., *Arginine-rich peptides: potential for intracellular delivery of macromolecules and the mystery of the translocation mechanisms.* International Journal of Pharmaceutics, 2002. 245(1-2): p. 1-7.

[102] Derossi, D., et al., *The third helix of the Antennapedia homeodomain translocates through biological membranes.* J Biol Chem, 1994. 269(14): p. 10444-50.

[103] Alves, I.D., et al., *Cell biology meets biophysics to unveil the different mechanisms of penetratin internalization in cells.* Biochim Biophys Acta, 2010. 1798(12): p. 2231-9.

[104] Herce, H.D. and A.E. Garcia, *Molecular dynamics simulations suggest a mechanism for translocation of the HIV-1 TAT peptide across lipid membranes.* Proceedings of the National Academy of Sciences of the United States of America, 2007. 104(52): p. 20805-20810.

[105] Padari, K., et al., *Cell transduction pathways of transportans.* Bioconjug Chem, 2005. 16(6): p. 1399-410.

[106] Yandek, L.E., et al., *Mechanism of the Cell-Penetrating Peptide Transportan 10 Permeation of Lipid Bilayers.* Biophysical Journal, 2007. 92(7): p. 2434-2444.

[107] Elmquist, A., M. Hansen, and Ü. Langel U, *Structure-activity relationship study of the cell-penetrating peptide pVEC.* Biochim Biophys Acta, 2006. 1758(6): p. 721-9.

[108] Banting, F.G., et al., *Pancreatic Extracts in the Treatment of Diabetes Mellitus.* Can Med Assoc J, 1922. 12(3): p. 141-6.

[109] Thomson, A.P., *THE CLINICAL USE OF INSULIN.* Br Med J, 1924. 1(3298): p. 457-60.

[110] Albericio, F., *Developments in peptide and amide synthesis.* Curr Opin Chem Biol, 2004. 8(3): p. 211-21.

[111] Merrifield, B., *Solid phase synthesis.* Science, 1986. 232(4748): p. 341-7.

[112] Lovshin, J.A. and D.J. Drucker, *Incretin-based therapies for type 2 diabetes mellitus.* Nature Reviews Endocrinology, 2009. 5(5): p. 262-269.

[113] Nguyen, L.T., E.F. Haney, and H.J. Vogel, *The expanding scope of antimicrobial peptide structures and their modes of action.* Trends in Biotechnology, 2011. 29(9): p. 464-72.

[114] Johnson, K.P., et al., *Copolymer 1 reduces relapse rate and improves disability in relapsing-remitting multiple sclerosis: results of a phase III multicenter, double-blind placebo-controlled trial. The Copolymer 1 Multiple Sclerosis Study Group.* Neurology, 1995. 45(7): p. 1268-76.

[115] Arnold, A.J. and A.D. Desmond, *Gonadotrophin hormone releasing analogues open new doors in cancer treatment.* Br Med J (Clin Res Ed), 1987. 295(6612): p. 1565.

[116] Furr, B.J. and R.I. Nicholson, *Use of analogues of luteinizing hormone-releasing hormone for the treatment of cancer.* J Reprod Fertil, 1982. 64(2): p. 529-39.

[117] Maurer, R., et al., *Opiate antagonistic properties of an octapeptide somatostatin analog.* Proc Natl Acad Sci USA, 1982. 79(15): p. 4815-7.

[118] DeFronzo, R.A., et al., *Effects of exenatide (exendin-4) on glycemic control and weight over 30 weeks in metformin-treated patients with type 2 diabetes.* Diabetes Care, 2005. 28(5): p. 1092-100.

[119] Neer, R.M., et al., *Effect of parathyroid hormone (1-34) on fractures and bone mineral density in postmenopausal women with osteoporosis.* N Engl J Med, 2001. 344(19): p. 1434-41.

[120] Kilby, J.M., et al., *Potent suppression of HIV-1 replication in humans by T-20, a peptide inhibitor of gp41-mediated virus entry.* Nat Med, 1998. 4(11): p. 1302-7.

[121] Naider, F. and J. Anglister, *Peptides in the treatment of AIDS.* Curr Opin Struct Biol, 2009. 19(4): p. 473-482.

[122] Chan, D.C. and P.S. Kim, *HIV entry and its inhibition.* Cell, 1998. 93(5): p. 681-4.

[123] Liu, S., S. Wu, and S. Jiang, *HIV entry inhibitors targeting gp41: from polypeptides to small-molecule compounds.* Curr Pharm Des, 2007. 13(2): p. 143-62.

[124] Wild, C., et al., *A synthetic peptide inhibitor of human immunodeficiency virus replication: correlation between solution structure and viral inhibition.* Proc Natl Acad Sci USA, 1992. 89(21): p. 10537-41.

[125] Lu, M. and P.S. Kim, *A trimeric structural subdomain of the HIV-1 transmembrane glycoprotein.* J Biomol Struct Dyn, 1997. 15(3): p. 465-71.

[126] Gaston, F., et al., *Development and characterization of peptidic fusion inhibitors derived from HIV-1 gp41 with partial D-amino acid substitutions.* ChemMedChem, 2009. 4(4): p. 570-81.

[127] Wexler-Cohen, Y. and Y. Shai, *Demonstrating the C-terminal boundary of the HIV 1 fusion conformation in a dynamic ongoing fusion process and implication for fusion inhibition.* FASEB J, 2007. 21(13): p. 3677-84.

[128] Dogo-Isonagie, C., et al., *Peptides from the second extracellular loop of the C-C chemokine receptor type 5 (CCR5) inhibit diverse strains of HIV-1.* J Biol Chem, 2012.

[129] Micewicz, E.D., et al., *Grifonin-1: a small HIV-1 entry inhibitor derived from the algal lectin, Griffithsin.* PLoS ONE, 2010. 5(12): p. e14360.

[130] Callebaut, C., et al., *Inhibition of HIV infection by pseudopeptides blocking viral envelope glycoprotein-mediated membrane fusion and cell death.* Virology, 1996. 218(1): p. 181-92.

[131] Krust, B., et al., *The anti-HIV pentameric pseudopeptide HB-19 is preferentially taken up in vivo by lymphoid organs where it forms a complex with nucleolin.* Proc Natl Acad Sci USA, 2001. 98(24): p. 14090-5.

[132] Kerr, J.F., C.M. Winterford, and B.V. Harmon, *Apoptosis. Its significance in cancer and cancer therapy.* Cancer, 1994. 73(8): p. 2013-26.

[133] Thornberry, N.A., et al., *A combinatorial approach defines specificities of members of the caspase family and granzyme B. Functional relationships established for key mediators of apoptosis.* J Biol Chem, 1997. 272(29): p. 17907-11.

[134] MacKenzie, S.H., J.L. Schipper, and A.C. Clark, *The potential for caspases in drug discovery.* Curr Opin Drug Discov Devel, 2010. 13(5): p. 568-76.

[135] Tang, Y., J.A. Wells, and M.R. Arkin, *Structural and enzymatic insights into caspase-2 protein substrate recognition and catalysis.* J Biol Chem, 2011. 286(39): p. 34147-54.

[136] Chang, C.y., et al., *Dissection of the LXXLL nuclear receptor-coactivator interaction motif using combinatorial peptide libraries: discovery of peptide antagonists of estrogen receptors alpha and beta.* Mol Cell Biol, 1999. 19(12): p. 8226-39.

[137] Petros, A.M., et al., *Rationale for Bcl-xL/Bad peptide complex formation from structure, mutagenesis, and biophysical studies.* Protein Sci, 2000. 9(12): p. 2528-34.

[138] Moarefi, I., et al., *{Activation of the Src-family tyrosine kinase Hck by SH3 domain displacement}.* Nature, 1997. 385: p. 650-653.

[139] Myslinski, J.M., et al., *Protein-ligand interactions: thermodynamic effects associated with increasing nonpolar surface area.* J Am Chem Soc, 2011. 133(46): p. 18518-21.

[140] Sabe, H., et al., *ArfGAP family proteins in cell adhesion, migration and tumor invasion.* Curr Opin Cell Biol, 2006. 18(5): p. 558-64.

[141] Onodera, Y., et al., *Expression of AMAP1, an ArfGAP, provides novel targets to inhibit breast cancer invasive activities.* EMBO J, 2005. 24(5): p. 963-973.

[142] Hashimoto, S., et al., *Targeting AMAP1 and cortactin binding bearing an atypical src homology 3/proline interface for prevention of breast cancer invasion and metastasis.* Proc Natl Acad Sci USA, 2006. 103(18): p. 7036-41.

[143] Selkoe, D.J., *Folding proteins in fatal ways.* Nature, 2003. 426(6968): p. 900-4.

[144] Wetzel, R., *Nucleation of huntingtin aggregation in cells.* Nat Chem Biol, 2006. 2(6): p. 297-8.

[145] Haass, C., *The molecular significance of amyloid beta-peptide for Alzheimer's disease.* Eur Arch Psychiatry Clin Neurosci, 1996. 246(3): p. 118-23.

[146] Soto, C., et al., *Inhibition of Alzheimer's amyloidosis by peptides that prevent beta-sheet conformation.* Biochem Biophys Res Commun, 1996. 226(3): p. 672-80.

[147] Soto, C., et al., *Beta-sheet breaker peptides inhibit fibrillogenesis in a rat brain model of amyloidosis: implications for Alzheimer's therapy.* Nat Med, 1998. 4(7): p. 822-6.

[148] Adessi, C., et al., *Pharmacological profiles of peptide drug candidates for the treatment of Alzheimer's disease.* J Biol Chem, 2003. 278(16): p. 13905-11.

[149] Bieler, S. and C. Soto, *Beta-sheet breakers for Alzheimer's disease therapy.* Curr Drug Targets, 2004. 5(6): p. 553-8.

[150] Tjernberg, L.O., et al., *Arrest of beta-amyloid fibril formation by a pentapeptide ligand.* J Biol Chem, 1996. 271(15): p. 8545-8.

[151] Permanne, B., et al., *Reduction of amyloid load and cerebral damage in a transgenic mouse model of Alzheimer's disease by treatment with a beta-sheet breaker peptide.* FASEB J, 2002. 16(8): p. 860-2.

[152] Frydman-Marom, A., et al., *The generic amyloid formation inhibition effect of a designed small aromatic β-breaking peptide.* Amyloid, 2011. 18(3): p. 119-27.

[153] Porat, Y., et al., *Inhibition of islet amyloid polypeptide fibril formation: a potential role for heteroaromatic interactions.* Biochemistry, 2004. 43(45): p. 14454-62.

Chapter 4

More Than a Simple Lock and Key Mechanism: Unraveling the Intricacies of Sperm-Zona Pellucida Binding

Kate A. Redgrove, R. John Aitken and Brett Nixon

Additional information is available at the end of the chapter

http://dx.doi.org/10.5772/50499

1. Introduction

Mammalian fertilization involves a concerted interplay between the male and female gametes that ultimately results in the creation of new life. However, despite the fundamental importance of gamete interaction, the precise molecular mechanisms that underpin and regulate this complex event remain to be fully elucidated. Such knowledge is crucial in our attempts to resolve the global problems of population control and infertility. The current world population has surpassed 7 billion people, and continues to grow at a rate of approximately 200 000 each day (UN, 2009). Alarmingly, the majority of this population growth is occurring in developing nations, and is driven in part by an unmet need for effective and accessible contraceptive technologies. Indeed, a recent study by the Global Health Council revealed that of the 205 million pregnancies recorded worldwide each year, 60-80 million of these are deemed to be unplanned or unwanted (Guttmacher, 2007). These concerning statistics highlight the inadequacies of our current armory of contraceptives and demonstrate the need for the development of novel methods for fertility control. By virtue of its specificity and its ability to be suppressed in both males and females, sperm interaction with the outer vestments of the oocyte, a structure known as the zona pellucida (ZP), represents an attractive target for the development of novel contraceptives. However, the realization of such technologies is predicated on a thorough understanding of the molecular mechanisms that underpin this intricate binding event.

Such knowledge will also contribute to the development of novel diagnostic and therapeutic strategies for the paradoxical increase in male infertility that is being experienced by Western countries. Indeed, male infertility has become a distressingly common condition affecting at least 1 in 20 men of reproductive age (McLachlan and de Kretser, 2001). In a vast majority

(>80%) of infertile patients sufficient numbers of spermatozoa are produced to achieve fertilization, however the functionality of these cells has become compromised, making defective sperm function the largest single defined cause of human infertility (Hull, et al., 1985, Ombelet, et al., 1997). Biologically, a major cause of impaired sperm function is a failure of these cells to recognize the surface of the egg. Defective sperm- zona pellucida interactions is thus a major cause of fertilization failure *in vitro* and bioassays of sperm- zona pellucida interaction are able to predict male infertility *in vivo* with great accuracy (Arslan, et al., 2006).

In this review we explore our current understanding of the mechanisms that are responsible for sperm- zona pellucida interactions. Consideration is given to well-established paradigms of receptor-ligand binding with an emphasis on the emerging evidence for models involving the participation of multimeric receptor complexes and the maturation events that promote their assembly.

2. Sperm-zona pellucida interactions

2.1. The mammalian zona pellucida

The zona pellucida (ZP) is a porous extracellular matrix that surrounds the oocyte (Dunbar, et al., 1994, Wassarman and Litscher, 2008). In the most widely accepted models of gamete interaction, the zona pellucida plays a critical role in tethering spermatozoa, and inducing the release of their acrosomal contents (Bleil and Wassarman, 1983). Binding to the zona pellucida is a highly selective and carefully regulated process that serves as an inter-species barrier to fertilization by preventing adherence of non-homologous sperm to eggs (Hardy and Garbers, 1994).

Although all mammalian eggs are enclosed in a zona pellucida matrix, it's thickness (~1-25μm) and protein content (~1-10ng) varies considerably for eggs derived from different species (Wassarman, 1988). In mice, the zona pellucida comprises three major sulfated glycoproteins designated ZP1 (200kDa), ZP2 (120kDa) and ZP3 (83kDa). Current evidence suggests that these proteins assemble into a non-covalently linked structure comprising ZP2-ZP3 dimers that polymerize into filaments and are cross-linked by ZP1 (Greve and Wassarman, 1985, Wassarman and Mortillo, 1991). In addition to orthologues of the three mouse zona pellucida proteins [hZP1 (100kDa), hZP2 (75kDa) and hZP3 (55kDa)], the human zona pellucida comprises a fourth glycoprotein, hZP4 (65kDa) (Bauskin, et al., 1999, Lefievre, et al., 2004), which is thought to be dysfunctional in the mouse (Lefievre, et al., 2004). The biological significance of the increased complexity in the zona pellucida of humans awaits further investigation. Given that the mouse remains the most widely studied model for understanding sperm- zona pellucida interaction, this species will serve as the focus for the following discussion.

2.2. The biochemistry of sperm-zona pellucida recognition

Sperm- zona pellucida interaction encompasses a complex sequence of events that relies on each gamete having achieved an appropriate level of maturity. Spermatozoa that approach the oocyte have undergone a behavioral and functional reprogramming event within the female reproductive tract, termed capacitation (see section 2.3.1.3), which ultimately endows the cells with the competence for fertilization. Notwithstanding recent evidence to the balance of evidence favors a model for sperm- zona pellucida interaction that involves three distinct stages: the first comprises primary binding of acrosome-intact spermatozoa to the zona pellucida, this is then followed by secondary binding of acrosome-reacted spermatozoa to the zona pellucida, and finally penetration of the acrosome-reacted sperm through the zona pellucida and into the perivitelline space (Florman and Storey, 1982, Inoue and Wolf, 1975, Saling, et al., 1979, Swenson and Dunbar, 1982).

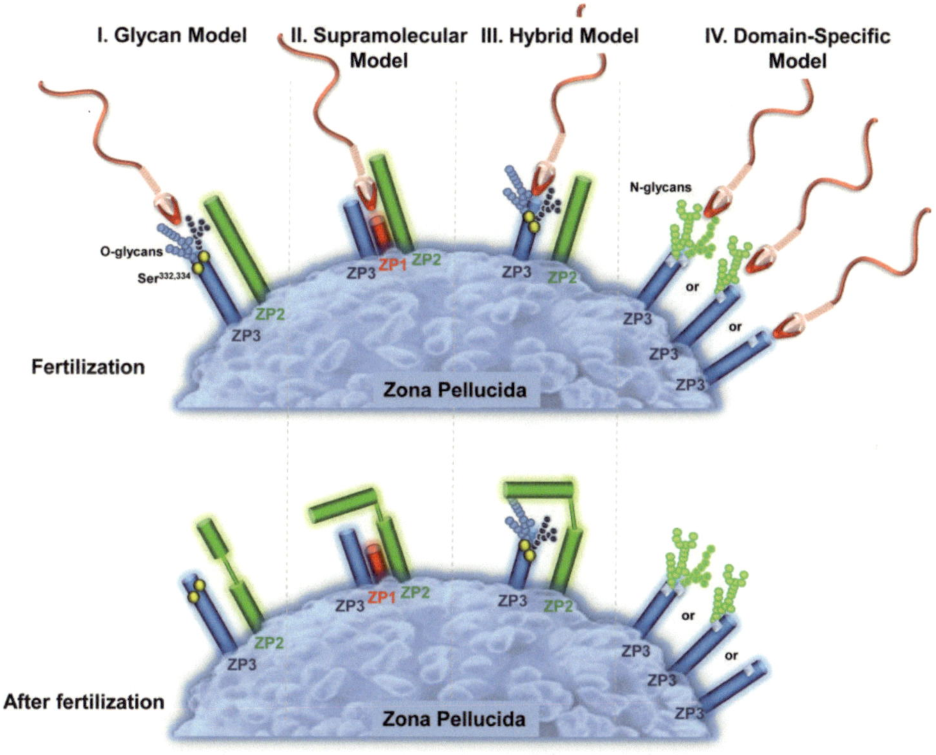

Figure 1. Putative models of sperm-zona pellucida binding. (I) The glycan model proposes that sperm binding is initiated via O-linked glycans that are attached at residues Ser^{332} and Ser^{334} of ZP3. After fertilization, these residues are deglycosylated thereby preventing further sperm adhesion. (ii) The supramolecular structure model is based on the premise that the physical structure of the matrix formed by the three zona pellucida glycoproteins is critical for the binding of sperm. Following fertilization, ZP2 is processed in such a way that it prevents further sperm adhesion. (iii) The hybrid model incorporates aspects of both the glycan model and the supramolecular model and proposes that O-linked glycosylation is a critical determinant of sperm recognition. However, the key O-glycans reside on residues other than Ser^{332} and Ser^{334}. Furthermore, the modification of ZP2 that accompanies fertilization renders these O-glycans inaccessible to sperm. (iv) In contrast, the domain-specific model proposes that sperm bind with a variety of N-linked glycans attached to ZP3 and/or the peptide backbone of the glycoprotein depending upon its glycosylation status. The concepts proposed in this figure are adapted from those of Visconti and Florman, 2010 and Clark, 2010.

The initial stages of primary binding involve a relatively loose, non-species specific attachment that serves to tether spermatozoa to the surface of the oocyte (Schmell and Gulyas, 1980, Swenson and Dunbar, 1982). This weak binding is rapidly followed (within 10 minutes) by an irreversible tight binding event (Bleil and Wassarman, 1983, Hartmann, et al., 1972) that resists physical manipulation (Hartmann, et al., 1972, Inoue and Wolf, 1975) and is commonly species-specific. In the mouse, this latter event appears to involve binding of the spermatozoon to ZP3. This model emerged from early experiments performed by Bleil and Wassarman using crudely purified native zona pellucida that demonstrated that mouse ZP3 is responsible for acting as both a primary sperm ligand, preferentially binding the plasma membrane overlying the acrosome of acrosome-intact sperm, as well as an inducer of the acrosome reaction (Bleil and Wassarman, 1980a, Bleil and Wassarman, 1980b, Bleil and Wassarman, 1986, Vazquez, et al., 1989, Yanagimachi, 1994b). Purified mouse ZP3 was also shown to competitively inhibit binding of spermatozoa to homologous eggs *in vitro* (Bleil and Wassarman, 1980a, Endo, et al., 1987, Florman, et al., 1984, Florman and Wassarman, 1985, Leyton and Saling, 1989). The bioactive component of ZP3 responsible for mediation of sperm binding was initially traced to specific O-linked carbohydrate moieties that decorate the protein (Florman and Wassarman, 1985, Litscher, et al., 1995). In support of this model, complete deglycosylation, or selective removal of O-linked oligosaccharides eliminated the ability of ZP3 to interact with spermatozoa (Florman and Wassarman, 1985). In addition, the O-linked oligosaccharides released by these procedures were able to bind directly to spermatozoa and competitively inhibit their ability to adhere to the zona pellucida (Florman and Wassarman, 1985). Furthermore, genetically engineered chimeric mouse oocytes expressing human ZP3, acquire the same O-linked glycans as mouse ZP3 and bind mouse, rather than human, spermatozoa (Rankin et al., 1996; Hoodbhoy and Dean, 2004). Mutagenesis studies of ZP3 suggested that that the key O-linked adhesion glycans for sperm are attached to either Ser^{332} and/or Ser^{334} residues (Chen, et al., 1998) located within the C-terminal portion of the ZP3 polypeptide chain.

Notwithstanding such compelling evidence in favor of this classical model it has increasingly been drawn into question by a number of recent observations from genetically manipulated mouse models. For instance, female mice bearing targeted deletions of key glycosyltransferase enzymes responsible for the addition of O-linked glycans produce oocytes that display normal sperm binding characteristics (Ellies, et al., 1998). Furthermore, in a series of elegant experiments, transgenic mice have been produced in which the putative sperm binding residues were mutated ($Ser^{329,\,333,\,334}\rightarrow$Ala, $Ser^{331}\rightarrow$Val, $Ser^{332}\rightarrow$Gly) to eliminate potential O-linked glycosylation sites at Ser^{332} and Ser^{334} (Gahlay et al. 2010). Females from these transgenic lines were shown to retain their fertility both *in vitro* and *in vivo*, and their oocytes maintained the ability to bind the same number of sperm as wild type mice, strongly suggesting that neither Ser^{332} nor Ser^{334} are critical for sperm- zona pellucida recognition. The latter findings are perhaps best explained by detailed glycoproteomic analyses that have revealed Ser^{332} and Ser^{334} are in fact unlikely to be glycosylated in mouse ZP3 (Boja et al. 2003; Chalabi et al. 2006).

These collective findings have led to the proposal of a number of alternative models of sperm- zona pellucida adhesion (Fig. 1), including the: (i) original glycan model that proposes the importance of O-linked glycosylation at Ser^{332} and Ser^{334}; (ii) a supramolecular structure model in which the sperm binding domain is formed by the complex of the three major zona pellucida glycoproteins and regulated by the cleavage status of ZP2 (Rankin et al. 2003), (iii) a hybrid model that incorporates elements of both former models by proposing that sperm bind to an O-glycan that is conjugated to ZP3 at a site other than Ser^{332} or Ser^{334} (Visconti and Florman, 2010) and that sperm access to this glycan is regulated by the proteolytic cleavage state of ZP2; (iv) domain specific model that envisages a dual adhesion system in which sperm protein(s) interact with the glycans and/or the protein backbone of ZP3 depending on its glycosylation state (Clark, 2011) and (v) a novel model in which gamete recognition is able to be resolved into at least two distinct binding events, the first of which involves adherence to oviductal glycoproteins that are peripherally associated with the egg coat prior to engaging with a ZP3-dependent ligand (Lyng and Shur, 2009) The evidence in support of each of these models of gamete interaction has been reviewed in depth previously (Dean 2004; Clark 2010, 2011; Visconti and Florman, 2010). What is clear from these studies is that the initiation of gamete interaction is not mediated by a simple lock and key mechanism involving a single receptor-ligand interaction. Rather it is likely that sperm engage in multiple binding events with a variety of ligands within the zona pellucida matrix. An advantage of this complex adhesion system is that it would enhance the opportunities of sperm to bind to the oocyte and thus maximize the chance of fertilization. It may also account for the myriad of sperm receptors that have been implicated in this process (see below).

2.3. Sperm receptor molecules involved in zona pellucida interaction

2.3.1. Acquisition of the ability to engage in sperm-zona pellucida interactions

Prior to interaction with the egg, the sperm cell must undergo a complex, multifaceted process of functional maturation (Fig. 2). This process begins in the testes where spermatogonial stem cells are dramatically remodeled during spermatogenesis to produce one of the most highly differentiated and specialized cells in the body, the spermatozoon. After their initial morphological differentiation, these cells are released from the germinal epithelium of the testes in a functionally immature state, incapable of movement or any of the complex array of cellular interactions that are required for fertilization (Hermo, et al., 2010a). In all mammalian species, the acquisition of functional competence occurs progressively during the cells descent through the epididymis, a long convoluted tubule that connects the testis to the vas deferens (Fig. 2B). A remarkable feature of epididymal maturation is that this process is driven entirely by extrinsic factors in the complete absence of nuclear gene transcription and significant protein translation within the spermatozoa (Engel, et al., 1973). The surface and intracellular changes associated with epididymal maturation prepare the spermatozoa for their final phase of maturation within the female reproductive tract, whereby they realize their potential to bind to the zona pellucida and ultimately fertilize the egg (Bailey, 2010, Fraser, 2010, Yanagimachi, 1994a).

2.3.1.1. Spermatogenesis

Spermatogenesis describes the process by which spermatozoa develop from undifferentiated germ cells within the seminiferous tubules of the testis. It is characterized by three functional stages: proliferation, meiosis and metamorphosis. During the proliferation phase, spermatogonial germ cells undergo several mitotic divisions in order to renew themselves in addition to producing spermatocytes (Brinster, 2002, de Rooij, 2001, Dym, 1994, Oatley and Brinster, 2006). These cells then undergo two meiotic divisions to form haploid spermatids. The latter then develop into spermatozoa via an extremely complex process of cytodifferentiation and metamorphosis. This includes structural modifications to the shape of their nucleus, compaction of the nuclear chromatin, formation of an acrosomal vesicle and establishment of a flagellum allowing for the subsequent

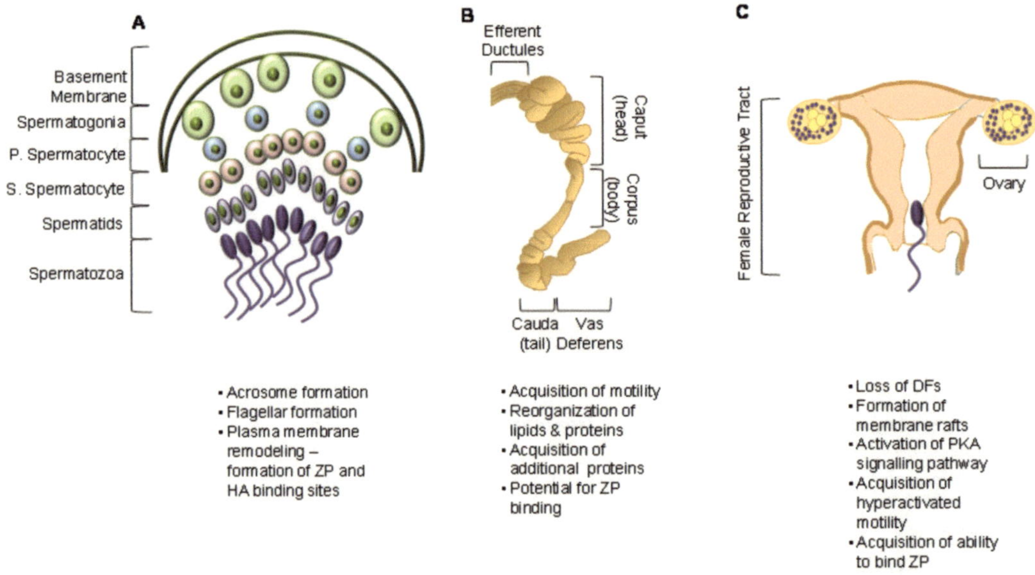

Figure 2. Acquisition of spermatozoa's ability to engage in interaction with the oocyte. (A) During spermatogenesis, primordial germ cells undergo several phases of mitotic and meiotic divisions in order to produce morphologically mature but functionally incompetent spermatozoa. Of particular importance is the process of spermiogensis, whereby spermatids undergo a process of cytodifferentiation that culminates in the production of spermatozoa. In the course of this dramatic transformation an acrosomal vesicle is formed in the anterior region of the sperm head and a flagellum develops posteriorly. The plasma membrane is also remodeled to produce zona pellucida (ZP) and hyaluronic acid (HA) binding sites. (B) Upon leaving the testis, spermatozoa traverse the epididymis and acquire the ability for forward progressive movement and to adhere to the zona pellucida surrounding the oocyte. These changes occur as a result of the reorganization of specific lipids and proteins. (C) However, it is not until the spermatozoa undergo a final phase of maturation termed 'capacitation' in the female reproductive tract that they realize the potential for zona pellucida interaction via the induction of hyperactivated motility along with the sequential loss of decapacitation factors (DFs), formation of membrane rafts and activation of key signaling cascades.

development of motility. The latter series of modifications that produce terminally differentiated spermatozoa from spermatids is referred to as spermiogenesis. Of particular importance to fertilization, is the formation of the acrosome during this stage. As seen by light microscopy, acrosomal development begins with the production of small proacrosome granules derived from the Golgi apparatus that lies adjacent to the early spermatid nucleus. These subsequently fuse together to form the acrosome, a large secretory vesicle that overlies the nucleus (Leblond and Clermont, 1952). There is also evidence to suggest that, in addition to the Golgi apparatus, the plasma membrane of the cell and endocytotic trafficking may also play a fundamental role in the formation of the this exocytotic vesicle (Ramalho-Santos, et al., 2001, West and Willison, 1996). Once formed, the acrosome remains associated with the nucleus of the spermatid, and subsequently the spermatozoa for the remainder of its life, and is of critical importance during fertilization due to its ability to aid in the penetration of the zona pellucida surrounding the ovulated oocyte. This function is, in turn, attributed to the hydrolytic enzymes enclosed within the acrosome. Notwithstanding recent evidence to the contrary, it is widely held that the release of these enzymes occurs upon engagement of sperm binding to the zona pellucida and facilitates localized digestion of the zona matrix, thereby facilitating sperm penetration through this barrier and providing access to the oocyte. The acrosomal enzymes are mostly derived from the lysosome, although several are unique to this organelle (Tulsiani, et al., 1998). In general terms, the acrosome can be divided into compartments, the first of which contains soluble proteins such as didpetididyl peptidase II and cystein-rich secretory protein 2 (Hardy, et al., 1991). The second compartment is known as the acrosomal matrix and contains the insoluble fraction of the enzymes including apexin (Kim, et al., 2001, Noland, et al., 1994, Westbrook-Case, et al., 1994), acrosin and acrosin-binding protein (Baba, et al., 1994b), and sp56, which has been previously implicated in the ability of sperm to interact with the zona pellucida (Buffone, et al., 2008a, Buffone, et al., 2008b).

In addition to the formation of the acrosome during spermiogenesis, the sperm develop a cytoplasmic droplet as well as undergoing plasma membrane remodeling events. The cytoplasmic droplet was first described by Retzius in 1909 as being a portion of germ cell cytoplasm that remains attached to the neck region of elongating spermatids. In most species, the cytoplasmic droplet migrates along the midpiece from the neck to annulus and is transiently retained by spermatozoa as they migrate through the epididymis (Cooper and Yeung, 2003), while in others it remains on the spermatozoa in the epididymis and is not shed until the time of ejaculation (Cooper, 2005, Harayama, et al., 1996, Kaplan, et al., 1984, Larsen, et al., 1980). The precise function of this residual cytoplasm remains elusive although its retention beyond ejaculation is associated with poor sperm function. For example, the cytoplasmic droplet on human spermatozoa is associated with poor sperm motility (Zini, et al., 1998), abnormal head and midpiece morphology (Gergely, et al., 1999, Gomez, et al., 1996, Huszar and Vigue, 1993), lower fertilizing capacity (Keating, et al., 1997) and reduced zona pellucida binding (Ergur, et al., 2002, Huszar, et al., 1994, Liu and Baker, 1992). The mechanism by which these abnormal sperm exhibit reduced function is attributed to disturbed membrane remodeling (Huszar, et al., 1997) and higher extents of lipid peroxidation (Aitken, et al., 1994, Huszar, et al., 1994, Ollero, et al., 2000). The latter is most likely due to the high levels of ROS produced by the cytoplasmic droplet itself (Aitken, et al., 1994, Gil-Guzman, et al., 2001, Gomez, et al., 1996, Huszar and Vigue, 1993, Ollero, et al., 2000), combined with the enriched polyunsaturated fatty acids derived from the membrane of the droplet (Huszar and Vigue, 1993, Ollero, et al., 2000). The plasma membrane remodeling event involves the formation of zona pellucida binding sites via protein transport, which is thought to be mediated by the molecular chaperone, HSPA2. In agreement with the observations discussed above, immature human sperm that fail to express HSPA2 display cytoplasmic retention and reduced zona pellucida binding (Huszar, et al., 2000). The sperm also develop the machinery necessary for functional motility during spermiogenesis. As the acrosome grows at one pole of the nuclear surface of round spermatids, paired centrioles migrate to the opposite pole where they initiate the formation of the flagellum. The flagellum consists of a neck piece, a mid piece, a principle piece and an endpiece (Fawcett, 1975, Katz, 1991). The motility apparatus of the flagellum consists of a central axoneme of nine microtubular doublets arranges to form a cylinder around a central pair of single microtubules (Fawcett, 1975).

In combination, these fundamental changes in structure and biochemisty result in terminally differentiated, highly polarized and morphologically mature spermatozoa. However, despite this level of specialization the spermatozoa that leave the testis are functionally incompetent, as yet unable to move forward progressively, nor interact with the zona pellucida and fertilize the oocyte. They must first traverse the epididymis, a highly convoluted tubule adjacent to the testis, during which time they undergo further biochemical and biophysical changes.

2.3.1.2. Epididymal maturation

Upon leaving the testes, the first region of the epididymis that immature sperm encounter is that of the caput (head). Within this region, the sperm are concentrated by a mechanism of resorption that rapidly removes almost all the testicular fluid/proteins that enter the epididymis. As they leave this environment and enter the corpus (body) epididymis, sperm begin to acquire their motility and fertilizing ability. These attributes continue to develop as the sperm move through the corpus, and reach an optimum level as they reach the cauda (tail) region where they are stored in a quiescent state prior to ejaculation (Fig. 2B) (Cornwall, 2009, Gatti, et al., 2004). Ground breaking research performed in the 1960's and 1970's provided the first evidence that the epididymis played an active role for the epididymis in sperm development (Bedford, 1963, Bedford, 1965, Bedford, 1967, Bedford, 1968, Orgebin-Crist, 1967a, Orgebin-Crist, 1967b, Orgebin-Crist, 1968, Orgebin-Crist, 1969). Most importantly, it was discovered that if sperm were held in the testis via ligation of the epididymal duct, they were unable to develop the ability to fertilize an ovum, and as such their maturation is not an intrinsic property (Cooper and Orgebin-Crist, 1975, Cooper and Orgebin-Crist, 1977).

Consistent with this notion, sperm maturation within the epididymis is not under genomic control, since the cells enter the ductal system in a transcriptionally inactive state with limited biosynthetic capacity (Eddy, 2002). Any subsequent molecular changes must therefore be driven by the dynamic intraluminal milieu in which they are bathed as they transit the length of the epididymal tubule (Cooper, 1986). This epididymal microenvironment is characterized by dramatic sequential changes in its composition, a reflection of segment-specific gene expression (Dube, et al., 2007, Jelinsky, et al., 2007, Jervis and Robaire, 2001, Johnston, et al., 2007) and protein secretion (Dacheux, et al., 2006, Dacheux, et al., 2009, Guyonnet, et al., 2011, Nixon, et al., 2002, Syntin, et al., 1996). The unique physiological compartments established by this activity are thought to have evolved to not only to support the maturation of spermatozoa, but to also to provide protection for the vulnerable cells during their transport and prolonged storage.

It is well established that as sperm descend through the epididymis they acquire the potential for forward motility (reviewed (Amann, et al., 1993, Cooper, 1993, Moore and Akhondi, 1996, Soler, et al., 1994). This progressive motion not only allows the sperm to negotiate the female reproductive tract, but has also been suggested to play a role in penetration of the oocytes outer protective barriers, including the cumulus oophorous and the zone pellucida. To date, the mechanisms underlying the acquisition of forward motility by cauda epididymal sperm have not been completely elucidated. However, a number of potential contributing factors have been identified. On a biochemical level, proteins from caput epididymal sperm contain a greater number of sulfhydryl groups than disulfide bonds. Importantly, the oxidation of these sulfhydryl groups during epididymal transit is correlated with stabilization of flagella, as well as the promotion of protein tyrosine phosphorylation on specific sperm proteins involved in key signaling pathways (Calvin and Bedford, 1971, Cornwall, et al., 1988, Seligman, et al., 2004). Additionally, there is also recent evidence to suggest that sperm isolated from the caput epididymis possess the ability to become motile, but that this activity is suppressed through the action of the cannaboid receptor CNR1, which upon engagement with its ligand, t ennocanaboid 2-arachidonoylglcerol, suppresses the capacity for motility (Cobellis, et al., 2010). Furthermore, changes in the luminal environment, as well as specific post-translational modification to sperm proteins have been shown to affect the motility status of these cells during their transit through the epididymis. In relation to the former, acidification of the luminal contents of the epididymis work to maintain sperm in an immotile state. This is finely regulated by epididymal clear cells which are capable of sensing a rise in luminal pH or bicarbonate concentrations via the sperm specific adenylyl cyclase (SACY)-dependent rise in cyclic-adenosinemonophosphate (cAMP) (Pastor-Soler, et al., 2003, Shum, et al., 2009). In terms of post-translational modifications, proteomic analyses of sperm proteins within the epididymis have identified a number of potential targets affected by changes in expression, disulfide bond status, proteolysis and alterations such as phosphorylation (Baker, et al., 2005). Finally, glycolysis plays an essential role as an energy pathway to fuel forward progressive movement in mouse spermatozoa. This is evidenced by the observation that male mice with genetic ablations of the sperm-specific forms of key glycolytic enzymes (glyceraldehydes 3-phosphate dehydrogenase S or phosphoglycerate kinase 2) are infertile or have very low fertility (Danshina, et al., 2010, Miki, et al., 2004). In part this can be explained by significantly decreased levels of ATP production (4 to 10-times lower than wildtype sperm) resulting in poor, or sluggish motility. Furthermore, the spermatogenic cell-specific type 7 hexokinase that is present in mouse spermatozoa undergoes cleavage of dilsulfide bonds during epididymal transit, resulting in increased hexokinase activity which, in turn, has been causally associated with the initiation of sperm motility (Nakamura, et al., 2008). This indicates that specific structural changes to proteins during epididymal maturation have functional consequences, improving sperm competence for motility, and subsequently their ability to engage in fertilization.

In addition to the maturation of the motility apparatus, the acquisition of zona pellucida binding is also temporally associated with the exposure of spermatozoa to two distinct subsets of macromolecular structures in the epididymal lumen: the first being amorphous chaperone-laden 'dense bodies' (Asquith, et al., 2005) and the second being membrane bound prostasome-like particles known as epididymosomes (Saez, et al., 2003). It has been suggested that these epididymal granules facilitate the transfer of proteins to the sperm surface during their transit of the organ (Asquith, et al., 2005, Saez, et al., 2003, Yano, et al., 2010). This is in keeping with the demonstration that biotinylated proteins are able to be transferred between epididymosomes and the sperm surface (Saez, et al., 2003). At present it remains to be determined how this transfer is mediated and the number of cargo proteins that are delivered to the maturing spermatozoa in this manner. Nevertheless, a number of proteins have been shown to be acquired by the sperm during epididymal transit. A non-exhaustive list of these proteins include HE5/CD52 (Kirchhoff and Hale, 1996), members of the ADAM family (Girouard, et al., 2011, Oh, et al., 2009), SPAM1 (Zhang and Martin-Deleon, 2003) and other hyaluronidases (Frenette and Sullivan, 2001, Legare, et al., 1999), macrophage migration inhibitory factor (MIF) (Eickhoff, et al., 2001, Frenette, et al., 2003, Girouard, et al., 2011) as well as a number of enzymes including aldose reductase and sorbitol dehydrogenase (Frenette, et al., 2004, Frenette, et al., 2006, Kobayashi, et al., 2002, Thimon, et al., 2008). Collectively these proteins are believed to participate in the modification of the sperm biochemistry and surface architecture conferring the potential to engage in oocyte interactions.

2.3.1.3. Capacitation

Although spermatozoa acquire the potential to fertilize an egg within the epididymis, the expression of this functional competence is suppressed until their release from this environment at the moment of ejaculation. Indeed they must first spend a period of time within the female reproductive tract (Austin, 1952, Chang, 1951) during which they undergo the final phase of post-testicular maturation, a process known as capacitation. Capacitation is characterized by a series of biochemical and biophysical alterations to the cell including changes in intracellular pH, remodeling of the cell surface architecture, changes in motility patterns and initiation of complex signal transduction pathways. These events have been correlated with a dramatic global up-regulation of tyrosine phosphorylation across a number of key proteins. The ensuing activation of these target proteins has, in turn, been causally linked to the initiation of hyperactivated motility, ability to recognize and adhere to the zona pellucida, and the ability to undergo acrosomal exocytosis (Nixon, et al., 2007). For the purpose of this review, focus will be placed on the molecular mechanisms that culminate in the ability of the sperm to interact with the zona matrix. Furthermore, as this is a cell-surface mediated event, discussion will be centered on the capacitation-associated pathways that mediate sperm surface remodeling.

One of the more widely accepted sequences for mammalian capacitation begins with the loss of surface-inhibitory factors, known as decapacitation factors. These factors mostly originate in the epididymis and accessory organs, and their removal from non-capacitated spermatozoa results in a rapid increase in their fertilizing ability (Fraser, 1984). Furthermore, as capacitation is a reversible process, addition of these decapacitation factors into a population of capacitating spermatozoa potently suppress their ability to recognize and fertilize an oocyte (Fraser, et al., 1990). A number of candidates with potential decapacitation activity have been identified including: DF glycoprotein (Fraser, 1998), phosphatidylethanolamine binding protein 1 (PEB1) (Gibbons, et al., 2005, Nixon, et al., 2006), sperm antigen 36, CRISP1 and plasma membrane fatty acid binding protein (Nixon, et al., 2006) and NYD-SP27 (Bi, et al., 2009). Following the release of these decapacitation factors, spermatozoa experience a dramatic efflux of cholesterol from the plasma membrane (Davis, 1981). This efflux appears to be driven by active sequestration upon exposure of the spermatozoa to an environment rich in appropriate cholesterol sinks (Davis, et al., 1979, Langlais, et al., 1988, Visconti, et al., 1999), and accounts for a striking increase in membrane fluidity. Bovine serum albumin is commonly used within *in vitro* capacitating media as a cholesterol acceptor, although analogous acceptor(s) are believed to be present within the female reproductive tract. Indeed, studies of human follicular fluid have identified the presence high concentrations of albumin and other cholesterol sinks (Langlais, et al., 1988). Cholesterol efflux from the plasma membrane has also been correlated with an influx of bicarbonate ions (HCO_3^-) into the cell (Boatman and Robbins, 1991, Chen, et al., 2000, Garty and Salomon, 1987, Okamura, et al., 1985). In addition to its key role in initiation of critical signal transduction cascades, HCO_3^- has itself been shown to have a more direct role in sperm surface remodeling via stimulation of phospholipid scramblase activity (Gadella and Harrison, 2000, Gadella and Harrison, 2002). The ensuing random translocation of phospholipids between the outer and inner leaflets of the bilayer serves to disrupt the characteristic membrane asymmetry, (Flesch, et al., 2001a). This redistribution of phospholipids has been suggested to prime the sperm plasma membrane for cholesterol efflux, thus rendering the cell more 'fusogenic' and responsive to zona pellucida glycoproteins (Harrison and Gadella, 2005).

A further consequence of capacitation-associated cholesterol efflux is the formation of membrane rafts and/or the polarized coalescence of these microdomains and their protein cargo into the anterior region of the sperm head, the precise location that mediate zona pellucida binding (Fig. 3). Membrane rafts are generally defined as small, heterogeneous domains that serve to compartmentalize cellular processes (Pike, 2006), and regulate the distribution of membrane proteins, the activation of receptors and initiation of signaling cascades (Brown and London, 1998, Brown and London, 2000, Simons and Ikonen, 1997, Simons and Toomre, 2000). Membrane rafts are highly stable structures due to the inflexible steroid backbone of cholesterol (Martinez-Seara, et al., 2008) and are therefore extremely resistant to solubilization by a number of non-ionic detergents (Schuck, et al., 2003). As such they are often referred to as detergent-resistant membranes (DRMs). However despite their stability, rafts remain highly dynamic entities and have been observed to display considerable lateral movement in various cell types as a response to physical stimuli or cellular activation events (Simons and Vaz, 2004). In sperm, membrane rafts have been identified by the presence of several somatic cell raft markers including G_{M1} gangliosides, flotillin and proteins that have raft affinity due to the presence of glycosylphophatidylinositol (GPI) anchors, including CD59 and SPAM1 (Nixon, et al., 2009, Sleight, et al., 2005, van Gestel, et al., 2005). Notably, the spatial distribution of membrane rafts within the sperm membrane is dramatically influenced by the capacitation status of the cells. Indeed, the uniform localization of rafts characteristically observed in non-capacitated spermatozoa is replaced by a pattern of confinement within the peri-acrosomal region of the sperm head following the induction of capacitation (Boerke, et al., 2008, Nixon, et al., 2009, Shadan, et al., 2004). This particularly interesting finding raises the possibility that membrane rafts are of significance in coordinating the functional competence of spermatozoa (Bou Khalil, et al., 2006). In keeping with this notion, recent studies have shown isolated DRMs are capable of binding to the zona pellucida of homologous oocytes with a high degree of affinity and specificity (Bou Khalil, et al., 2006, Nixon, et al., 2009, Nixon, et al., 2011) and that these membrane fractions contain a number of key molecules that have been previously implicated in sperm-zona pellucida interactions (Bou Khalil, et al., 2006, Nixon, et al., 2009, Nixon, et al., 2011, Sleight, et al., 2005). Taken together, such findings encourage speculation that sperm membrane rafts may serve as platforms that act to spatially constrain key zona pellucida recognition molecules and deliver them to their site of action on the anterior region of the sperm head during capacitation (Nixon, et al., 2009, Nixon, et al., 2011). Consistent with this notion, elegant real time tracking studies have demonstrated that cholesterol efflux initiates diffusion (and possibly formation) of novel membrane raft-like structures containing zona-binding molecules over the acrosome of live spermatozoa. Furthermore, following head-to-head agglutination spermatozoa show contact-induced coalescence of G_{M1} gangliosides suggestive of a specific mechanosensitive response that concentrates important molecules to the appropriate site on the sperm surface to mediate zona binding (Jones, et al., 2010).

In addition to stimulating the loss of cholesterol from the plasma membrane, and promoting aggregation of membrane rafts, the elevation of intracellular HCO_3^- also activates a unique form of soluble adenylyl cyclase (SACY), which synthesizes cAMP from adenine triphosphate (ATP) (Aitken, et al., 1998, White and Aitken, 1989). Calcium has also been shown to coordinate with bicarbonate to stimulate SACY, although the precise mechanism that underpins this interaction remains to be elucidated (Carlson, et al., 2007, Litvin, et al., 2003). The importance of SACY has been demonstrated by the fact that sperm from *Sacy*-null male mice display limited motility (Esposito, et al., 2004). Furthermore, inhibition of SACY activity in wildtype mice results in the obstruction of capacitation-associated tyrosine phosphorylation and *in vitro* fertilization (Hess, et al., 2005). In addition to SACY, intracellular levels of cAMP are also regulated by cAMP phosphodiesterases (PDEs) that degrade cAMP to 5′-AMP (Fig. 3). The initial production of cAMP activates protein kinase A (PKA) through association with the regulatory subunits of the enzyme, promoting dissociation and activation of the catalytic subunits that in turn catalyze the phosphorylation of serine/threonine residues (Urner and Sakkas, 2003). Activation of PKA

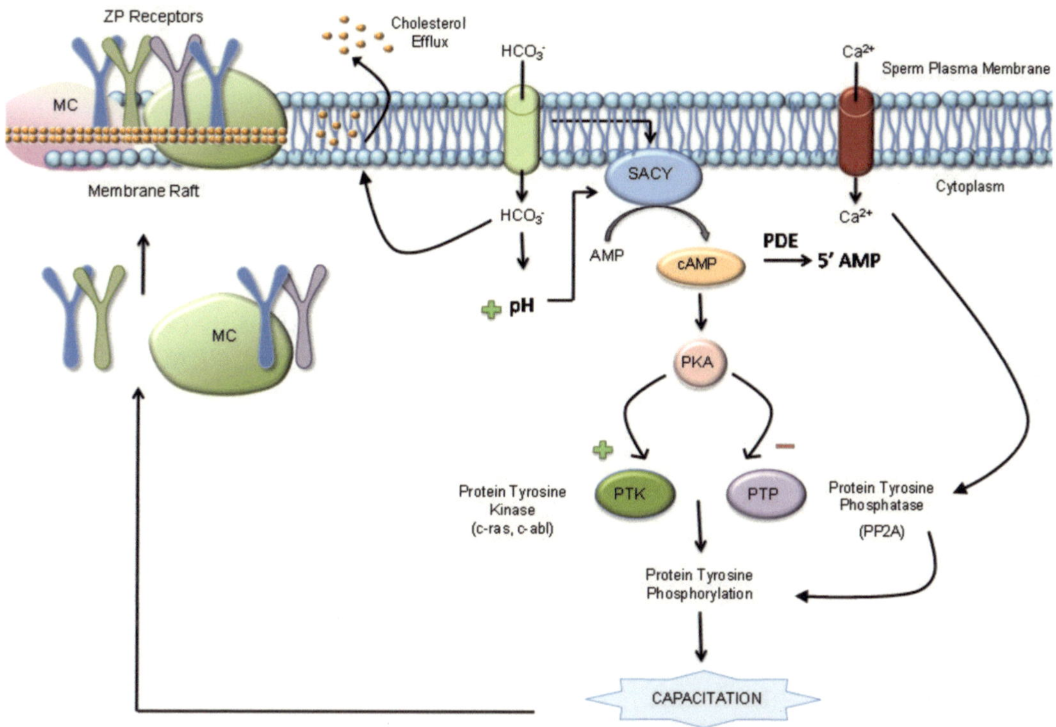

Figure 3. Model of mammalian sperm capacitation. Cholesterol efflux during the early phases of capacitation increases plasma membrane fluidity, facilitating the entry of bicarbonate (HCO_3^-) and calcium ions (Ca^{2+}) into the sperm cytosol through specific membrane channels. Cholesterol is preferentially lost from non-membrane raft portions of the plasma membrane, and appears to promote a polarized redistribution of membrane rafts to the anterior region of the sperm head. This event may serve to reposition key zona pellucida receptor molecules and enable their surface presentation and / or assembly into functional zona pellucida receptor complexes in this region of the sperm head. There is compelling evidence that such dramatic membrane remodeling events may be augmented by the action of molecular chaperones that are themselves activated during capacitation. This activation appears to be underpinned by a complex signaling cascade involving cross-talk between several pathways. In the most well characterized of these, a sperm specific form of soluble adenylyl cyclase (SACY) is activated by increases in intracellular bicarbonate, calcium and pH, leading to the production of the second messenger cyclic AMP (cAMP). cAMP, in turn, initiates the activation of protein kinase A (PKA), which then simultaneously inhibits the activity of protein tyrosine phosphatases (PTP) and activates protein tyrosine kinases (PTK). This dual regulation results in a global increase in protein tyrosine phosphorylation across a myriad of proteins, including a subset of molecular chaperones, and culminates in the functional activation of the cell. Calcium regulated adenylyl cyclases, phosphodiesterases (PDE), tyrosine kinases and tyrosine phosphatases have also been implicated in various aspects of capacitation associated cell signaling in the spermatozoa of a number of mammalian species.

also results in the induction of tyrosine phosphorylation across a number of substrates, most likely through activation of an intermediary protein tyrosine kinase (PTK) and/or inhibition of protein tyrosine phosphatases (PTP), or both. Of the potential candidates, inhibitory studies have implicated the promiscuous SRC kinase-family of PTKs in driving the increase in phosphotyrosine content (Baker, et al., 2006), especially in human spermatozoa (Lawson, et al., 2008, Mitchell, et al., 2008). However, more recent work has demonstrated that the suppression of capacitation-associated parameters induced by SRC kinase inhibitors is able to be overcome by incubation of sperm in the presence of Ser/Thr phosphatase inhibitors. In addition, sperm from *Src*-null mice contained similar levels of capacitation-associated tyrosine phosphorylation as wild-type sperm. These data indicate that SRC is not directly involved in capacitation-associated changes in tyrosine phosphorylation in mouse spermatozoa. They also provide evidence that capacitation is regulated by two parallel pathways, one requiring activation of PKA and another involving inactivation of Ser/Thr phosphatases, such as PP2A (Krapf, et al., 2010). Other potential candidates include c-ras which has been identified in human sperm (Naz, et al., 1992a), as well as c-abl which has been studied in both mouse (Baker, et al., 2009) and human models (Naz, 1998). It is important to note, that while the above canonical pathway is the primary pathway thought to induce capacitation, there is evidence to suggest that there is significant cross-talk with other signaling pathways. For instance, it has been demonstrated that a subset of the targets for capacitation associated protein tyrosine phosphorylation are activated by the extracellular signal-regulated kinase (ERK) module of the mitogen-activated protein kinase (MAPK) pathway. Interestingly, inhibition of several elements of this pathway results in suppression of sperm surface phosphotyrosine expression and a concomitant reduction in sperm-zona pellucida interactions (Nixon, et al., 2010).

Irrespective of the mechanisms, capacitation-associated tyrosine phosphorylation has been causally related to the induction of hyperactivated motility, increasing the ability of sperm to bind to the zona pellucida, priming of the cells for acrosomal exocytosis and ultimately enhancing their capacity to fertilize an oocyte (Leclerc, et al., 1997, Sakkas, et al., 2003, Urner and Sakkas, 2003, Visconti, et al., 1995b). The diversity of functions regulated by phosphorylation is consistent with the demonstration that this process occurs in a specific sequence within different compartments of the sperm cell, and is altered again upon binding to the zona pellucida (Sakkas, et al., 2003). In mouse spermatozoa, overt capacitation-associated increases in protein tyrosine phosphorylation have been documented in the flagellum, with principal piece phosphorylation preceding that of the midpiece. Several targets have been identified including aldolase A, NADH dehydrogenase, acrosin binding protein (sp32), proteasome subunit alpha type 6B, and voltage-dependent anion channel 2 among others (Arcelay, et al., 2008). In human spermatozoa however, this increase appears to be restricted to the principal piece, with evidence that both A-kinase anchor protein (AKAP) 3 and AKAP4 are targets (Ficarro, et al., 2003, Sakkas, et al., 2003). The tyrosine phosphorylation of proteins in the sperm flagellum has been causally related to the induction of hyperactivated motility (Mahony and Gwathmey, 1999, Nassar, et al., 1999, Si and Okuno, 1999), a vigorous pattern of motility that is required for spermatozoa to penetrate through the cumulus cell layer and the zona pellucida in order to reach the inner membrane of the oocyte. In addition, to the increased phosphorylation, hyperactivation requires the alkalinization of the sperm and is also calcium-dependent. The calcium required for the induction of hyperactivation can be mobilized into sperm from the external milieu by plasma membrane channel, and can also be released from intracellular stores, including the redundant nuclear envelope located at the base of the sperm flagellum, or the acrosome (Costello, et al., 2009, Herrick, et al., 2005, Ho and Suarez, 2003). Of particular importance in importing calcium into sperm are the CATSPER (cation channel, sperm associated) family of calcium channel proteins, which are sensitive to intracellular alkalinization, and thus are critical for capacitation (Kirichok, et al., 2006, Lobley, et al., 2003, Qi, et al., 2007, Quill, et al., 2001, Ren, et al., 2001). Male mice null for each of the four individual *Catsper* genes have been shown to be infertile as they are incapable of the hyperactivated motility required for zona pellucida penetration (Carlson, et al., 2005, Jin, et al., 2007, Qi, et al., 2007, Quill, et al., 2001, Ren, et al., 2001).

In addition to the more widely studied phosphorylation of flagellum proteins, capacitation-associated increases in tyrosine phosphorylation have also been reported in an alternate set of proteins located in the sperm head (Asquith, et al., 2004, Flesch, et al., 2001b, Tesarik, et al., 1993, Urner, et al., 2001). Although these proteins represent only a minor proportion of the total pool of phosphorylation substrates in mouse spermatozoa, their importance has been highlighted by the observation that they are expressed on the surface of live, capacitated spermatozoa in a position compatible with a role in mediation of sperm-zona pellucida interactions (Asquith, et al., 2004, Piehler, et al., 2006). Furthermore, these phosphoproteins are present on virtually all sperm that are competent to adhere to the zona pellucida opposed to less than one quarter of sperm in the free swimming population. Although such findings invite speculation that a subset of proteins targeted for phosphotyrosine residues may directly participate sperm-zona pellucida adhesion, this conclusion is at odds with the fact that pre-incubation of sperm with anti-phosphotyrosine antibodies has no discernible effect on their subsequent fertilizing ability (Asquith, et al., 2004). Rather it has been suggested that, following their activation via phosphorylation, these proteins play an indirect role by mediating sperm surface remodeling to render cells competent to engage in zona pellucida adhesion (Fig. 3). In agreement with this proposal, a subset of phosphorylated proteins have been identified in the mouse as the molecular chaperone proteins heat shock protein (HSP) 60 (HSPD1) and endoplasmin (HSP90B1) (Asquith, et al., 2004). Such proteins have well-characterized roles in the folding and trafficking proteins, the assembly of multi-protein structures, and the translocation of proteins across membranes (Nixon, et al., 2005) In addition to mice, a similar cohort of molecular chaperone proteins have also been detected on the surface of sperm from other species including bull (Kamaruddin, et al., 2004), boar (Spinaci, et al., 2005) and human (Miller, et al., 1992, Naaby-Hansen and Herr, 2010), although their phosphorylation status in these species is less clear.

Maturational Phase	Changes contributing to acquisition of zona pellucida binding ability	References
Spermatogenesis	• Primordial germ cells undergo multiple stages of mitotic and meiotic divisions, followed by a process of cytodifferentiation which results in a highly polarized cell • In early spermatids the Golgi apparatus is transformed into the acrosome • The flagellum is formed to provide sperm with the ability for forward progressive movement • Expression of the molecular chaperone in elongating spermatids is correlated with plasma membrane remodeling that results in the formation of zona pellucida and hyaluronic acid binding sites. These HA binding sites are thought to be responsible for the sperm to penetrate the cumulus cell layer surrounding the oocyte	(Berruti and Paiardi, 2011, Hermo, et al., 2010b, Hermo, et al., 2010c, Huszar, et al., 2007)
Epididymal Transit	• Lipid architecture is remodeled in preparation for the formation of membrane rafts during capacitation • Protein architecture is altered. Existing proteins are unmasked or undergo post-translational modifications, or alternatively novel proteins are integrated into the plasma membrane via epididymosomes and intraluminal fluid • Motility machinery is matured in preparation for acquisition of motility • Upon reaching the cauda epididymis spermatozoa are capable of a sinusoidal movement pattern characterized by a symmetrical tail motion at high frequency and low amplitude • Increase in ability to recognize and interact with zona pellucida	(Cooper, 1986, Cooper and Orgebin-Crist, 1975, Dacheux and Paquignon, 1980, Jones, 1998, Jones, et al., 2007)
Capacitation	• Loss of specific decapacitation factors (DFs) allows freshly ejaculated spermatozoa to commence capacitation • Cholesterol efflux from the plasma membrane increases membrane fluidity promoting lateral movement of integral proteins, as well as the formation of membrane rafts • Influx of HCO_3^- activates key signaling cascades whereby SACY stimulates cAMP and in turn PKA. This results in increased tyrosine phosphorylation of specific sperm proteins • In the tail, AKAPs become activated via this phosphorylation and induce a hyperactivated form of motility which allows the sperm to navigate through the oviduct to the site of ovulation. • Key zona pellucida recognition molecules aggregate to the apical region of the sperm head, using membrane rafts as a platform to mediate zona pellucida interaction	(Fraser, 1984, Jones, et al., 2010, Nixon, et al., 2009, Nixon, et al., 2011, Sleight, et al., 2005, Suarez, 2008, Visconti, et al., 1995a)

Table 1. Summary of specific biochemical- and biophysical-changes that occur during mammalian sperm maturation.

Although the precise role that these surface expressed chaperones play in preparing the sperm for their interaction with the oocyte remains to be established, one possibility is that they promote the presentation and/or assembly of oocyte receptor complex(es) on the sperm surface (Asquith, et al., 2004) (Fig. 3). This notion is supported by the observation that a subset of chaperones have been shown to be the subject of dynamic redistribution during capacitation, leading to their exposure on the anterior region of the sperm head (Asquith, et al., 2005, Dun, et al., 2011). Despite this relocation, a direct role for the chaperones in the mediation of sperm-zona pellucida interactions has been discounted on the basis that anti-chaperone antibodies consistently fail to compromise sperm-zona pellucida adhesion (Asquith, et al., 2005, Dun, et al., 2011, Walsh, et al., 2008). The chaperones do however form stable interactions with a number of putative zona pellucida adhesion molecules which, as discussed below (see Section 2.3.2), appears to indicate that they play an indirect role in gamete interaction. Whether a similar role extends to molecular chaperones in the spermatozoa of other species, such as our own, remains somewhat more controversial. A study by Mitchell *et al* (2007) failed to localize any of the prominent chaperones to the sperm surface, nor secure evidence for the capacitation-associated phosphorylation of these chaperone proteins (Mitchell, et al., 2007). However, a more recent study by Naaby-Hansen and Herr (2009) demonstrated the expression of seven members from four different chaperone families on the surface of human spermatozoa. They also demonstrated that inhibition of several isoforms of HSPA2 results in decreased fertilization rates *in vitro* (Naaby-Hansen and Herr, 2010). These studies are supported by earlier work which suggests that the absence of HSPA2 is correlated with decreased ability of sperm to bind to the zona pellucida (Huszar, et al., 2007).

2.3.2. *Zona pellucida receptor candidates*

Consistent with the apparent complexity of the zona pellucida ligands to which spermatozoa bind, a plethora of candidates have been proposed to act as primary receptors capable of interacting with the carbohydrate moieties and or protein present within the zona pellucida matrix. In most species the list is constantly being refined as new candidates emerge and others are disproven through, for example, the production of knockout models bearing targeted deletions of the putative receptors. Consistent with the notion that primary sperm- zona pellucida interaction involves engagement with specific carbohydrate structures on ZP3, a number of the identified sperm receptors possess lectin-like affinity for specific sugar residues (McLeskey, et al., 1998, Topfer-Petersen, 1999, Wassarman, 1992). In the mouse, the most widely studied model, these receptors include, but are not limited to: β-1,4-galatosyltransferase (GalT1) (Lopez, et al., 1985, Nixon, et al., 2001, Shur and Bennett, 1979, Shur and Hall, 1982a), ZP3R (or sp56) (Bookbinder, et al., 1995, Cheng, et al., 1994, Cohen and Wassarman, 2001), α-D-mannosidase (Cornwall, et al., 1991) and zonadhesin (Gao and Garbers, 1998, Tardif and Cormier, 2011, Topfer-Petersen, et al., 1998) (see Table 1). However, despite the wealth of knowledge accumulated about each of these putative zona pellucida receptors it is now apparent that none are uniquely capable of directing sperm- zona pellucida adhesion. For example, the targeted disruption of GalT1 in knockout mice fails to result in infertility (Lu, et al., 1997). Although sperm from GalT1 null mice bind poorly to ZP3 and fail to undergo a zona-induced acrosome reaction, they retain the ability to bind to the ovulated egg coat *in vitro* (Lu and Shur, 1997). In a similar vein, a number of zona pellucida binding molecules have been identified in human spermatozoa, including sperm autoantigenic protein 17 (SPA17) (Grizzi, et al., 2003), fucosyltransferase 5 (FUT5) (Chiu, et al., 2003a, Chiu, et al., 2004), and mannose binding receptor (Rosano, et al., 2007). However, further analyses of these receptor molecules have compromised their status as being the single molecule responsible for zona pellucida interaction (see Table 2). In fact prevailing evidence now strongly suggests that no individual receptor is exclusively responsible for regulating gamete interaction. Underscoring the amazing complexity of this interaction, it has instead been proposed to rely on the coordinated action of several zona receptor molecules, which may be assembled into a functional multimeric complex.

Candidate (synonyms)	Species	Evidence	References
Angiotensin-converting enzyme (ACE)	Mouse Rat Horse Human	• Testis-specific form is found within developing spermatids and mature sperm • ACE KO mice are infertile due to defective transport in the oviducts as well as decreased zona pellucida binding • Play significant role in re-distribution of ADAM3 to the sperm surface	(Esther, et al., 1996, Foresta, et al., 1991, Kohn, et al., 1995, Langford, et al., 1993, Sibony, et al., 1993)
A disintegrin and metalloproteinase (ADAMs)	Mouse Rat Pig Human	• Family of transmembrane proteins that have varying roles in maturation of spermatozoa • ADAM3 has important role in zona pellucida binding • ADAM2 KO mice show strong suppression of zona pellucida binding and difficulty in moving through female reproductive tract, due to absence of ADAM3 in these mice • ADAM1a KO mice are fertile, but show decreased levels of ADAM3 on the sperm surface • ADAM1b KO mice are fertile	(Kim, et al., 2004, Kim, et al., 2006a, Kim, et al., 2006b, Nishimura, et al., 2004, Nishimura, et al., 2007, Yamaguchi, et al., 2009)
α-D-mannosidase (MAN2B2)	Mouse Rat Hamster Human	• Integral plasma membrane protein that may facilitate sperm-zona pellucida binding by adhering to mannose-containing zona pellucida oligosaccharides	(Cornwall, et al., 1991, Pereira, et al., 1998, Tulsiani, et al., 1993, Tulsiani, et al., 1989, Yoshida-Komiya, et al., 1999),

Candidate (synonyms)	Species	Evidence	References
		• Pre-incubation of sperm with either D-mannose or anti-MAN2B2 antibody elicits a dose-dependent inhibition of zona pellucida binding	
Arylsulfatase A (AS-A; ARSA)	Mouse Human Boar	• Acquired onto the sperm surface during epididymal transit • Addition of exogenous ARSA, or anti-ARSA antibodies inhibit zona pellucida binding in a dose-dependent manner • ARSA-null males are fertile but fertility decreases with age	(Carmona, et al., 2002, Hess, et al., 1996, Tantibhedhyangkul, et al., 2002, Weerachatyanukul, et al., 2003)
Calmegin (CLGN)/Calnexin/Calspernin (CALR3)	Mouse	• CLGN- and CALR3-deficient mice are infertile due to defective sperm migration from uterus into the oviduct, as well as defective zona pellucidabinding • CLGN is required for ADAM1a/ADAM2 dimerization • CALR3 is required for ADAM3 maturation	(Ikawa, et al., 2001, Ikawa, et al., 2011, Yamagata, et al., 2002)
GalT1 (β-1,4-galactosyltransferase; GAlTase; GALT; B4GALT1)	Mouse Rat Human Guinea Pig Rabbit Bull Boar Stallion	• Transmembrane protein located on the sperm head overlying the intact acrosome • Transgenic mice overexpressing GalTase are hypersensitive to ZP3 and undergo precocious acrosome reactions • Sperm from mice bearing targeted deletions in GalTase are unable to bind ZP3 or undergo ZP3-dependent acrosomal exocytosis • GalTase-null sperm retain ability to bind to zona pellucida	(Lopez, et al., 1985, Lopez and Shur, 1987, Shi, et al., 2004, Shur and Hall, 1982a, Shur and Hall, 1982b)
Fertization antigen 1 (FA1)	Mouse Human Bull	• Localized to the postacrosomal region of sperm head • Anti-FA-1 antibodies have been implicated in immune infertility in humans • No recorded knockout	(Coonrod, et al., 1994, Menge, et al., 1999, Naz, et al., 1992b, Naz, et al., 1984, Naz and Zhu, 1998)

Candidate (synonyms)	Species	Evidence	References
Fucosyltransferase 5 (FUT5)	Human	• Localized to the acrosomal region of the sperm head • Pre-treatment of sperm with antibodies directed against FUT5 inhibits zona pellucida binding	(Chiu, et al., 2003b, Chiu, et al., 2004)
Milk fat globule-EGF factor 8 (MFGE8; p47; SED1)	Mouse Boar	• Protein is applied to the sperm acrosome during epididymal transit • Binds specifically to the zona pellucida of unfertilized, but not fertilized eggs • Recombinant MFGE8 and anti-MFGE8 antibodies competitively inhibits zona pellucida binding • MFGE8 null males are subfertile and their sperm are unable to bind to the zona pellucida *in vitro*	(Ensslin, et al., 1995, Ensslin and Shur, 2003)
Proacrosin (acrosin)	Mouse Boar	• Localizes to acrosome and inner acrosomal membrane • Mediates secondary zona pellucida binding via interaction with ZP2 • Binding to zona pellucida is non-enzymatic and thought to involve recognition of polysulfate groups on zona pellucida glycoproteins • Acrosin null males are fertile but displaycompromised zona pellucida penetration	(Baba, et al., 1994a, Baba, et al., 1994b, Howes, et al., 2001, Howes and Jones, 2002, Moreno, et al., 1998, Urch and Patel, 1991)
Sperm adhesion molecule 1 (SPAM1; PH-20)	All mammals	• Widely conserved sperm surface protein • Localized to plasma membrane over anterior region of sperm head • Possesses hyaluronidase activity that aids in the digestion of cumulus cells • Relocalizes to inner acrosomal membrane following acrosome reaction; potentially participates in secondary zona pellucida binding • SPAM1 null males are fertile although their sperm areless efficient in cumulus cell dispersal	(Baba, et al., 2002, Hunnicutt, et al., 1996a, Hunnicutt, et al., 1996b, Lin, et al., 1994, Morales, et al., 2004, Myles and Primakoff, 1997)

Candidate (synonyms)	Species	Evidence	References
Sperm autoantigenic protein 17 (SPA17; SP17)	Mouse Rabbit Human Primates	• Highly conserved protein localized to the acrosome and fibrous sheath • Has been implicated in regulation of sperm maturation, capacitation, acrosomal exocytosis and zona pellucida binding • Shown to bind to specific mannose components of the zona pellucida	(Chiriva-Internati, et al., 2009, Grizzi, et al., 2003, Yamasaki, et al., 1995)
Spermadhesins (AWN; AQN-1; AQN-3)	Boar Stallion Bull	• Are major components of seminal plasma • May be involved in several sequential steps of fertilization through multifuncational ability to bind to carbohydrates, sulfated glycosaminoglycans, phospholipids and protease inhibitors	(Petrunkina, et al., 2000, Sinowatz, et al., 1995, Topfer-Petersen, et al., 1998)
Sulfogalactosylglycerolipid (SGG)	Mouse Rat Human Boar	• SGG is a major sperm sulfoglycolipid that putatively facilitates uptake of sulfolipid-immobilizing protein-1 (SLIP1) and ARSA • Following capacitation, SGG is predominantly found in membrane rafts, microdomains that possess zona pellucida affinity • Pre-incubation of sperm with monovalent anti-SGG Fab fragments significantly inhibits zona pellucida binding	(Bou Khalil, et al., 2006, Kornblatt, 1979, Tanphaichitr, et al., 1990, Tanphaichitr, et al., 1993, Weerachatyanukul, et al., 2001, White, et al., 2000)
Zonadhesin (ZAN)	Mouse Hamster Rabbit Boar Bull Horse Primates	• Localizes to the apical region of the sperm head following spermatogenesis and epididymal maturation • Features a mosaic protein architecture with several domains that potentially enable the protein to participate in multiple cell adhesion processes including zona pellucida binding	(Bi, et al., 2003, Gasper and Swanson, 2006, Hardy and Garbers, 1994, Hardy and Garbers, 1995, Herlyn and Zischler, 2008, Hickox, et al., 2001, Olson, et al., 2004, Tardif, et al., 2010)

Candidate (synonyms)	Species	Evidence	References
		• Appears to confer species specificity to sperm-zona pellucida adhesion in that sperm from *Zan* -/- males are able to bind promiscuously to the zona pellucida of non-homologous species	
ZP3R (sp56)	Mouse	• Localized to the surface of the sperm head • Pre-incubation of sperm with anti-ZP3R antibodies blocks zona pellucida binding • Pre-treatment of sperm with recombinant ZP3R inhibits fertilization *in vivo* • EM localizes ZP3R within acrosomal matrix, but the protein appears to undergo a capacitation-associated relocation to the surface of the anterior region of the sperm head • *ZP3r* -/- males are fertile and their spermatozoa retain their ability to bind zonae of unfertilized eggs and undergo acrosomal exocytosis	(Hardy, et al., 2004, Muro, et al., 2012, Wassarman, 2009)

Table 2. Putative sperm- zona pellucida receptor candidates

2.4. Toward an integrated model of sperm- zona pellucida interaction

2.4.1. Multimeric protein complexes in zona pellucida binding

Despite decades of research, the specific molecular mechanisms that drive the initial interaction between the male and female gametes remain elusive. As stated previously, a myriad of diverse candidate molecules have been proposed as putative mediators of sperm binding to the zona matrix (Table 1). Regardless of this, prevailing evidence now indicates that none are uniquely responsible for directing or maintaining this interaction (Nixon, et al., 2007). Indeed, the classical model of a simple lock and key mechanism that prevailed in this field of research for several decades has been largely disproven. The fact that spermatozoa contain a multiplicity of zona pellucida receptor candidates allows for a level of functional redundancy commensurate with the overall importance of this fundamental cellular interaction. It also accounts for the succession of both low affinity and high affinity interactions (Thaler and Cardullo, 1996, Thaler and Cardullo, 2002) that characterize gamete interaction. Although the biochemical basis of this multifaceted adhesion process remains obscure, it is unlikely that it could be regulated by the activity of a single receptor.

Furthermore, mammalian spermatozoa undergo considerable changes in their already complex surface architecture during epididymal transit and the capacitation process in the female reproductive tract. Prior to these events, the cells are unable to recognize or bind to the zona pellucida. A simple lock and key mechanism involving a constitutively expressed surface receptor does not account for the need to undergo such radical alterations prior to obtaining affinity for the zonae.. Collectively, these data have led to an alternative hypothesis that sperm maturation leads to the surface expression and/or assembly of multimeric complex(es) compromising a multitude of zona pellucida receptors.

The concept that multimeric protein complexes are capable of regulating cell-cell interactions draws on an extensive body of literature. It is well known for instance that the human genome codes for in excess of 500 000 different proteins, of which an estimated 80% function as part of multimeric protein complexes, as opposed to individual proteins (Berggard, et al., 2007). In addition, there are many documented examples of cell-cell adhesion events that require the formation of multimeric protein complexes. As a case in point, β-catenin is well-known to form a complex with several other adhesion proteins, such as cadherin, at sites of cell-cell contact. Interestingly, the formation of these complexes is tightly regulated by phosphorylation and dephosphorylation of the N-terminus of β-catenin (Maher, et al., 2009). Tight junctions have also been shown to rely heavily on the formation of specific protein complexes, comprising transmembrane and membrane-associated proteins (Shen, et al., 2008). Studies with migrating cells, and other cell types that interact in fluid, dynamic environments similar to that in which gametes bind, have illustrated that they most likely rely on the sequential receptor-ligand interactions that are coordinated through the formation of protein adhesion complexes (Sackstein, 2005). In a situation analogous to that recorded in spermatozoa, recent work in cancer cell biology has described the importance of molecular chaperone complexes in increasing the migration and invasiveness of specific cancer types. Breast cancer in particular relies heavily on the action of HSP90α in order to invade other cell types. In this case, HSP90α is excreted by the cancer cell in order to act as a mediator between a complex of co-chaperones outside the cell, including HSP70, HSP40, Hop (HSP70/HSP90 organizing protein) and p23, subsequently activating MMP-2 (matrix metalloproteinase 2) (Eustace, et al., 2004, McCready, et al., 2010, Sims, et al., 2011). MMP-2 then acts to degrade proteins in the extracellular matrix of target cells, thus increasing the invasive ability of the malignant cancer cells (Folgueras, et al., 2004, Jezierska and Motyl, 2009).

The concept of a multimeric zona pellucida receptor complex in spermatozoa was originally proposed by Asquith *et al* in mouse spermatozoa (Asquith, et al., 2004). This work demonstrated the preferential tyrosine phosphorylation of a specific subset of molecular chaperones during capacitation. A finding that generated considerable interest was that this modification, coincided with the translocation of the chaperones the surface of the sperm head in the precise region that mediates zona pellucida binding. However, the failure of either anti-phosphotyrosine or anti-chaperone antibodies to compromise sperm- zona pellucida interactions led to the proposal that these chaperones may have an indirect role in zona pellucida interaction by virtue of their ability to coordinate the assembly of a zona pellucida receptor complex during capacitation. A key observation in support of this model is that the chaperones, along with numerous putative zona pellucida receptors, partition into lipid microdomains or DRMs (discussed in Section 2.3.1.3). It is proposed that these microdomains may serve as platforms to recruit chaperone clients proteins and/or enhance productive interactions between these two classes of proteins (Nixon, et al., 2009). Indeed, independent evidence indicates that chaperones do form stable protein complexes within membrane rafts during the capacitation of mouse spermatozoa. For instance, Han *et al* (2011) have recently revealed that the molecular chaperones, HSPA5 and calnexin, associate with a number of client proteins to form a stable supramolecular complex on the surface of mouse spermatozoa. These client proteins include ADAM7 (a disintegrin and metalloprotease 7), a protease that is transferred to the sperm surface via epididymosomes as the cells transit through the epididymis (Oh et al. 2009) and belongs to a family of proteases that have been implicated in sperm migration in the female reproductive tract and adhesion to the zona pellucida (Muro and Okabe 2011) (Cho, et al., 1998, Shamsadin, et al., 1999, Yanagimachi, 2009). Interesting the HSPA5/calnexin/ADAM7 complex resides within DRMs (membrane rafts) and its assembly is promoted by sperm capacitation (Han et al. 2011). In addition, recent work performed by Dun *et al* (2011) demonstrated the presence of a number of high molecular weight protein complexes expressed on the surface of capacitated mouse sperm utilizing the technique of Blue Native PAGE (Dun, et al., 2011). Of particular interest was the identification of the chaperonin-containing TCP-1 complex (CCT/TRiC) and its ability to form a stable complex with zona pellucida binding protein 2 (ZPBP2). In addition to independent evidence that ZPBP2 participates in zona pellucida binding (Lin, et al., 2007) the CCT/TRiC / ZPBP2 complex was also shown to display affinity for homologous zonae. Importantly, a complex of similar size and compromising the same combination of the CCT/TRiC / ZPBP2 complex was also recently identified via application of the same methodology in human spermatozoa and again shown to participate in zona pellucida interaction in this species (Redgrove, et al., 2011). The conservation of this complex implies that it may be involved in mediation of non-species specific initial interactions, which are relatively weak and forgiving of species barriers. The same may also be true of the 20S proteasome complex that has been shown to display a high level of conservation among the spermatozoa of different species. For instance, the proteasome complex has been described in the spermatozoa of pig, mouse and human and, in each of these species, it has been implicated in zonae interactions (Morales, et al., 2003, Pasten, et al., 2005, Yi, et al., 2010, Zimmerman, et al., 2011). Although this is a constitutively expressed complex, there is evidence that certain subunits of the complex may be subjected to post-translational modifications, including tyrosine phosphorylation, during capacitation (Redgrove et al., 2011). In this context it is noteworthy that the tyrosine phosphorylation of similar proteasome subunits has been shown to influence the substrate specificity of the complex in other cell types (Bose et al., 1999; Castano et al., 1996; Mason et al., 1996; Wehren et al., 1996). Taken together, these findings raise the possibility the proteasome complex may be activated during sperm maturation in preparation for its functional role(s) in sperm–oocyte interactions. These roles appear to extend beyond that of zona pellucida recognition (Zimmerman, et al., 2011) to include regulation of the acrosome reaction in addition to penetration of the zona matrix (Kong, et al., 2009, Sutovsky, et al., 2004), (Morales, et al., 2003).

Interestingly, the indirect role of molecular chaperones in sperm- zona pellucida interactions appears to extend beyond the capacitation-associated remodeling of the sperm surface. Indeed, chaperones such as calmegin, calspernin, calnexin, and HSPA2 have been implicated in additional remodeling events during spermatogenesis and epididymal maturation. With respect to calspernin and calmegin, it has been shown that mice lacking these genes are incapable of binding to the zona pellucida, a defect that is attributable to the role these chaperones play in the maturation of ADAM3 (a protein required for fertilization), as well as the dimerization of an ADAM1 / ADAM2 heterodimer (Ikawa, et al., 2011). In contrast, calnexin has a primary role in retaining unfolded or unassembled N-linked glycoproteins in the ER (Sitia and Braakman, 2003). Importantly however, calnexin has also been shown to be present on the surface of mouse spermatozoa where it partitions into membrane rafts (Nixon, et al., 2009, Stein, et al., 2006). In addition to these lectin-like chaperones, testis-specific HSPA2 has been shown to be essential in several stages of spermatogenesis (Govin, et al., 2006) and, in the human, it has a prominent role in plasma membrane remodeling through the formation of zona pellucida and hyaluronic acid binding sites (Huszar, et al., 2007, Huszar, et al., 2006).

3. Summary

For decades, researchers have strived to find the key molecule on the sperm surface that is responsible for directing its binding to the zona pellucida in a cell and specifies specific manner. However, this premise of a simple lock and key mechanism has been increasingly drawn into question since it fails to account for the myriad of potential receptor molecules that have been identified over the intervening years and the fact that sperm- zona pellucida binding can be resolved into a number of sequential recognition events of varying affinity. Instead, owing largely to the application of elegant genetic manipulation strategies, it is now apparent that the interaction between the two gametes relies on an intricate interplay between a multitude of receptors and their complementary ligands, none of which are uniquely responsible. Such a level of functional redundancy is commensurate with the overall importance that this interaction holds in the initiation of a new life.

An important question that arises from this work is how the activity of such a diverse array of receptors is coordinated to ensure they are presented in the correct sequence to enable productive interactions with the zonae. One possibility is that the zona pellucida binding proteins are organized into functional receptor complexes that are assembled on the anterior region of the sperm head during the different phases of sperm maturation. Such a model may account for the need for the dramatic membrane remodeling events that accompany epididymal maturation and capacitation. Until recently a major challenge to this model has been the lack of direct evidence that sperm harbor multimeric protein complexes on their surface. However, through the application of a variety of novel techniques, independent laboratories have now verified that sperm do express high molecular weight protein complexes on their surface, a subset of which possess affinity for homologous zonae. Furthermore, there is compelling evidence that the assembly and / or surface presentation of these complexes is regulated by the capacitation status of the cells (Dun, et al., 2011, Han, et al., 2010, Morales, et al., 2003, Redgrove, et al., 2011, Sutovsky, et al., 2004).

The conservation of complexes such as the 20S proteasome and CCT/TRiC implies that they are not involved in high-affinity species specific binding to homologous zonae. Rather they may mediate the initial loose tethering of sperm to the zona pellucida and / or downstream events in the fertilization cascade. It is therefore considered likely that the higher affinity, species-specific zona pellucida interactions that follow are executed by additional protein complexes that have been shown to reside in human and mouse spermatozoa (Dun, et al., 2011, Redgrove, et al., 2011) but have yet to be characterised. The proteomic profiling and functional characterization of these additional multiprotein complexes therefore promises to shed new light on the intricacies of sperm-egg interactions.

Author details

Kate A. Redgrove, R. John Aitken and Brett Nixon
Reproductive Science Group, University of Newcastle, Australia

4. References

Aitken, J., Krausz, C. and Buckingham, D. (1994). "Relationships between biochemical markers for residual sperm cytoplasm, reactive oxygen species generation, and the presence of leukocytes and precursor germ cells in human sperm suspensions." *Mol Reprod Dev* 39(3): pp. 268-79, ISSN 1040-452X

Aitken, R. J., Harkiss, D., Knox, W., Paterson, M. and Irvine, D. S. (1998). "A novel signal transduction cascade in capacitating human spermatozoa characterised by a redox-regulated, cAMP-mediated induction of tyrosine phosphorylation." *J Cell Sci* 111 (Pt 5)(pp. 645-56, ISSN 0021-9533

Amann, R. P., Hammerstedt, R. H. and Veeramachaneni, D. N. (1993). "The epididymis and sperm maturation: a perspective." *Reprod Fertil Dev* 5(4): pp. 361-81, ISSN 1031-3613

Arcelay, E., Salicioni, A. M., Wertheimer, E. and Visconti, P. E. (2008). "Identification of proteins undergoing tyrosine phosphorylation during mouse sperm capacitation." *Int J Dev Biol* 52(5-6): pp. 463-72, ISSN 0214-6282

Arslan, M., Morshedi, M., Arslan, E. O., Taylor, S., Kanik, A., Duran, H. E. and Oehninger, S. (2006). "Predictive value of the hemizona assay for pregnancy outcome in patients undergoing controlled ovarian hyperstimulation with intrauterine insemination." *Fertil Steril* 85(6): pp. 1697-707, ISSN 1556-5653

Asquith, K. L., Baleato, R. M., McLaughlin, E. A., Nixon, B. and Aitken, R. J. (2004). "Tyrosine phosphorylation activates surface chaperones facilitating sperm-zona recognition." *J Cell Sci* 117(Pt 16): pp. 3645-57, ISSN 0021-9533

Asquith, K. L., Harman, A. J., McLaughlin, E. A., Nixon, B. and Aitken, R. J. (2005). "Localization and significance of molecular chaperones, heat shock protein 1, and tumor rejection antigen gp96 in the male reproductive tract and during capacitation and acrosome reaction." *Biol Reprod* 72(2): pp. 328-37, ISSN 0006-3363

Austin, C. R. (1952). "The capacitation of the mammalian sperm." *Nature* 170(4321): pp. 326, ISSN 0028-0836

Baba, D., Kashiwabara, S., Honda, A., Yamagata, K., Wu, Q., Ikawa, M., Okabe, M. and Baba, T. (2002). "Mouse sperm lacking cell surface hyaluronidase PH-20 can pass through the layer of cumulus cells and fertilize the egg." *J Biol Chem* 277(33): pp. 30310-4, ISSN 0021-9258

Baba, T., Azuma, S., Kashiwabara, S. and Toyoda, Y. (1994a). "Sperm from mice carrying a targeted mutation of the acrosin gene can penetrate the oocyte zona pellucida and effect fertilization." *J Biol Chem* 269(50): pp. 31845-9, ISSN 0021-9258

Baba, T., Niida, Y., Michikawa, Y., Kashiwabara, S., Kodaira, K., Takenaka, M., Kohno, N., Gerton, G. L. and Arai, Y. (1994b). "An acrosomal protein, sp32, in mammalian sperm is a binding protein specific for two proacrosins and an acrosin intermediate." *J Biol Chem* 269(13): pp. 10133-40, ISSN 0021-9258

Bailey, J. L. (2010). "Factors regulating sperm capacitation." *Syst Biol Reprod Med* 56(5): pp. 334-48, ISSN 1939-6376

Baker, M. A., Hetherington, L. and Aitken, R. J. (2006). "Identification of SRC as a key PKA-stimulated tyrosine kinase involved in the capacitation-associated hyperactivation of murine spermatozoa." *J Cell Sci* 119(Pt 15): pp. 3182-92, ISSN 0021-9533

Baker, M. A., Hetherington, L., Curry, B. and Aitken, R. J. (2009). "Phosphorylation and consequent stimulation of the tyrosine kinase c-Abl by PKA in mouse spermatozoa; its implications during capacitation." *Dev Biol* 333(1): pp. 57-66, ISSN 1095-564X

Baker, M. A., Witherdin, R., Hetherington, L., Cunningham-Smith, K. and Aitken, R. J. (2005). "Identification of post-translational modifications that occur during sperm maturation using difference in two-dimensional gel electrophoresis." *Proteomics* 5(4): pp. 1003-12, ISSN 1615-9853

Bauskin, A. R., Franken, D. R., Eberspaecher, U. and Donner, P. (1999). "Characterization of human zona pellucida glycoproteins." *Mol Hum Reprod* 5(6): pp. 534-40, ISSN 1360-9947

Bedford, J. M. (1963). "Morphological changes in rabbit spermatozoa during passage through the epididymis." *J Reprod Fertil* 5(pp. 169-77, ISSN 0022-4251

Bedford, J. M. (1965). "Changes in fine structure of the rabbit sperm head during passage through the epididymis." *J Anat* 99(Pt 4): pp. 891-906, ISSN 0021-8782

Bedford, J. M. (1967). "Effects of duct ligation on the fertilizing ability of spermatozoa from different regions of the rabbit epididymis." *J Exp Zool* 166(2): pp. 271-81, ISSN 0022-104X

Bedford, J. M. (1968). "Ultrastructural changes in the sperm head during fertilization in the rabbit." *Am J Anat* 123(2): pp. 329-58, ISSN 0002-9106

Berggard, T., Linse, S. and James, P. (2007). "Methods for the detection and analysis of protein-protein interactions." *Proteomics* 7(16): pp. 2833-42, ISSN 1615-9853

Berruti, G. and Paiardi, C. (2011). "Acrosome biogenesis: Revisiting old questions to yield new insights." *Spermatogenesis* 1(2): pp. 95-98, ISSN 2156-5562

Bi, M., Hickox, J. R., Winfrey, V. P., Olson, G. E. and Hardy, D. M. (2003). "Processing, localization and binding activity of zonadhesin suggest a function in sperm adhesion to the zona pellucida during exocytosis of the acrosome." *Biochem J* 375(Pt 2): pp. 477-88, ISSN 1470-8728

Bi, Y., Xu, W. M., Wong, H. Y., Zhu, H., Zhou, Z. M., Chan, H. C. and Sha, J. H. (2009). "NYD-SP27, a novel intrinsic decapacitation factor in sperm." *Asian J Androl* 11(2): pp. 229-39, ISSN 1008-682X

Bleil, J. D. and Wassarman, P. M. (1980a). "Mammalian sperm-egg interaction: identification of a glycoprotein in mouse egg zonae pellucidae possessing receptor activity for sperm." *Cell* 20(3): pp. 873-82, ISSN 0092-8674

Bleil, J. D. and Wassarman, P. M. (1980b). "Structure and function of the zona pellucida: identification and characterization of the proteins of the mouse oocyte's zona pellucida." *Dev Biol* 76(1): pp. 185-202, ISSN 0012-1606

Bleil, J. D. and Wassarman, P. M. (1983). "Sperm-egg interactions in the mouse: sequence of events and induction of the acrosome reaction by a zona pellucida glycoprotein." *Dev Biol* 95(2): pp. 317-24, ISSN 0012-1606

Bleil, J. D. and Wassarman, P. M. (1986). "Autoradiographic visualization of the mouse egg's sperm receptor bound to sperm." *J Cell Biol* 102(4): pp. 1363-71, ISSN 0021-9525

Boatman, D. E. and Robbins, R. S. (1991). "Bicarbonate: carbon-dioxide regulation of sperm capacitation, hyperactivated motility, and acrosome reactions." *Biol Reprod* 44(5): pp. 806-13, ISSN 0006-3363

Boerke, A., Tsai, P. S., Garcia-Gil, N., Brewis, I. A. and Gadella, B. M. (2008). "Capacitation-dependent reorganization of microdomains in the apical sperm head plasma membrane: functional relationship with zona binding and the zona-induced acrosome reaction." *Theriogenology* 70(8): pp. 1188-96, ISSN 0093-691X

Boja, E. S., Hoodbhoy, T., Fales, H. M. and Dean, J. (2003). "Structural characterization of native mouse zona pellucida proteins using mass spectrometry." *J Biol Chem* 278(36): pp. 34189-202, ISSN 0021-9258

Bookbinder, L. H., Cheng, A. and Bleil, J. D. (1995). "Tissue- and species-specific expression of sp56, a mouse sperm fertilization protein." *Science* 269(5220): pp. 86-9, ISSN 0036-8075

Bose, S., Mason, G. G. and Rivett, A. J. (1999). "Phosphorylation of proteasomes in mammalian cells." *Mol Biol Rep* 26(1-2): pp. 11-4, ISSN 0301-4851

Bou Khalil, M., Chakrabandhu, K., Xu, H., Weerachatyanukul, W., Buhr, M., Berger, T., Carmona, E., Vuong, N., Kumarathasan, P., Wong, P. T., Carrier, D. and Tanphaichitr, N. (2006). "Sperm capacitation induces an increase in lipid rafts having zona pellucida binding ability and containing sulfogalactosylglycerolipid." *Dev Biol* 290(1): pp. 220-35, ISSN 0012-1606

Brinster, R. L. (2002). "Germline stem cell transplantation and transgenesis." *Science* 296(5576): pp. 2174-6, ISSN 1095-9203

Brown, D. A. and London, E. (1998). "Functions of lipid rafts in biological membranes." *Annu Rev Cell Dev Biol* 14(pp. 111-36, ISSN 1081-0706

Brown, D. A. and London, E. (2000). "Structure and function of sphingolipid- and cholesterol-rich membrane rafts." *J Biol Chem* 275(23): pp. 17221-4, ISSN 0021-9258

Buffone, M. G., Foster, J. A. and Gerton, G. L. (2008a). "The role of the acrosomal matrix in fertilization." *Int J Dev Biol* 52(5-6): pp. 511-22, ISSN 0214-6282

Buffone, M. G., Zhuang, T., Ord, T. S., Hui, L., Moss, S. B. and Gerton, G. L. (2008b). "Recombinant mouse sperm ZP3-binding protein (ZP3R/sp56) forms a high order oligomer that binds eggs and inhibits mouse fertilization in vitro." *J Biol Chem* 283(18): pp. 12438-45, ISSN 0021-9258

Calvin, H. I. and Bedford, J. M. (1971). "Formation of disulphide bonds in the nucleus and accessory structures of mammalian spermatozoa during maturation in the epididymis." *J Reprod Fertil Suppl* 13(pp. Suppl 13:65-75, ISSN 0449-3087

Carlson, A. E., Hille, B. and Babcock, D. F. (2007). "External Ca2+ acts upstream of adenylyl cyclase SACY in the bicarbonate signaled activation of sperm motility." *Dev Biol* 312(1): pp. 183-92, ISSN 1095-564X

Carlson, A. E., Quill, T. A., Westenbroek, R. E., Schuh, S. M., Hille, B. and Babcock, D. F. (2005). "Identical phenotypes of CatSper1 and CatSper2 null sperm." *J Biol Chem* 280(37): pp. 32238-44, ISSN 0021-9258

Carmona, E., Weerachatyanukul, W., Xu, H., Fluharty, A., Anupriwan, A., Shoushtarian, A., Chakrabandhu, K. and Tanphaichitr, N. (2002). "Binding of arylsulfatase A to mouse sperm inhibits gamete interaction and induces the acrosome reaction." *Biol Reprod* 66(6): pp. 1820-7, ISSN 0006-3363

Castano, J. G., Mahillo, E., Arizti, P. and Arribas, J. (1996). "Phosphorylation of C8 and C9 subunits of the multicatalytic proteinase by casein kinase II and identification of the C8 phosphorylation sites by direct mutagenesis." *Biochemistry* 35(12): pp. 3782-9, ISSN 0006-2960

Chalabi, S., Panico, M., Sutton-Smith, M., Haslam, S. M., Patankar, M. S., Lattanzio, F. A., Morris, H. R., Clark, G. F. and Dell, A. (2006). "Differential O-glycosylation of a conserved domain expressed in murine and human ZP3." *Biochemistry* 45(2): pp. 637-47, ISSN 0006-2960

Chang, M. C. (1951). "Fertilizing capacity of spermatozoa deposited into the fallopian tubes." *Nature* 168(4277): pp. 697-8, ISSN 0028-0836

Chen, J., Litscher, E. S. and Wassarman, P. M. (1998). "Inactivation of the mouse sperm receptor, mZP3, by site-directed mutagenesis of individual serine residues located at the combining site for sperm." *Proc Natl Acad Sci U S A* 95(11): pp. 6193-7, ISSN 0027-8424

Chen, Y., Cann, M. J., Litvin, T. N., Iourgenko, V., Sinclair, M. L., Levin, L. R. and Buck, J. (2000). "Soluble adenylyl cyclase as an evolutionarily conserved bicarbonate sensor." *Science* 289(5479): pp. 625-8, ISSN 0036-8075

Cheng, A., Le, T., Palacios, M., Bookbinder, L. H., Wassarman, P. M., Suzuki, F. and Bleil, J. D. (1994). "Sperm-egg recognition in the mouse: characterization of sp56, a sperm protein having specific affinity for ZP3." *J Cell Biol* 125(4): pp. 867-78, ISSN 0021-9525

Chiriva-Internati, M., Gagliano, N., Donetti, E., Costa, F., Grizzi, F., Franceschini, B., Albani, E., Levi-Setti, P. E., Gioia, M., Jenkins, M., Cobos, E. and Kast, W. M. (2009). "Sperm protein 17 is expressed in the sperm fibrous sheath." *J Transl Med* 7(pp. 61, ISSN 1479-5876

Chiu, P. C., Koistinen, R., Koistinen, H., Seppala, M., Lee, K. F. and Yeung, W. S. (2003a). "Binding of zona binding inhibitory factor-1 (ZIF-1) from human follicular fluid on spermatozoa." *J Biol Chem* 278(15): pp. 13570-7, ISSN 0021-9258

Chiu, P. C., Koistinen, R., Koistinen, H., Seppala, M., Lee, K. F. and Yeung, W. S. (2003b). "Zona-binding inhibitory factor-1 from human follicular fluid is an isoform of glycodelin." *Biol Reprod* 69(1): pp. 365-72, ISSN 0006-3363

Chiu, P. C., Tsang, H. Y., Koistinen, R., Koistinen, H., Seppala, M., Lee, K. F. and Yeung, W. S. (2004). "The contribution of D-mannose, L-fucose, N-acetylglucosamine, and selectin residues on the binding of glycodelin isoforms to human spermatozoa." *Biol Reprod* 70(6): pp. 1710-9, ISSN 0006-3363

Cho, C., Bunch, D. O., Faure, J. E., Goulding, E. H., Eddy, E. M., Primakoff, P. and Myles, D. G. (1998). "Fertilization defects in sperm from mice lacking fertilin beta." *Science* 281(5384): pp. 1857-9, ISSN 0036-8075

Clark, G. F. (2010). "The mammalian zona pellucida: a matrix that mediates both gamete binding and immune recognition?" *Syst Biol Reprod Med* 56(5): pp. 349-64, ISSN 1939-6376

Clark, G. F. (2011a). "The molecular basis of mouse sperm-zona pellucida binding: a still unresolved issue in developmental biology." *Reproduction* 142(3): pp. 377-81, ISSN 1741-7899

Clark, G. F. (2011b). "Molecular models for mouse sperm-oocyte binding." *Glycobiology* 21(1): pp. 3-5, ISSN 1460-2423

Cobellis, G., Ricci, G., Cacciola, G., Orlando, P., Petrosino, S., Cascio, M. G., Bisogno, T., De Petrocellis, L., Chioccarelli, T., Altucci, L., Fasano, S., Meccariello, R., Pierantoni, R., Ledent, C. and Di Marzo, V. (2010). "A gradient of 2-arachidonoylglycerol regulates mouse epididymal sperm cell start-up." *Biol Reprod* 82(2): pp. 451-8, ISSN 1529-7268

Cohen, N. and Wassarman, P. M. (2001). "Association of egg zona pellucida glycoprotein mZP3 with sperm protein sp56 during fertilization in mice." *Int J Dev Biol* 45(3): pp. 569-76, ISSN 0214-6282

Coonrod, S. A., Westhusin, M. E. and Naz, R. K. (1994). "Monoclonal antibody to human fertilization antigen-1 (FA-1) inhibits bovine fertilization in vitro: application in immunocontraception." *Biol Reprod* 51(1): pp. 14-23, ISSN 0006-3363

Cooper, T. G. (1993). "The human epididymis--is it necessary?" *Int J Androl* 16(4): pp. 245-300, ISSN 0105-6263

Cooper, T. G. (2005). "Cytoplasmic droplets: the good, the bad or just confusing?" *Hum Reprod* 20(1): pp. 9-11, ISSN 0268-1161

Cooper, T. G. and Orgebin-Crist, M. C. (1975). "The effect of epididymal and testicular fluids on the fertilising capacity of testicular and epididymal spermatozoa." *Andrologia* 7(2): pp. 85-93, ISSN 0303-4569

Cooper, T. G. and Orgebin-Crist, M. C. (1977). "Effect of aging on the fertilizing capacity of testicular spermatozoa from the rabbit." *Biol Reprod* 16(2): pp. 258-66, ISSN 0006-3363

Cooper, T. G. and Yeung, C. H. (2003). "Acquisition of volume regulatory response of sperm upon maturation in the epididymis and the role of the cytoplasmic droplet." *Microsc Res Tech* 61(1): pp. 28-38, ISSN 1059-910X

Cornwall, G. A. (2009). "New insights into epididymal biology and function." *Hum Reprod Update* 15(2): pp. 213-27, ISSN 1460-2369

Cornwall, G. A., Tulsiani, D. R. and Orgebin-Crist, M. C. (1991). "Inhibition of the mouse sperm surface alpha-D-mannosidase inhibits sperm-egg binding in vitro." *Biol Reprod* 44(5): pp. 913-21, ISSN 0006-3363

Cornwall, G. A., Vindivich, D., Tillman, S. and Chang, T. S. (1988). "The effect of sulfhydryl oxidation on the morphology of immature hamster epididymal spermatozoa induced to acquire motility in vitro." *Biol Reprod* 39(1): pp. 141-55, ISSN 0006-3363

Costello, S., Michelangeli, F., Nash, K., Lefievre, L., Morris, J., Machado-Oliveira, G., Barratt, C., Kirkman-Brown, J. and Publicover, S. (2009). "Ca2+-stores in sperm: their identities and functions." *Reproduction* 138(3): pp. 425-37, ISSN 1741-7899

Dacheux, J. L., Belghazi, M., Lanson, Y. and Dacheux, F. (2006). "Human epididymal secretome and proteome." *Mol Cell Endocrinol* 250(1-2): pp. 36-42, ISSN 0303-7207

Dacheux, J. L., Belleannee, C., Jones, R., Labas, V., Belghazi, M., Guyonnet, B., Druart, X., Gatti, J. L. and Dacheux, F. (2009). "Mammalian epididymal proteome." *Mol Cell Endocrinol* 306(1-2): pp. 45-50, ISSN 1872-8057

Dacheux, J. L. and Paquignon, M. (1980). "Relations between the fertilizing ability, motility and metabolism of epididymal spermatozoa." *Reprod Nutr Dev* 20(4A): pp. 1085-99, ISSN 0181-1916

Danshina, P. V., Geyer, C. B., Dai, Q., Goulding, E. H., Willis, W. D., Kitto, G. B., McCarrey, J. R., Eddy, E. M. and O'Brien, D. A. (2010). "Phosphoglycerate kinase 2 (PGK2) is essential for sperm function and male fertility in mice." *Biol Reprod* 82(1): pp. 136-45, ISSN 1529-7268

Davis, B. K. (1981). "Timing of fertilization in mammals: sperm cholesterol/phospholipid ratio as a determinant of the capacitation interval." *Proc Natl Acad Sci U S A* 78(12): pp. 7560-4, ISSN 0027-8424

Davis, B. K., Byrne, R. and Hungund, B. (1979). "Studies on the mechanism of capacitation. II. Evidence for lipid transfer between plasma membrane of rat sperm and serum albumin during capacitation in vitro." *Biochim Biophys Acta* 558(3): pp. 257-66, ISSN 0006-3002

de Rooij, D. G. (2001). "Proliferation and differentiation of spermatogonial stem cells." *Reproduction* 121(3): pp. 347-54, ISSN 1470-1626.

Dean, J. (2004). "Reassessing the molecular biology of sperm-egg recognition with mouse genetics." *Bioessays* 26(1): pp. 29-38, ISSN 0265-9247

Dube, E., Chan, P. T., Hermo, L. and Cyr, D. G. (2007). "Gene expression profiling and its relevance to the blood-epididymal barrier in the human epididymis." *Biol Reprod* 76(6): pp. 1034-44, ISSN 0006-3363

Dun, M. D., Smith, N. D., Baker, M. A., Lin, M., Aitken, R. J. and Nixon, B. (2011). "The chaperonin containing TCP1 complex (CCT/TRiC) is involved in mediating sperm-oocyte interaction." *J Biol Chem* pp. ISSN 1083-351X

Dunbar, B. S., Avery, S., Lee, V., Prasad, S., Schwahn, D., Schwoebel, E., Skinner, S. and Wilkins, B. (1994). "The mammalian zona pellucida: its biochemistry, immunochemistry, molecular biology, and developmental expression." *Reprod Fertil Dev* 6(3): pp. 331-47, ISSN 1031-3613

Dym, M. (1994). "Spermatogonial stem cells of the testis." *Proc Natl Acad Sci U S A* 91(24): pp. 11287-9, ISSN 0027-8424

Eddy, E. M. (2002). "Male germ cell gene expression." *Recent Prog Horm Res* 57(pp. 103-28, ISSN 0079-9963

Eickhoff, R., Wilhelm, B., Renneberg, H., Wennemuth, G., Bacher, M., Linder, D., Bucala, R., Seitz, J. and Meinhardt, A. (2001). "Purification and characterization of macrophage migration inhibitory factor as a secretory protein from rat epididymis: evidences for alternative release and transfer to spermatozoa." *Mol Med* 7(1): pp. 27-35, ISSN 1076-1551

Ellies, L. G., Tsuboi, S., Petryniak, B., Lowe, J. B., Fukuda, M. and Marth, J. D. (1998). "Core 2 oligosaccharide biosynthesis distinguishes between selectin ligands essential for leukocyte homing and inflammation." *Immunity* 9(6): pp. 881-90, ISSN 1074-7613

Endo, Y., Mattei, P., Kopf, G. S. and Schultz, R. M. (1987). "Effects of a phorbol ester on mouse eggs: dissociation of sperm receptor activity from acrosome reaction-inducing activity of the mouse zona pellucida protein, ZP3." *Dev Biol* 123(2): pp. 574-7, ISSN 0012-1606

Engel, J. C., Bernard, E. A. and Wassermann, G. F. (1973). "Protein synthesis by isolated spermatozoa from cauda and caput epididymis of rat." *Acta Physiol Lat Am* 23(5): pp. 358-62, ISSN 0001-6764

Ensslin, M., Calvete, J. J., Thole, H. H., Sierralta, W. D., Adermann, K., Sanz, L. and Topfer-Petersen, E. (1995). "Identification by affinity chromatography of boar sperm membrane-associated proteins bound to immobilized porcine zona pellucida. Mapping of the phosphorylethanolamine-binding region of spermadhesin AWN." *Biol Chem Hoppe Seyler* 376(12): pp. 733-8, ISSN 0177-3593

Ensslin, M. A. and Shur, B. D. (2003). "Identification of mouse sperm SED1, a bimotif EGF repeat and discoidin-domain protein involved in sperm-egg binding." *Cell* 114(4): pp. 405-17, ISSN 0092-8674

Ergur, A. R., Dokras, A., Giraldo, J. L., Habana, A., Kovanci, E. and Huszar, G. (2002). "Sperm maturity and treatment choice of in vitro fertilization (IVF) or intracytoplasmic sperm injection: diminished sperm HspA2 chaperone levels predict IVF failure." *Fertil Steril* 77(5): pp. 910-8, ISSN 0015-0282

Esposito, G., Jaiswal, B. S., Xie, F., Krajnc-Franken, M. A., Robben, T. J., Strik, A. M., Kuil, C., Philipsen, R. L., van Duin, M., Conti, M. and Gossen, J. A. (2004). "Mice deficient for soluble adenylyl cyclase are infertile because of a severe sperm-motility defect." *Proc Natl Acad Sci U S A* 101(9): pp. 2993-8, ISSN 0027-8424

Esther, C. R., Jr., Howard, T. E., Marino, E. M., Goddard, J. M., Capecchi, M. R. and Bernstein, K. E. (1996). "Mice lacking angiotensin-converting enzyme have low blood pressure, renal pathology, and reduced male fertility." *Lab Invest* 74(5): pp. 953-65, ISSN 0023-6837

Eustace, B. K., Sakurai, T., Stewart, J. K., Yimlamai, D., Unger, C., Zehetmeier, C., Lain, B., Torella, C., Henning, S. W., Beste, G., Scroggins, B. T., Neckers, L., Ilag, L. L. and Jay, D.

G. (2004). "Functional proteomic screens reveal an essential extracellular role for hsp90 alpha in cancer cell invasiveness." *Nat Cell Biol* 6(6): pp. 507-14, ISSN 1465-7392

Fawcett, D. W. (1975). "Gametogenesis in the male: prospects for its control." *Symp Soc Dev Biol* 33): pp. 25-53,

Ficarro, S., Chertihin, O., Westbrook, V. A., White, F., Jayes, F., Kalab, P., Marto, J. A., Shabanowitz, J., Herr, J. C., Hunt, D. F. and Visconti, P. E. (2003). "Phosphoproteome analysis of capacitated human sperm. Evidence of tyrosine phosphorylation of a kinase-anchoring protein 3 and valosin-containing protein/p97 during capacitation." *J Biol Chem* 278(13): pp. 11579-89, ISSN 0021-9258

Flesch, F. M., Brouwers, J. F., Nievelstein, P. F., Verkleij, A. J., van Golde, L. M., Colenbrander, B. and Gadella, B. M. (2001a). "Bicarbonate stimulated phospholipid scrambling induces cholesterol redistribution and enables cholesterol depletion in the sperm plasma membrane." *J Cell Sci* 114(Pt 19): pp. 3543-55, ISSN 0021-9533

Flesch, F. M., Wijnand, E., van de Lest, C. H., Colenbrander, B., van Golde, L. M. and Gadella, B. M. (2001b). "Capacitation dependent activation of tyrosine phosphorylation generates two sperm head plasma membrane proteins with high primary binding affinity for the zona pellucida." *Mol Reprod Dev* 60(1): pp. 107-15, ISSN 1040-452X

Florman, H. M., Bechtol, K. B. and Wassarman, P. M. (1984). "Enzymatic dissection of the functions of the mouse egg's receptor for sperm." *Dev Biol* 106(1): pp. 243-55, ISSN 0012-1606

Florman, H. M. and Storey, B. T. (1982). "Mouse gamete interactions: the zona pellucida is the site of the acrosome reaction leading to fertilization in vitro." *Dev Biol* 91(1): pp. 121-30, ISSN 0012-1606

Florman, H. M. and Wassarman, P. M. (1985). "O-linked oligosaccharides of mouse egg ZP3 account for its sperm receptor activity." *Cell* 41(1): pp. 313-24, ISSN 0092-8674

Folgueras, A. R., Pendas, A. M., Sanchez, L. M. and Lopez-Otin, C. (2004). "Matrix metalloproteinases in cancer: from new functions to improved inhibition strategies." *Int J Dev Biol* 48(5-6): pp. 411-24, ISSN 0214-6282

Foresta, C., Mioni, R., Rossato, M., Varotto, A. and Zorzi, M. (1991). "Evidence for the involvement of sperm angiotensin converting enzyme in fertilization." *Int J Androl* 14(5): pp. 333-9, ISSN 0105-6263

Fraser, L. R. (1984). "Mouse sperm capacitation in vitro involves loss of a surface-associated inhibitory component." *J Reprod Fertil* 72(2): pp. 373-84, ISSN 0022-4251

Fraser, L. R. (1998). "Interactions between a decapacitation factor and mouse spermatozoa appear to involve fucose residues and a GPI-anchored receptor." *Mol Reprod Dev* 51(2): pp. 193-202, ISSN 1040-452X

Fraser, L. R. (2010). "The "switching on" of mammalian spermatozoa: molecular events involved in promotion and regulation of capacitation." *Mol Reprod Dev* 77(3): pp. 197-208, ISSN 1098-2795

Fraser, L. R., Harrison, R. A. and Herod, J. E. (1990). "Characterization of a decapacitation factor associated with epididymal mouse spermatozoa." *J Reprod Fertil* 89(1): pp. 135-48, ISSN 0022-4251

Frenette, G., Lessard, C., Madore, E., Fortier, M. A. and Sullivan, R. (2003). "Aldose reductase and macrophage migration inhibitory factor are associated with epididymosomes and spermatozoa in the bovine epididymis." *Biol Reprod* 69(5): pp. 1586-92, ISSN 0006-3363

Frenette, G., Lessard, C. and Sullivan, R. (2004). "Polyol pathway along the bovine epididymis." *Mol Reprod Dev* 69(4): pp. 448-56, ISSN 1040-452X

Frenette, G. and Sullivan, R. (2001). "Prostasome-like particles are involved in the transfer of P25b from the bovine epididymal fluid to the sperm surface." *Mol Reprod Dev* 59(1): pp. 115-21, ISSN 1040-452X

Frenette, G., Thabet, M. and Sullivan, R. (2006). "Polyol pathway in human epididymis and semen." *J Androl* 27(2): pp. 233-9, ISSN 0196-3635

Gadella, B. M. and Harrison, R. A. (2000). "The capacitating agent bicarbonate induces protein kinase A-dependent changes in phospholipid transbilayer behavior in the sperm plasma membrane." *Development* 127(11): pp. 2407-20, ISSN 0950-1991

Gadella, B. M. and Harrison, R. A. (2002). "Capacitation induces cyclic adenosine 3',5'-monophosphate-dependent, but apoptosis-unrelated, exposure of aminophospholipids at the apical head plasma membrane of boar sperm cells." *Biol Reprod* 67(1): pp. 340-50, ISSN 0006-3363

Gahlay, G., Gauthier, L., Baibakov, B., Epifano, O. and Dean, J. (2010). "Gamete recognition in mice depends on the cleavage status of an egg's zona pellucida protein." *Science* 329(5988): pp. 216-9, ISSN 1095-9203

Gao, Z. and Garbers, D. L. (1998). "Species diversity in the structure of zonadhesin, a sperm-specific membrane protein containing multiple cell adhesion molecule-like domains." *J Biol Chem* 273(6): pp. 3415-21, ISSN 0021-9258

Garty, N. B. and Salomon, Y. (1987). "Stimulation of partially purified adenylate cyclase from bull sperm by bicarbonate." *FEBS Lett* 218(1): pp. 148-52, ISSN 0014-5793

Gasper, J. and Swanson, W. J. (2006). "Molecular population genetics of the gene encoding the human fertilization protein zonadhesin reveals rapid adaptive evolution." *Am J Hum Genet* 79(5): pp. 820-30, ISSN 0002-9297

Gatti, J. L., Castella, S., Dacheux, F., Ecroyd, H., Metayer, S., Thimon, V. and Dacheux, J. L. (2004). "Post-testicular sperm environment and fertility." *Anim Reprod Sci* 82-83(pp. 321-39, ISSN 0378-4320

Gergely, A., Kovanci, E., Senturk, L., Cosmi, E., Vigue, L. and Huszar, G. (1999). "Morphometric assessment of mature and diminished-maturity human spermatozoa: sperm regions that reflect differences in maturity." *Hum Reprod* 14(8): pp. 2007-14, ISSN 0268-1161

Gibbons, R., Adeoya-Osiguwa, S. A. and Fraser, L. R. (2005). "A mouse sperm decapacitation factor receptor is phosphatidylethanolamine-binding protein 1." *Reproduction* 130(4): pp. 497-508, ISSN 1470-1626

Gil-Guzman, E., Ollero, M., Lopez, M. C., Sharma, R. K., Alvarez, J. G., Thomas, A. J., Jr. and Agarwal, A. (2001). "Differential production of reactive oxygen species by subsets of human spermatozoa at different stages of maturation." *Hum Reprod* 16(9): pp. 1922-30, ISSN 0268-1161

Girouard, J., Frenette, G. and Sullivan, R. (2011). "Comparative proteome and lipid profiles of bovine epididymosomes collected in the intraluminal compartment of the caput and cauda epididymidis." *Int J Androl* 34(5 Pt 2): pp. e475-86, ISSN 1365-2605

Gomez, E., Buckingham, D. W., Brindle, J., Lanzafame, F., Irvine, D. S. and Aitken, R. J. (1996). "Development of an image analysis system to monitor the retention of residual cytoplasm by human spermatozoa: correlation with biochemical markers of the cytoplasmic space, oxidative stress, and sperm function." *J Androl* 17(3): pp. 276-87, ISSN 0196-3635

Govin, J., Caron, C., Escoffier, E., Ferro, M., Kuhn, L., Rousseaux, S., Eddy, E. M., Garin, J. and Khochbin, S. (2006). "Post-meiotic shifts in HSPA2/HSP70.2 chaperone activity during mouse spermatogenesis." *J Biol Chem* 281(49): pp. 37888-92, ISSN 0021-9258

Greve, J. M. and Wassarman, P. M. (1985). "Mouse egg extracellular coat is a matrix of interconnected filaments possessing a structural repeat." *J Mol Biol* 181(2): pp. 253-64, ISSN 0022-2836

Grizzi, F., Chiriva-Internati, M., Franceschini, B., Hermonat, P. L., Soda, G., Lim, S. H. and Dioguardi, N. (2003). "Immunolocalization of sperm protein 17 in human testis and ejaculated spermatozoa." *J Histochem Cytochem* 51(9): pp. 1245-8, 0022-1554 (Print)
0022-1554 (Linking).

Guyonnet, B., Dacheux, F., Dacheux, J. L. and Gatti, J. L. (2011). "The epididymal transcriptome and proteome provide some insights into new epididymal regulations." *J Androl* 32(6): pp. 651-64, ISSN 1939-4640

Han, C., Park, I., Lee, B., Jin, S., Choi, H., Kwon, J. T., Kwon, Y. I., Kim do, H., Park, Z. Y. and Cho, C. (2010). "Identification of heat shock protein 5, calnexin and integral membrane protein 2B as Adam7-interacting membrane proteins in mouse sperm." *J Cell Physiol* 226(5): pp. 1186-95, ISSN 1097-4652

Harayama, H., Shibukawa, T., Miyake, M., Kannan, Y. and Kato, S. (1996). "Fructose stimulates shedding of cytoplasmic droplets from epididymal boar spermatozoa." *Reprod Fertil Dev* 8(7): pp. 1039-43, ISSN 1031-3613

Hardy, C. M., Clydesdale, G. and Mobbs, K. J. (2004). "Development of mouse-specific contraceptive vaccines: infertility in mice immunized with peptide and polyepitope antigens." *Reproduction* 128(4): pp. 395-407, ISSN 1470-1626

Hardy, D. M. and Garbers, D. L. (1994). "Species-specific binding of sperm proteins to the extracellular matrix (zona pellucida) of the egg." *J Biol Chem* 269(29): pp. 19000-4, ISSN 0021-9258

Hardy, D. M. and Garbers, D. L. (1995). "A sperm membrane protein that binds in a species-specific manner to the egg extracellular matrix is homologous to von Willebrand factor." *J Biol Chem* 270(44): pp. 26025-8, ISSN 0021-9258

Hardy, D. M., Oda, M. N., Friend, D. S. and Huang, T. T., Jr. (1991). "A mechanism for differential release of acrosomal enzymes during the acrosome reaction." *Biochem J* 275 (Pt 3)(pp. 759-66, ISSN 0264-6021

Harrison, R. A. and Gadella, B. M. (2005). "Bicarbonate-induced membrane processing in sperm capacitation." *Theriogenology* 63(2): pp. 342-51, ISSN 0093-691X

Hartmann, J. F., Gwatkin, R. B. and Hutchison, C. F. (1972). "Early contact interactions between mammalian gametes in vitro: evidence that the vitellus influences adherence between sperm and zona pellucida." *Proc Natl Acad Sci U S A* 69(10): pp. 2767-9, ISSN 0027-8424

Herlyn, H. and Zischler, H. (2008). "The molecular evolution of sperm zonadhesin." *Int J Dev Biol* 52(5-6): pp. 781-90, ISSN 0214-6282

Hermo, L., Pelletier, R. M., Cyr, D. G. and Smith, C. E. (2010a). "Surfing the wave, cycle, life history, and genes/proteins expressed by testicular germ cells. Part 1: background to spermatogenesis, spermatogonia, and spermatocytes." *Microsc Res Tech* 73(4): pp. 241-78, ISSN 1097-0029

Hermo, L., Pelletier, R. M., Cyr, D. G. and Smith, C. E. (2010b). "Surfing the wave, cycle, life history, and genes/proteins expressed by testicular germ cells. Part 2: changes in spermatid organelles associated with development of spermatozoa." *Microsc Res Tech* 73(4): pp. 279-319, ISSN 1097-0029

Hermo, L., Pelletier, R. M., Cyr, D. G. and Smith, C. E. (2010c). "Surfing the wave, cycle, life history, and genes/proteins expressed by testicular germ cells. Part 5: intercellular junctions and contacts between germs cells and Sertoli cells and their regulatory interactions, testicular cholesterol, and genes/proteins associated with more than one germ cell generation." *Microsc Res Tech* 73(4): pp. 409-94, ISSN 1097-0029

Herrick, S. B., Schweissinger, D. L., Kim, S. W., Bayan, K. R., Mann, S. and Cardullo, R. A. (2005). "The acrosomal vesicle of mouse sperm is a calcium store." *J Cell Physiol* 202(3): pp. 663-71, ISSN 0021-9541

Hess, B., Saftig, P., Hartmann, D., Coenen, R., Lullmann-Rauch, R., Goebel, H. H., Evers, M., von Figura, K., D'Hooge, R., Nagels, G., De Deyn, P., Peters, C. and Gieselmann, V. (1996). "Phenotype of arylsulfatase A-deficient mice: relationship to human metachromatic leukodystrophy." *Proc Natl Acad Sci U S A* 93(25): pp. 14821-6, ISSN 0027-8424

Hess, K. C., Jones, B. H., Marquez, B., Chen, Y., Ord, T. S., Kamenetsky, M., Miyamoto, C., Zippin, J. H., Kopf, G. S., Suarez, S. S., Levin, L. R., Williams, C. J., Buck, J. and Moss, S. B. (2005). "The "soluble" adenylyl cyclase in sperm mediates multiple signaling events required for fertilization." *Dev Cell* 9(2): pp. 249-59, ISSN 1534-5807

Hickox, J. R., Bi, M. and Hardy, D. M. (2001). "Heterogeneous processing and zona pellucida binding activity of pig zonadhesin." *J Biol Chem* 276(44): pp. 41502-9, ISSN 0021-9258

Ho, H. C. and Suarez, S. S. (2003). "Characterization of the intracellular calcium store at the base of the sperm flagellum that regulates hyperactivated motility." *Biol Reprod* 68(5): pp. 1590-6, ISSN 0006-3363

Hoodbhoy, T. and Dean, J. (2004). "Insights into the molecular basis of sperm-egg recognition in mammals." *Reproduction* 127(4): pp. 417-22, ISSN 1470-1626

Howes, E., Pascall, J. C., Engel, W. and Jones, R. (2001). "Interactions between mouse ZP2 glycoprotein and proacrosin; a mechanism for secondary binding of sperm to the zona pellucida during fertilization." *J Cell Sci* 114(Pt 22): pp. 4127-36, ISSN 0021-9533

Howes, L. and Jones, R. (2002). "Interactions between zona pellucida glycoproteins and sperm proacrosin/acrosin during fertilization." *J Reprod Immunol* 53(1-2): pp. 181-92, ISSN 0165-0378

Hull, M. G., Glazener, C. M., Kelly, N. J., Conway, D. I., Foster, P. A., Hinton, R. A., Coulson, C., Lambert, P. A., Watt, E. M. and Desai, K. M. (1985). "Population study of causes, treatment, and outcome of infertility." *Br Med J (Clin Res Ed)* 291(6510): pp. 1693-7, ISSN 0267-0623

Hunnicutt, G. R., Mahan, K., Lathrop, W. F., Ramarao, C. S., Myles, D. G. and Primakoff, P. (1996a). "Structural relationship of sperm soluble hyaluronidase to the sperm membrane protein PH-20." *Biol Reprod* 54(6): pp. 1343-9, ISSN 0006-3363

Hunnicutt, G. R., Primakoff, P. and Myles, D. G. (1996b). "Sperm surface protein PH-20 is bifunctional: one activity is a hyaluronidase and a second, distinct activity is required in secondary sperm-zona binding." *Biol Reprod* 55(1): pp. 80-6, ISSN 0006-3363

Huszar, G., Jakab, A., Sakkas, D., Ozenci, C. C., Cayli, S., Delpiano, E. and Ozkavukcu, S. (2007). "Fertility testing and ICSI sperm selection by hyaluronic acid binding: clinical and genetic aspects." *Reprod Biomed Online* 14(5): pp. 650-63, ISSN 1472-6483

Huszar, G., Ozkavukcu, S., Jakab, A., Celik-Ozenci, C., Sati, G. L. and Cayli, S. (2006). "Hyaluronic acid binding ability of human sperm reflects cellular maturity and fertilizing potential: selection of sperm for intracytoplasmic sperm injection." *Curr Opin Obstet Gynecol* 18(3): pp. 260-7, ISSN 1040-872X

Huszar, G., Sbracia, M., Vigue, L., Miller, D. J. and Shur, B. D. (1997). "Sperm plasma membrane remodeling during spermiogenetic maturation in men: relationship among plasma membrane beta 1,4-galactosyltransferase, cytoplasmic creatine phosphokinase, and creatine phosphokinase isoform ratios." *Biol Reprod* 56(4): pp. 1020-4, ISSN 0006-3363

Huszar, G., Stone, K., Dix, D. and Vigue, L. (2000). "Putative creatine kinase M-isoform in human sperm is identifiedas the 70-kilodalton heat shock protein HspA2." *Biol Reprod* 63(3): pp. 925-32, ISSN 0006-3363

Huszar, G. and Vigue, L. (1993). "Incomplete development of human spermatozoa is associated with increased creatine phosphokinase concentration and abnormal head morphology." *Mol Reprod Dev* 34(3): pp. 292-8, ISSN 1040-452X

Huszar, G., Vigue, L. and Oehninger, S. (1994). "Creatine kinase immunocytochemistry of human sperm-hemizona complexes: selective binding of sperm with mature creatine kinase-staining pattern." *Fertil Steril* 61(1): pp. 136-42, ISSN 0015-0282

Ikawa, M., Nakanishi, T., Yamada, S., Wada, I., Kominami, K., Tanaka, H., Nozaki, M., Nishimune, Y. and Okabe, M. (2001). "Calmegin is required for fertilin alpha/beta heterodimerization and sperm fertility." *Dev Biol* 240(1): pp. 254-61, ISSN 0012-1606

Ikawa, M., Tokuhiro, K., Yamaguchi, R., Benham, A. M., Tamura, T., Wada, I., Satouh, Y., Inoue, N. and Okabe, M. (2011). "Calsperin is a testis-specific chaperone required for sperm fertility." *J Biol Chem* 286(7): pp. 5639-46, ISSN 1083-351X

Inoue, M. and Wolf, D. P. (1975). "Fertilization-associated changes in the murine zona pellucida: a time sequence study." *Biol Reprod* 13(5): pp. 546-51, ISSN 0006-3363

Jelinsky, S. A., Turner, T. T., Bang, H. J., Finger, J. N., Solarz, M. K., Wilson, E., Brown, E. L., Kopf, G. S. and Johnston, D. S. (2007). "The rat epididymal transcriptome: comparison of segmental gene expression in the rat and mouse epididymides." *Biol Reprod* 76(4): pp. 561-70, ISSN 0006-3363

Jervis, K. M. and Robaire, B. (2001). "Dynamic changes in gene expression along the rat epididymis." *Biol Reprod* 65(3): pp. 696-703, ISSN 0006-3363

Jezierska, A. and Motyl, T. (2009). "Matrix metalloproteinase-2 involvement in breast cancer progression: a mini-review." *Med Sci Monit* 15(2): pp. RA32-40, ISSN 1643-3750

Jin, J., Jin, N., Zheng, H., Ro, S., Tafolla, D., Sanders, K. M. and Yan, W. (2007). "Catsper3 and Catsper4 are essential for sperm hyperactivated motility and male fertility in the mouse." *Biol Reprod* 77(1): pp. 37-44, ISSN 0006-3363

Johnston, D. S., Turner, T. T., Finger, J. N., Owtscharuk, T. L., Kopf, G. S. and Jelinsky, S. A. (2007). "Identification of epididymis-specific transcripts in the mouse and rat by transcriptional profiling." *Asian J Androl* 9(4): pp. 522-7, ISSN 1008-682X

Jones, R. (1998). "Plasma membrane structure and remodelling during sperm maturation in the epididymis." *J Reprod Fertil Suppl* 53(pp. 73-84, ISSN 0449-3087

Jones, R., Howes, E., Dunne, P. D., James, P., Bruckbauer, A. and Klenerman, D. (2010). "Tracking diffusion of GM1 gangliosides and zona pellucida binding molecules in sperm plasma membranes following cholesterol efflux." *Dev Biol* 339(2): pp. 398-406, ISSN 1095-564X

Jones, R., James, P. S., Howes, L., Bruckbauer, A. and Klenerman, D. (2007). "Supramolecular organization of the sperm plasma membrane during maturation and capacitation." *Asian J Androl* 9(4): pp. 438-44, ISSN 1008-682X

Kamaruddin, M., Kroetsch, T., Basrur, P. K., Hansen, P. J. and King, W. A. (2004). "Immunolocalization of heat shock protein 70 in bovine spermatozoa." *Andrologia* 36(5): pp. 327-34, ISSN 0303-4569

Kaplan, M., Russell, L. D., Peterson, R. N. and Martan, J. (1984). "Boar sperm cytoplasmic droplets: their ultrastructure, their numbers in the epididymis and at ejaculation and their removal during isolation of sperm plasma membranes." *Tissue Cell* 16(3): pp. 455-68, ISSN 0040-8166

Katz, D. F. (1991). "Characteristics of sperm motility." *Ann N Y Acad Sci* 637(pp. 409-23, ISSN 0077-8923

Keating, J., Grundy, C. E., Fivey, P. S., Elliott, M. and Robinson, J. (1997). "Investigation of the association between the presence of cytoplasmic residues on the human sperm midpiece and defective sperm function." *J Reprod Fertil* 110(1): pp. 71-7, ISSN 0022-4251

Kim, E., Nishimura, H., Iwase, S., Yamagata, K., Kashiwabara, S. and Baba, T. (2004). "Synthesis, processing, and subcellular localization of mouse ADAM3 during spermatogenesis and epididymal sperm transport." *J Reprod Dev* 50(5): pp. 571-8, ISSN 0916-8818

Kim, E., Yamashita, M., Nakanishi, T., Park, K. E., Kimura, M., Kashiwabara, S. and Baba, T. (2006a). "Mouse sperm lacking ADAM1b/ADAM2 fertilin can fuse with the egg plasma membrane and effect fertilization." *J Biol Chem* 281(9): pp. 5634-9, ISSN 0021-9258

Kim, K. S., Foster, J. A. and Gerton, G. L. (2001). "Differential release of guinea pig sperm acrosomal components during exocytosis." *Biol Reprod* 64(1): pp. 148-56, ISSN 0006-3363

Kim, T., Oh, J., Woo, J. M., Choi, E., Im, S. H., Yoo, Y. J., Kim, D. H., Nishimura, H. and Cho, C. (2006b). "Expression and relationship of male reproductive ADAMs in mouse." *Biol Reprod* 74(4): pp. 744-50, ISSN 0006-3363

Kirchhoff, C. and Hale, G. (1996). "Cell-to-cell transfer of glycosylphosphatidylinositol-anchored membrane proteins during sperm maturation." *Mol Hum Reprod* 2(3): pp. 177-84, ISSN 1360-9947

Kirichok, Y., Navarro, B. and Clapham, D. E. (2006). "Whole-cell patch-clamp measurements of spermatozoa reveal an alkaline-activated Ca2+ channel." *Nature* 439(7077): pp. 737-40, ISSN 1476-4687

Kobayashi, T., Kaneko, T., Iuchi, Y., Matsuki, S., Takahashi, M., Sasagawa, I., Nakada, T. and Fujii, J. (2002). "Localization and physiological implication of aldose reductase and sorbitol dehydrogenase in reproductive tracts and spermatozoa of male rats." *J Androl* 23(5): pp. 674-83, ISSN 0196-3635

Kohn, F. M., Miska, W. and Schill, W. B. (1995). "Release of angiotensin-converting enzyme (ACE) from human spermatozoa during capacitation and acrosome reaction." *J Androl* 16(3): pp. 259-65, ISSN 0196-3635

Kong, M., Diaz, E. S. and Morales, P. (2009). "Participation of the human sperm proteasome in the capacitation process and its regulation by protein kinase A and tyrosine kinase." *Biol Reprod* 80(5): pp. 1026-35, ISSN 0006-3363

Kornblatt, M. J. (1979). "Synthesis and turnover of sulfogalactoglycerolipid, a membrane lipid, during spermatogenesis." *Can J Biochem* 57(3): pp. 255-8, ISSN 0008-4018

Krapf, D., Arcelay, E., Wertheimer, E. V., Sanjay, A., Pilder, S. H., Salicioni, A. M. and Visconti, P. E. (2010). "Inhibition of Ser/Thr phosphatases induces capacitation-associated signaling in the presence of Src kinase inhibitors." *J Biol Chem* 285(11): pp. 7977-85, ISSN 1083-351X

Langford, K. G., Zhou, Y., Russell, L. D., Wilcox, J. N. and Bernstein, K. E. (1993). "Regulated expression of testis angiotensin-converting enzyme during spermatogenesis in mice." *Biol Reprod* 48(6): pp. 1210-8, ISSN 0006-3363

Langlais, J., Kan, F. W., Granger, L., Raymond, L., Bleau, G. and Roberts, K. D. (1988). "Identification of sterol acceptors that stimulate cholesterol efflux from human spermatozoa during in vitro capacitation." *Gamete Res* 20(2): pp. 185-201, ISSN 0148-7280

Larsen, R. E., Shope, R. E., Jr., Leman, A. D. and Kurtz, H. J. (1980). "Semen changes in boars after experimental infection with pseudorabies virus." *Am J Vet Res* 41(5): pp. 733-39, ISSN 0002-9645

Lawson, C., Goupil, S. and Leclerc, P. (2008). "Increased activity of the human sperm tyrosine kinase SRC by the cAMP-dependent pathway in the presence of calcium." *Biol Reprod* 79(4): pp. 657-66, ISSN 0006-3363

Leblond, C. P. and Clermont, Y. (1952). "Spermiogenesis of rat, mouse, hamster and guinea pig as revealed by the periodic acid-fuchsin sulfurous acid technique." *Am J Anat* 90(2): pp. 167-215, ISSN 0002-9106

Leclerc, P., de Lamirande, E. and Gagnon, C. (1997). "Regulation of protein-tyrosine phosphorylation and human sperm capacitation by reactive oxygen derivatives." *Free Radic Biol Med* 22(4): pp. 643-56, ISSN 0891-5849

Lefievre, L., Conner, S. J., Salpekar, A., Olufowobi, O., Ashton, P., Pavlovic, B., Lenton, W., Afnan, M., Brewis, I. A., Monk, M., Hughes, D. C. and Barratt, C. L. (2004). "Four zona pellucida glycoproteins are expressed in the human." *Hum Reprod* 19(7): pp. 1580-6, ISSN 0268-1161

Legare, C., Berube, B., Boue, F., Lefievre, L., Morales, C. R., El-Alfy, M. and Sullivan, R. (1999). "Hamster sperm antigen P26h is a phosphatidylinositol-anchored protein." *Mol Reprod Dev* 52(2): pp. 225-33, ISSN 1040-452X

Leyton, L. and Saling, P. (1989). "Evidence that aggregation of mouse sperm receptors by ZP3 triggers the acrosome reaction." *J Cell Biol* 108(6): pp. 2163-8, ISSN 0021-9525

Lin, Y., Mahan, K., Lathrop, W. F., Myles, D. G. and Primakoff, P. (1994). "A hyaluronidase activity of the sperm plasma membrane protein PH-20 enables sperm to penetrate the cumulus cell layer surrounding the egg." *J Cell Biol* 125(5): pp. 1157-63, ISSN 0021-9525

Lin, Y. N., Roy, A., Yan, W., Burns, K. H. and Matzuk, M. M. (2007). "Loss of zona pellucida binding proteins in the acrosomal matrix disrupts acrosome biogenesis and sperm morphogenesis." *Mol Cell Biol* 27(19): pp. 6794-805, ISSN 0270-7306

Litscher, E. S., Juntunen, K., Seppo, A., Penttila, L., Niemela, R., Renkonen, O. and Wassarman, P. M. (1995). "Oligosaccharide constructs with defined structures that inhibit binding of mouse sperm to unfertilized eggs in vitro." *Biochemistry* 34(14): pp. 4662-9, ISSN 0006-2960

Litvin, T. N., Kamenetsky, M., Zarifyan, A., Buck, J. and Levin, L. R. (2003). "Kinetic properties of "soluble" adenylyl cyclase. Synergism between calcium and bicarbonate." *J Biol Chem* 278(18): pp. 15922-6, ISSN 0021-9258

Liu, D. Y. and Baker, H. W. (1992). "Morphology of spermatozoa bound to the zona pellucida of human oocytes that failed to fertilize in vitro." *J Reprod Fertil* 94(1): pp. 71-84, ISSN 0022-4251

Lobley, A., Pierron, V., Reynolds, L., Allen, L. and Michalovich, D. (2003). "Identification of human and mouse CatSper3 and CatSper4 genes: characterisation of a common interaction domain and evidence for expression in testis." *Reprod Biol Endocrinol* 1(pp. 53, ISSN 1477-7827

Lopez, L. C., Bayna, E. M., Litoff, D., Shaper, N. L., Shaper, J. H. and Shur, B. D. (1985). "Receptor function of mouse sperm surface galactosyltransferase during fertilization." *J Cell Biol* 101(4): pp. 1501-10, ISSN 0021-9525

Lopez, L. C. and Shur, B. D. (1987). "Redistribution of mouse sperm surface galactosyltransferase after the acrosome reaction." *J Cell Biol* 105(4): pp. 1663-70, ISSN 0021-9525

Lu, Q., Hasty, P. and Shur, B. D. (1997). "Targeted mutation in beta1,4-galactosyltransferase leads to pituitary insufficiency and neonatal lethality." *Dev Biol* 181(2): pp. 257-67, ISSN 0012-1606

Lu, Q. and Shur, B. D. (1997). "Sperm from beta 1,4-galactosyltransferase-null mice are refractory to ZP3-induced acrosome reactions and penetrate the zona pellucida poorly." *Development* 124(20): pp. 4121-31, ISSN 0950-1991

Lyng, R. and Shur, B. D. (2009). "Mouse oviduct-specific glycoprotein is an egg-associated ZP3-independent sperm-adhesion ligand." *J Cell Sci* 122(Pt 21): pp. 3894-906, ISSN 1477-9137

Maher, M. T., Flozak, A. S., Stocker, A. M., Chenn, A. and Gottardi, C. J. (2009). "Activity of the beta-catenin phosphodestruction complex at cell-cell contacts is enhanced by cadherin-based adhesion." *J Cell Biol* 186(2): pp. 219-28, ISSN 1540-8140

Mahony, M. C. and Gwathmey, T. (1999). "Protein tyrosine phosphorylation during hyperactivated motility of cynomolgus monkey (Macaca fascicularis) spermatozoa." *Biol Reprod* 60(5): pp. 1239-43, ISSN 0006-3363

Martinez-Seara, H., Rog, T., Pasenkiewicz-Gierula, M., Vattulainen, I., Karttunen, M. and Reigada, R. (2008). "Interplay of unsaturated phospholipids and cholesterol in membranes: effect of the double-bond position." *Biophys J* 95(7): pp. 3295-305, ISSN 1542-0086

McCready, J., Sims, J. D., Chan, D. and Jay, D. G. (2010). "Secretion of extracellular hsp90alpha via exosomes increases cancer cell motility: a role for plasminogen activation." *BMC Cancer* 10(pp. 294, ISSN 1471-2407

McLachlan, R. I. and de Kretser, D. M. (2001). "Male infertility: the case for continued research." *Med J Aust* 174(3): pp. 116-7, ISSN 0025-729X

McLeskey, S. B., Dowds, C., Carballada, R., White, R. R. and Saling, P. M. (1998). "Molecules involved in mammalian sperm-egg interaction." *Int Rev Cytol* 177(pp. 57-113, ISSN 0074-7696

Menge, A. C., Christman, G. M., Ohl, D. A. and Naz, R. K. (1999). "Fertilization antigen-1 removes antisperm autoantibodies from spermatozoa of infertile men and results in increased rates of acrosome reaction." *Fertil Steril* 71(2): pp. 256-60, ISSN 0015-0282

Miki, K., Qu, W., Goulding, E. H., Willis, W. D., Bunch, D. O., Strader, L. F., Perreault, S. D., Eddy, E. M. and O'Brien, D. A. (2004). "Glyceraldehyde 3-phosphate dehydrogenase-S, a sperm-specific glycolytic enzyme, is required for sperm motility and male fertility." *Proc Natl Acad Sci U S A* 101(47): pp. 16501-6, ISSN 0027-8424

Miller, D., Brough, S. and al-Harbi, O. (1992). "Characterization and cellular distribution of human spermatozoal heat shock proteins." *Hum Reprod* 7(5): pp. 637-45, ISSN 0268-1161

Mitchell, L. A., Nixon, B. and Aitken, R. J. (2007). "Analysis of chaperone proteins associated with human spermatozoa during capacitation." *Mol Hum Reprod* 13(9): pp. 605-13, ISSN 1360-9947

Mitchell, L. A., Nixon, B., Baker, M. A. and Aitken, R. J. (2008). "Investigation of the role of SRC in capacitation-associated tyrosine phosphorylation of human spermatozoa." *Mol Hum Reprod* 14(4): pp. 235-43, ISSN 1460-2407

Moore, H. D. and Akhondi, M. A. (1996). "In vitro maturation of mammalian spermatozoa." *Rev Reprod* 1(1): pp. 54-60, ISSN 1359-6004

Morales, C. R., Badran, H., El-Alfy, M., Men, H., Zhang, H. and Martin-DeLeon, P. A. (2004). "Cytoplasmic localization during testicular biogenesis of the murine mRNA for Spam1

(PH-20), a protein involved in acrosomal exocytosis." *Mol Reprod Dev* 69(4): pp. 475-82, ISSN 1040-452X

Morales, P., Kong, M., Pizarro, E. and Pasten, C. (2003). "Participation of the sperm proteasome in human fertilization." *Hum Reprod* 18(5): pp. 1010-7, 0268-1161 (Print)
0268-1161 (Linking).

Moreno, R. D., Sepulveda, M. S., de Ioannes, A. and Barros, C. (1998). "The polysulphate binding domain of human proacrosin/acrosin is involved in both the enzyme activation and spermatozoa-zona pellucida interaction." *Zygote* 6(1): pp. 75-83, ISSN 0967-1994

Muro, Y., Buffone, M. G., Okabe, M. and Gerton, G. L. (2012). "Function of the acrosomal matrix: zona pellucida 3 receptor (ZP3R/sp56) is not essential for mouse fertilization." *Biol Reprod* 86(1): pp. 1-6, ISSN 1529-7268

Muro, Y. and Okabe, M. (2011). "Mechanisms of fertilization--a view from the study of gene-manipulated mice." *J Androl* 32(3): pp. 218-25, ISSN 1939-4640

Myles, D. G. and Primakoff, P. (1997). "Why did the sperm cross the cumulus? To get to the oocyte. Functions of the sperm surface proteins PH-20 and fertilin in arriving at, and fusing with, the egg." *Biol Reprod* 56(2): pp. 320-7, ISSN 0006-3363

Naaby-Hansen, S. and Herr, J. C. (2010). "Heat shock proteins on the human sperm surface." *J Reprod Immunol* 84(1): pp. 32-40, ISSN 1872-7603

Nakamura, N., Miranda-Vizuete, A., Miki, K., Mori, C. and Eddy, E. M. (2008). "Cleavage of disulfide bonds in mouse spermatogenic cell-specific type 1 hexokinase isozyme is associated with increased hexokinase activity and initiation of sperm motility." *Biol Reprod* 79(3): pp. 537-45, ISSN 0006-3363

Nassar, A., Mahony, M., Morshedi, M., Lin, M. H., Srisombut, C. and Oehninger, S. (1999). "Modulation of sperm tail protein tyrosine phosphorylation by pentoxifylline and its correlation with hyperactivated motility." *Fertil Steril* 71(5): pp. 919-23, ISSN 0015-0282

Naz, R. K. (1998). "c-Abl proto-oncoprotein is expressed and tyrosine phosphorylated in human sperm cell." *Mol Reprod Dev* 51(2): pp. 210-7, ISSN 1040-452X

Naz, R. K., Ahmad, K. and Kaplan, P. (1992a). "Expression and function of ras proto-oncogene proteins in human sperm cells." *J Cell Sci* 102 (Pt 3)(pp. 487-94, ISSN 0021-9533

Naz, R. K., Brazil, C. and Overstreet, J. W. (1992b). "Effects of antibodies to sperm surface fertilization antigen-1 on human sperm-zona pellucida interaction." *Fertil Steril* 57(6): pp. 1304-10, ISSN 0015-0282

Naz, R. K., Rosenblum, B. B. and Menge, A. C. (1984). "Characterization of a membrane antigen from rabbit testis and sperm isolated by using monoclonal antibodies and effect of its antiserum on fertility." *Proc Natl Acad Sci U S A* 81(3): pp. 857-61, ISSN 0027-8424

Naz, R. K. and Zhu, X. (1998). "Recombinant fertilization antigen-1 causes a contraceptive effect in actively immunized mice." *Biol Reprod* 59(5): pp. 1095-100, ISSN 0006-3363

Nishimura, H., Kim, E., Nakanishi, T. and Baba, T. (2004). "Possible function of the ADAM1a/ADAM2 Fertilin complex in the appearance of ADAM3 on the sperm surface." *J Biol Chem* 279(33): pp. 34957-62, ISSN 0021-9258

Nishimura, H., Myles, D. G. and Primakoff, P. (2007). "Identification of an ADAM2-ADAM3 complex on the surface of mouse testicular germ cells and cauda epididymal sperm." *J Biol Chem* 282(24): pp. 17900-7, ISSN 0021-9258

Nixon, B., Aitken, R. J. and McLaughlin, E. A. (2007). "New insights into the molecular mechanisms of sperm-egg interaction." *Cell Mol Life Sci* 64(14): pp. 1805-23, 1420-682X (Print)

1420-682X (Linking).

Nixon, B., Asquith, K. L. and John Aitken, R. (2005). "The role of molecular chaperones in mouse sperm-egg interactions." *Mol Cell Endocrinol* 240(1-2): pp. 1-10, ISSN 0303-7207

Nixon, B., Bielanowicz, A., Anderson, A. L., Walsh, A., Hall, T., McCloghry, A. and Aitken, R. J. (2010). "Elucidation of the signaling pathways that underpin capacitation-associated surface phosphotyrosine expression in mouse spermatozoa." *J Cell Physiol* 224(1): pp. 71-83, ISSN 1097-4652

Nixon, B., Bielanowicz, A., McLaughlin, E. A., Tanphaichitr, N., Ensslin, M. A. and Aitken, R. J. (2009). "Composition and significance of detergent resistant membranes in mouse spermatozoa." *J Cell Physiol* 218(1): pp. 122-34, ISSN 1097-4652

Nixon, B., Jones, R. C., Hansen, L. A. and Holland, M. K. (2002). "Rabbit epididymal secretory proteins. I. Characterization and hormonal regulation." *Biol Reprod* 67(1): pp. 133-9, ISSN 0006-3363

Nixon, B., Lu, Q., Wassler, M. J., Foote, C. I., Ensslin, M. A. and Shur, B. D. (2001). "Galactosyltransferase function during mammalian fertilization." *Cells Tissues Organs* 168(1-2): pp. 46-57, ISSN 1422-6405

Nixon, B., MacIntyre, D. A., Mitchell, L. A., Gibbs, G. M., O'Bryan, M. and Aitken, R. J. (2006). "The identification of mouse sperm-surface-associated proteins and characterization of their ability to act as decapacitation factors." *Biol Reprod* 74(2): pp. 275-87, ISSN 0006-3363

Nixon, B., Mitchell, L. A., Anderson, A. L., McLaughlin, E. A., O'Bryan M, K. and Aitken, R. J. (2011). "Proteomic and functional analysis of human sperm detergent resistant membranes." *J Cell Physiol* 226(10): pp. 2651-65, ISSN 1097-4652

Noland, T. D., Friday, B. B., Maulit, M. T. and Gerton, G. L. (1994). "The sperm acrosomal matrix contains a novel member of the pentaxin family of calcium-dependent binding proteins." *J Biol Chem* 269(51): pp. 32607-14, ISSN 0021-9258.

Oatley, J. M. and Brinster, R. L. (2006). "Spermatogonial stem cells." *Methods Enzymol* 419(pp. 259-82, ISSN 0076-6879

Oh, J. S., Han, C. and Cho, C. (2009). "ADAM7 is associated with epididymosomes and integrated into sperm plasma membrane." *Mol Cells* 28(5): pp. 441-6, ISSN 0219-1032

Okamura, N., Tajima, Y., Soejima, A., Masuda, H. and Sugita, Y. (1985). "Sodium bicarbonate in seminal plasma stimulates the motility of mammalian spermatozoa through direct activation of adenylate cyclase." *J Biol Chem* 260(17): pp. 9699-705, ISSN 0021-9258

Ollero, M., Powers, R. D. and Alvarez, J. G. (2000). "Variation of docosahexaenoic acid content in subsets of human spermatozoa at different stages of maturation: implications for sperm lipoperoxidative damage." *Mol Reprod Dev* 55(3): pp. 326-34, ISSN 1040-452X

Olson, G. E., Winfrey, V. P., Bi, M., Hardy, D. M. and NagDas, S. K. (2004). "Zonadhesin assembly into the hamster sperm acrosomal matrix occurs by distinct targeting strategies during spermiogenesis and maturation in the epididymis." *Biol Reprod* 71(4): pp. 1128-34, ISSN 0006-3363

Ombelet, W., Wouters, E., Boels, L., Cox, A., Janssen, M., Spiessens, C., Vereecken, A., Bosmans, E. and Steeno, O. (1997). "Sperm morphology assessment: diagnostic potential and comparative analysis of strict or WHO criteria in a fertile and a subfertile population." *Int J Androl* 20(6): pp. 367-72, ISSN 0105-6263

Orgebin-Crist, M. C. (1967a). "Fertility in does inseminated with epididymal spermatozoa." *J Reprod Fertil* 14(2): pp. 346-7, ISSN 0022-4251

Orgebin-Crist, M. C. (1967b). "Sperm maturation in rabbit epididymis." *Nature* 216(5117): pp. 816-8, ISSN 0028-0836

Orgebin-Crist, M. C. (1968). "Maturation of spermatozoa in the rabbit epididymis: delayed fertilization in does inseminated with epididymal spermatozoa." *J Reprod Fertil* 16(1): pp. 29-33, ISSN 0022-4251

Orgebin-Crist, M. C. (1969). "Studies on the function of the epididymis." *Biol Reprod* 1(pp. Suppl 1:155-75, ISSN 0006-3363

Pasten, C., Morales, P. and Kong, M. (2005). "Role of the sperm proteasome during fertilization and gamete interaction in the mouse." *Mol Reprod Dev* 71(2): pp. 209-19, ISSN 1040-452X

Pastor-Soler, N., Beaulieu, V., Litvin, T. N., Da Silva, N., Chen, Y., Brown, D., Buck, J., Levin, L. R. and Breton, S. (2003). "Bicarbonate-regulated adenylyl cyclase (sAC) is a sensor that regulates pH-dependent V-ATPase recycling." *J Biol Chem* 278(49): pp. 49523-9, ISSN 0021-9258

Pereira, B. M., Abou-Haila, A. and Tulsiani, D. R. (1998). "Rat sperm surface mannosidase is first expressed on the plasma membrane of testicular germ cells." *Biol Reprod* 59(6): pp. 1288-95, ISSN 0006-3363

Petrunkina, A. M., Harrison, R. A. and Topfer-Petersen, E. (2000). "Only low levels of spermadhesin AWN are detectable on the surface of live ejaculated boar spermatozoa." *Reprod Fertil Dev* 12(7-8): pp. 361-71, ISSN 1031-3613

Piehler, E., Petrunkina, A. M., Ekhlasi-Hundrieser, M. and Topfer-Petersen, E. (2006). "Dynamic quantification of the tyrosine phosphorylation of the sperm surface proteins during capacitation." *Cytometry A* 69(10): pp. 1062-70, ISSN 1552-4922

Pike, L. J. (2006). "Rafts defined: a report on the Keystone Symposium on Lipid Rafts and Cell Function." *J Lipid Res* 47(7): pp. 1597-8, ISSN 0022-2275

Qi, H., Moran, M. M., Navarro, B., Chong, J. A., Krapivinsky, G., Krapivinsky, L., Kirichok, Y., Ramsey, I. S., Quill, T. A. and Clapham, D. E. (2007). "All four CatSper ion channel proteins are required for male fertility and sperm cell hyperactivated motility." *Proc Natl Acad Sci U S A* 104(4): pp. 1219-23, ISSN 0027-8424

Quill, T. A., Ren, D., Clapham, D. E. and Garbers, D. L. (2001). "A voltage-gated ion channel expressed specifically in spermatozoa." *Proc Natl Acad Sci U S A* 98(22): pp. 12527-31, ISSN 0027-8424

Ramalho-Santos, J., Moreno, R. D., Wessel, G. M., Chan, E. K. and Schatten, G. (2001). "Membrane trafficking machinery components associated with the mammalian acrosome during spermiogenesis." *Exp Cell Res* 267(1): pp. 45-60, ISSN 0014-4827

Rankin, T. L., Coleman, J. S., Epifano, O., Hoodbhoy, T., Turner, S. G., Castle, P. E., Lee, E., Gore-Langton, R. and Dean, J. (2003). "Fertility and taxon-specific sperm binding persist after replacement of mouse sperm receptors with human homologs." *Dev Cell* 5(1): pp. 33-43, ISSN 1534-5807

Redgrove, K. A., Anderson, A. L., Dun, M. D., McLaughlin, E. A., O'Bryan, M. K., Aitken, R. J. and Nixon, B. (2011). "Involvement of multimeric protein complexes in mediating the capacitation-dependent binding of human spermatozoa to homologous zonae pellucidae." *Dev Biol* 356(2): pp. 460-74, ISSN 1095-564X

Ren, D., Navarro, B., Perez, G., Jackson, A. C., Hsu, S., Shi, Q., Tilly, J. L. and Clapham, D. E. (2001). "A sperm ion channel required for sperm motility and male fertility." *Nature* 413(6856): pp. 603-9, ISSN 0028-0836

Rosano, G., Caille, A. M., Gallardo-Rios, M. and Munuce, M. J. (2007). "D-Mannose-binding sites are putative sperm determinants of human oocyte recognition and fertilization." *Reprod Biomed Online* 15(2): pp. 182-90, ISSN 1472-6483

Sackstein, R. (2005). "The lymphocyte homing receptors: gatekeepers of the multistep paradigm." *Curr Opin Hematol* 12(6): pp. 444-50, ISSN 1065-6251

Saez, F., Frenette, G. and Sullivan, R. (2003). "Epididymosomes and prostasomes: their roles in posttesticular maturation of the sperm cells." *J Androl* 24(2): pp. 149-54, ISSN 0196-3635

Sakkas, D., Leppens-Luisier, G., Lucas, H., Chardonnens, D., Campana, A., Franken, D. R. and Urner, F. (2003). "Localization of tyrosine phosphorylated proteins in human sperm and relation to capacitation and zona pellucida binding." *Biol Reprod* 68(4): pp. 1463-9, ISSN 0006-3363

Saling, P. M., Sowinski, J. and Storey, B. T. (1979). "An ultrastructural study of epididymal mouse spermatozoa binding to zonae pellucidae in vitro: sequential relationship to the acrosome reaction." *J Exp Zool* 209(2): pp. 229-38, ISSN 0022-104X

Schmell, E. D. and Gulyas, B. J. (1980). "Mammalian sperm-egg recognition and binding in vitro. I. Specificity of sperm interactions with live and fixed eggs in homologous and heterologous inseminations of hamster, mouse, and guinea pig oocytes." *Biol Reprod* 23(5): pp. 1075-85, ISSN 0006-3363

Schuck, S., Honsho, M., Ekroos, K., Shevchenko, A. and Simons, K. (2003). "Resistance of cell membranes to different detergents." *Proc Natl Acad Sci U S A* 100(10): pp. 5795-800, ISSN 0027-8424

Seligman, J., Zipser, Y. and Kosower, N. S. (2004). "Tyrosine phosphorylation, thiol status, and protein tyrosine phosphatase in rat epididymal spermatozoa." *Biol Reprod* 71(3): pp. 1009-15, ISSN 0006-3363

Shadan, S., James, P. S., Howes, E. A. and Jones, R. (2004). "Cholesterol efflux alters lipid raft stability and distribution during capacitation of boar spermatozoa." *Biol Reprod* 71(1): pp. 253-65, ISSN 0006-3363

Shamsadin, R., Adham, I. M., Nayernia, K., Heinlein, U. A., Oberwinkler, H. and Engel, W. (1999). "Male mice deficient for germ-cell cyritestin are infertile." *Biol Reprod* 61(6): pp. 1445-51, ISSN 0006-3363

Shen, L., Weber, C. R. and Turner, J. R. (2008). "The tight junction protein complex undergoes rapid and continuous molecular remodeling at steady state." *J Cell Biol* 181(4): pp. 683-95, ISSN 1540-8140

Shi, S., Williams, S. A., Seppo, A., Kurniawan, H., Chen, W., Ye, Z., Marth, J. D. and Stanley, P. (2004). "Inactivation of the Mgat1 gene in oocytes impairs oogenesis, but embryos lacking complex and hybrid N-glycans develop and implant." *Mol Cell Biol* 24(22): pp. 9920-9, ISSN 0270-7306

Shum, W. W., Da Silva, N., Brown, D. and Breton, S. (2009). "Regulation of luminal acidification in the male reproductive tract via cell-cell crosstalk." *J Exp Biol* 212(Pt 11): pp. 1753-61, ISSN 0022-0949

Shur, B. D. and Bennett, D. (1979). "A specific defect in galactosyltransferase regulation on sperm bearing mutant alleles of the T/t locus." *Dev Biol* 71(2): pp. 243-59, ISSN 0012-1606

Shur, B. D. and Hall, N. G. (1982a). "A role for mouse sperm surface galactosyltransferase in sperm binding to the egg zona pellucida." *J Cell Biol* 95(2 Pt 1): pp. 574-9, ISSN 0021-9525

Shur, B. D. and Hall, N. G. (1982b). "Sperm surface galactosyltransferase activities during in vitro capacitation." *J Cell Biol* 95(2 Pt 1): pp. 567-73, ISSN 0021-9525

Si, Y. and Okuno, M. (1999). "Role of tyrosine phosphorylation of flagellar proteins in hamster sperm hyperactivation." *Biol Reprod* 61(1): pp. 240-6, ISSN 0006-3363

Sibony, M., Gasc, J. M., Soubrier, F., Alhenc-Gelas, F. and Corvol, P. (1993). "Gene expression and tissue localization of the two isoforms of angiotensin I converting enzyme." *Hypertension* 21(6 Pt 1): pp. 827-35, ISSN 0194-911X

Simons, K. and Ikonen, E. (1997). "Functional rafts in cell membranes." *Nature* 387(6633): pp. 569-72, ISSN 0028-0836

Simons, K. and Toomre, D. (2000). "Lipid rafts and signal transduction." *Nat Rev Mol Cell Biol* 1(1): pp. 31-9, ISSN 1471-0072

Simons, K. and Vaz, W. L. (2004). "Model systems, lipid rafts, and cell membranes." *Annu Rev Biophys Biomol Struct* 33(pp. 269-95, ISSN 1056-8700

Sims, J. D., McCready, J. and Jay, D. G. (2011). "Extracellular heat shock protein (Hsp)70 and Hsp90alpha assist in matrix metalloproteinase-2 activation and breast cancer cell migration and invasion." *PLoS One* 6(4): pp. e18848, ISSN 1932-6203

Sinowatz, F., Amselgruber, W., Topfer-Petersen, E., Calvete, J. J., Sanz, L. and Plendl, J. (1995). "Immunohistochemical localization of spermadhesin AWN in the porcine male genital tract." *Cell Tissue Res* 282(1): pp. 175-9, ISSN 0302-766X

Sitia, R. and Braakman, I. (2003). "Quality control in the endoplasmic reticulum protein factory." *Nature* 426(6968): pp. 891-4, ISSN 1476-4687

Sleight, S. B., Miranda, P. V., Plaskett, N. W., Maier, B., Lysiak, J., Scrable, H., Herr, J. C. and Visconti, P. E. (2005). "Isolation and proteomic analysis of mouse sperm detergent-resistant membrane fractions: evidence for dissociation of lipid rafts during capacitation." *Biol Reprod* 73(4): pp. 721-9, ISSN 0006-3363

Soler, C., Yeung, C. H. and Cooper, T. G. (1994). "Development of sperm motility patterns in the murine epididymis." *Int J Androl* 17(5): pp. 271-8, ISSN 0105-6263

Spinaci, M., Volpe, S., Bernardini, C., De Ambrogi, M., Tamanini, C., Seren, E. and Galeati, G. (2005). "Immunolocalization of heat shock protein 70 (Hsp 70) in boar spermatozoa and its role during fertilization." *Mol Reprod Dev* 72(4): pp. 534-41, ISSN 1040-452X

Stein, K. K., Go, J. C., Lane, W. S., Primakoff, P. and Myles, D. G. (2006). "Proteomic analysis of sperm regions that mediate sperm-egg interactions." *Proteomics* 6(12): pp. 3533-43, ISSN 1615-9853

Suarez, S. S. (2008). "Control of hyperactivation in sperm." *Hum Reprod Update* 14(6): pp. 647-57, ISSN 1460-2369

Sutovsky, P., Manandhar, G., McCauley, T. C., Caamano, J. N., Sutovsky, M., Thompson, W. E. and Day, B. N. (2004). "Proteasomal interference prevents zona pellucida penetration and fertilization in mammals." *Biol Reprod* 71(5): pp. 1625-37, ISSN 0006-3363

Swenson, C. E. and Dunbar, B. S. (1982). "Specificity of sperm-zona interaction." *J Exp Zool* 219(1): pp. 97-104, ISSN 0022-104X

Syntin, P., Dacheux, F., Druart, X., Gatti, J. L., Okamura, N. and Dacheux, J. L. (1996). "Characterization and identification of proteins secreted in the various regions of the adult boar epididymis." *Biol Reprod* 55(5): pp. 956-74, ISSN 0006-3363

Tanphaichitr, N., Smith, J. and Kates, M. (1990). "Levels of sulfogalactosylglycerolipid in capacitated motile and immotile mouse spermatozoa." *Biochem Cell Biol* 68(2): pp. 528-35, ISSN 0829-8211

Tanphaichitr, N., Smith, J., Mongkolsirikieart, S., Gradil, C. and Lingwood, C. A. (1993). "Role of a gamete-specific sulfoglycolipid immobilizing protein on mouse sperm-egg binding." *Dev Biol* 156(1): pp. 164-75, ISSN 0012-1606

Tantibhedhyangkul, J., Weerachatyanukul, W., Carmona, E., Xu, H., Anupriwan, A., Michaud, D. and Tanphaichitr, N. (2002). "Role of sperm surface arylsulfatase A in mouse sperm-zona pellucida binding." *Biol Reprod* 67(1): pp. 212-9, ISSN 0006-3363

Tardif, S. and Cormier, N. (2011). "Role of zonadhesin during sperm-egg interaction: a species-specific acrosomal molecule with multiple functions." *Mol Hum Reprod* 17(11): pp. 661-8, ISSN 1460-2407

Tardif, S., Wilson, M. D., Wagner, R., Hunt, P., Gertsenstein, M., Nagy, A., Lobe, C., Koop, B. F. and Hardy, D. M. (2010). "Zonadhesin is essential for species specificity of sperm adhesion to the egg zona pellucida." *J Biol Chem* 285(32): pp. 24863-70, ISSN 1083-351X

Tesarik, J., Moos, J. and Mendoza, C. (1993). "Stimulation of protein tyrosine phosphorylation by a progesterone receptor on the cell surface of human sperm." *Endocrinology* 133(1): pp. 328-35, ISSN 0013-7227

Thaler, C. D. and Cardullo, R. A. (1996). "The initial molecular interaction between mouse sperm and the zona pellucida is a complex binding event." *J Biol Chem* 271(38): pp. 23289-97, ISSN 0021-9258

Thaler, C. D. and Cardullo, R. A. (2002). "Distinct membrane fractions from mouse sperm bind different zona pellucida glycoproteins." *Biol Reprod* 66(1): pp. 65-9, ISSN 0006-3363

Thimon, V., Frenette, G., Saez, F., Thabet, M. and Sullivan, R. (2008). "Protein composition of human epididymosomes collected during surgical vasectomy reversal: a proteomic and genomic approach." *Hum Reprod* 23(8): pp. 1698-707, ISSN 1460-2350

Topfer-Petersen, E. (1999). "Carbohydrate-based interactions on the route of a spermatozoon to fertilization." *Hum Reprod Update* 5(4): pp. 314-29, ISSN 1355-4786

Topfer-Petersen, E., Romero, A., Varela, P. F., Ekhlasi-Hundrieser, M., Dostalova, Z., Sanz, L. and Calvete, J. J. (1998). "Spermadhesins: a new protein family. Facts, hypotheses and perspectives." *Andrologia* 30(4-5): pp. 217-24, ISSN 0303-4569

Tulsiani, D. R., Abou-Haila, A., Loeser, C. R. and Pereira, B. M. (1998). "The biological and functional significance of the sperm acrosome and acrosomal enzymes in mammalian fertilization." *Exp Cell Res* 240(2): pp. 151-64, ISSN 0014-4827

Tulsiani, D. R., Skudlarek, M. D., Nagdas, S. K. and Orgebin-Crist, M. C. (1993). "Purification and characterization of rat epididymal-fluid alpha-D-mannosidase: similarities to sperm plasma-membrane alpha-D-mannosidase." *Biochem J* 290 (Pt 2)(pp. 427-36, ISSN 0264-6021

Tulsiani, D. R., Skudlarek, M. D. and Orgebin-Crist, M. C. (1989). "Novel alpha-D-mannosidase of rat sperm plasma membranes: characterization and potential role in sperm-egg interactions." *J Cell Biol* 109(3): pp. 1257-67, ISSN 0021-9525

UN (2009). "World population to exceed 9 billion by 2050." pp.

Urch, U. A. and Patel, H. (1991). "The interaction of boar sperm proacrosin with its natural substrate, the zona pellucida, and with polysulfated polysaccharides." *Development* 111(4): pp. 1165-72, ISSN 0950-1991

Urner, F., Leppens-Luisier, G. and Sakkas, D. (2001). "Protein tyrosine phosphorylation in sperm during gamete interaction in the mouse: the influence of glucose." *Biol Reprod* 64(5): pp. 1350-7, ISSN 0006-3363

Urner, F. and Sakkas, D. (2003). "Protein phosphorylation in mammalian spermatozoa." *Reproduction* 125(1): pp. 17-26, ISSN 1470-1626

van Gestel, R. A., Brewis, I. A., Ashton, P. R., Helms, J. B., Brouwers, J. F. and Gadella, B. M. (2005). "Capacitation-dependent concentration of lipid rafts in the apical ridge head area of porcine sperm cells." *Mol Hum Reprod* 11(8): pp. 583-90, ISSN 1360-9947

Vazquez, M. H., Phillips, D. M. and Wassarman, P. M. (1989). "Interaction of mouse sperm with purified sperm receptors covalently linked to silica beads." *J Cell Sci* 92 (Pt 4)(pp. 713-22, ISSN 0021-9533

Visconti, P. E., Bailey, J. L., Moore, G. D., Pan, D., Olds-Clarke, P. and Kopf, G. S. (1995a). "Capacitation of mouse spermatozoa. I. Correlation between the capacitation state and protein tyrosine phosphorylation." *Development* 121(4): pp. 1129-37, ISSN 0950-1991

Visconti, P. E. and Florman, H. M. (2010). "Mechanisms of sperm-egg interactions: between sugars and broken bonds." *Sci Signal* 3(142): pp. pe35, ISSN 1937-9145

Visconti, P. E., Moore, G. D., Bailey, J. L., Leclerc, P., Connors, S. A., Pan, D., Olds-Clarke, P. and Kopf, G. S. (1995b). "Capacitation of mouse spermatozoa. II. Protein tyrosine phosphorylation and capacitation are regulated by a cAMP-dependent pathway." *Development* 121(4): pp. 1139-50, ISSN 0950-1991

Visconti, P. E., Ning, X., Fornes, M. W., Alvarez, J. G., Stein, P., Connors, S. A. and Kopf, G. S. (1999). "Cholesterol efflux-mediated signal transduction in mammalian sperm: cholesterol release signals an increase in protein tyrosine phosphorylation during mouse sperm capacitation." *Dev Biol* 214(2): pp. 429-43, ISSN 0012-1606

Walsh, A., Whelan, D., Bielanowicz, A., Skinner, B., Aitken, R. J., O'Bryan, M. K. and Nixon, B. (2008). "Identification of the molecular chaperone, heat shock protein 1 (chaperonin 10), in the reproductive tract and in capacitating spermatozoa in the male mouse." *Biol Reprod* 78(6): pp. 983-93, ISSN 0006-3363

Wassarman, P. M. (1988). "Zona pellucida glycoproteins." *Annu Rev Biochem* 57(pp. 415-42, ISSN 0066-4154

Wassarman, P. M. (1992). "Mouse gamete adhesion molecules." *Biol Reprod* 46(2): pp. 186-91, ISSN 0006-3363

Wassarman, P. M. (2009). "Mammalian fertilization: the strange case of sperm protein 56." *Bioessays* 31(2): pp. 153-8, ISSN 1521-1878

Wassarman, P. M. and Litscher, E. S. (2008). "Mammalian fertilization: the egg's multifunctional zona pellucida." *Int J Dev Biol* 52(5-6): pp. 665-76, ISSN 0214-6282

Wassarman, P. M. and Mortillo, S. (1991). "Structure of the mouse egg extracellular coat, the zona pellucida." *Int Rev Cytol* 130(pp. 85-110, ISSN 0074-7696

Weerachatyanukul, W., Rattanachaiyanont, M., Carmona, E., Furimsky, A., Mai, A., Shoushtarian, A., Sirichotiyakul, S., Ballakier, H., Leader, A. and Tanphaichitr, N. (2001). "Sulfogalactosylglycerolipid is involved in human gamete interaction." *Mol Reprod Dev* 60(4): pp. 569-78, ISSN 1040-452X

Weerachatyanukul, W., Xu, H., Anupriwan, A., Carmona, E., Wade, M., Hermo, L., da Silva, S. M., Rippstein, P., Sobhon, P., Sretarugsa, P. and Tanphaichitr, N. (2003). "Acquisition of arylsulfatase A onto the mouse sperm surface during epididymal transit." *Biol Reprod* 69(4): pp. 1183-92, ISSN 0006-3363

Wehren, A., Meyer, H. E., Sobek, A., Kloetzel, P. M. and Dahlmann, B. (1996). "Phosphoamino acids in proteasome subunits." *Biol Chem* 377(7-8): pp. 497-503, ISSN 1431-6730

West, A. P. and Willison, K. R. (1996). "Brefeldin A and mannose 6-phosphate regulation of acrosomic related vesicular trafficking." *Eur J Cell Biol* 70(4): pp. 315-21, ISSN 0171-9335

Westbrook-Case, V. A., Winfrey, V. P. and Olson, G. E. (1994). "Characterization of two antigenically related integral membrane proteins of the guinea pig sperm periacrosomal plasma membrane." *Mol Reprod Dev* 39(3): pp. 309-21, ISSN 1040-452X

White, D., Weerachatyanukul, W., Gadella, B., Kamolvarin, N., Attar, M. and Tanphaichitr, N. (2000). "Role of sperm sulfogalactosylglycerolipid in mouse sperm-zona pellucida binding." *Biol Reprod* 63(1): pp. 147-55, ISSN 0006-3363

White, D. R. and Aitken, R. J. (1989). "Relationship between calcium, cyclic AMP, ATP, and intracellular pH and the capacity of hamster spermatozoa to express hyperactivated motility." *Gamete Res* 22(2): pp. 163-77, ISSN 0148-7280

Yamagata, K., Nakanishi, T., Ikawa, M., Yamaguchi, R., Moss, S. B. and Okabe, M. (2002). "Sperm from the calmegin-deficient mouse have normal abilities for binding and fusion to the egg plasma membrane." *Dev Biol* 250(2): pp. 348-57, ISSN 0012-1606

Yamaguchi, R., Muro, Y., Isotani, A., Tokuhiro, K., Takumi, K., Adham, I., Ikawa, M. and Okabe, M. (2009). "Disruption of ADAM3 impairs the migration of sperm into oviduct in mouse." *Biol Reprod* 81(1): pp. 142-6, ISSN 0006-3363

Yamasaki, N., Richardson, R. T. and O'Rand, M. G. (1995). "Expression of the rabbit sperm protein Sp17 in COS cells and interaction of recombinant Sp17 with the rabbit zona pellucida." *Mol Reprod Dev* 40(1): pp. 48-55, ISSN 1040-452X

Yanagimachi, R. (1994a). "Fertility of mammalian spermatozoa: its development and relativity." *Zygote* 2(4): pp. 371-2, ISSN 0967-1994

Yanagimachi, R. (2009). "Germ cell research: a personal perspective." *Biol Reprod* 80(2): pp. 204-18, ISSN 0006-3363

Yano, R., Matsuyama, T., Kaneko, T., Kurio, H., Murayama, E., Toshimori, K. and Iida, H. (2010). "Bactericidal/Permeability-increasing protein is associated with the acrosome region of rodent epididymal spermatozoa." *J Androl* 31(2): pp. 201-14, ISSN 1939-4640

Yi, Y. J., Manandhar, G., Sutovsky, M., Zimmerman, S. W., Jonakova, V., van Leeuwen, F. W., Oko, R., Park, C. S. and Sutovsky, P. (2010). "Interference with the 19S proteasomal regulatory complex subunit PSMD4 on the sperm surface inhibits sperm-zona pellucida penetration during porcine fertilization." *Cell Tissue Res* 341(2): pp. 325-40, ISSN 1432-0878

Yoshida-Komiya, H., Tulsiani, D. R., Hirayama, T. and Araki, Y. (1999). "Mannose-binding molecules of rat spermatozoa and sperm-egg interaction." *Zygote* 7(4): pp. 335-46, ISSN 0967-1994

Zhang, H. and Martin-Deleon, P. A. (2003). "Mouse epididymal Spam1 (pH-20) is released in the luminal fluid with its lipid anchor." *J Androl* 24(1): pp. 51-8, ISSN 0196-3635

Zimmerman, S. W., Manandhar, G., Yi, Y. J., Gupta, S. K., Sutovsky, M., Odhiambo, J. F., Powell, M. D., Miller, D. J. and Sutovsky, P. (2011). "Sperm proteasomes degrade sperm receptor on the egg zona pellucida during mammalian fertilization." *PLoS One* 6(2): pp. e17256, ISSN 1932-6203

Zini, A., O'Bryan, M. K., Israel, L. and Schlegel, P. N. (1998). "Human sperm NADH and NADPH diaphorase cytochemistry: correlation with sperm motility." *Urology* 51(3): pp. 464-8, ISSN 0090-4295

Chapter 5

Modulation of Gene Expression by RNA Binding Proteins: mRNA Stability and Translation

Kotb Abdelmohsen

Additional information is available at the end of the chapter

http://dx.doi.org/10.5772/48485

1. Introduction

Regulation of gene expression is an essential process through which mammalian cells counter the changes in their microenvironment. These changes drive cells to respond to different stimuli that trigger cellular re-programming towards proliferation, differentiation, development, apoptosis, senescence, carcinogenesis, etc. Once mRNAs are transcribed they are subjected to posttranscriptional events that regulate mRNA metabolism including stability and translation. These two processes normally dictate the protein levels encoded by mRNA. RNA-binding proteins (RPBs) that bind mature mRNA sequences normally have an important regulatory effect on the mRNA.

RBPs are also named mRNA turnover and translation regulator RBPs (TTR-RBPs) since they are capable of regulating both mRNA stability and translation. This family includes numerous members such as Hu proteins [HuA (HuR), HuB, HuC, and HuD] known to bind AU-rich sequences in the 3′ untranslated region (3′UTR) to enhance mRNA translation or to increase its stability [1, 2]. Other RBPs such as T-cell intracellular antigen 1 (TIA-1), TIA-1-related (TIAR), tristetraprolin (TTP), fragile X mental retardation protein (FMRP), polypyrimidine tract-binding protein (PTB), CUG triple repeats RNA-binding protein (CUGBP), nucleolin, and heterogeneous nuclear ribonucleoproteins (hnRNP) A1, A2, and C1/C2 have been shown to influence mRNA stability or translation through interaction with the 3′UTR, CR or the 5′UTR [3-9].

Hu proteins are among the RBPs that are well characterized. While HuR is ubiquitously expressed, HuB, HuC and HuD are primarily neuronal [10]. HuR, also known as embryonic lethal, abnormal vision, Drosophila-like 1 (ELAV L1), binds mRNAs bearing AU- and U-rich sequences, which are considered binding signatures, or RNA-recognition motifs (RRMs) found in numerous mRNAs [11]. HuR binds target mRNA to enhance its stability and/or translation. These targets are involved in several processes such as cell growth, survival, proliferation, stress response, senescence and carcinogenesis [2, 12-17].

The RBP AU-binding factor 1 (AUF1), also known as heterogeneous nuclear ribonucleoprotein D (hnRNPD), is known to bind AU-rich sequences mostly in the 3'UTR of target mRNA. AUF1 belongs to a large family that includes several hnRNPs such as hnRNNP A, B, C, D, E, F, H, I, K, L, M, Q, R and U. AUF1 promotes the degradation of several target transcripts. However, it was also found to enhance the stability and translation of some mRNAs [18-21]. AUF1 is alternatively spliced and all known four isoforms (p37, p40, p42, p45) bind mRNAs but with different binding affinities [22]. AUF1 is thought to recruit mRNAs to the exosome and proteasome for degradation [23, 24]. Target mRNAs are implicated in several processes such as cell cycle, stress response, apoptosis, and carcinogenesis [21].

TIA-1 and TIAR RBPs bind AU/U-rich sequences in the 3'UTR of target transcripts and suppress mRNA translation [25]. However, they can also modulate translation through 5' terminal oligopyrimidine tracts (5'TOP) in response to changes in the cellular environment [26]. Under stress conditions, these proteins are thought to halt mRNA translation in RNA-protein aggregations known as stress granules [27].

The RBP nuclear factor 90 (NF90) interacts with many RNAs bearing AU-rich sequences. NF90 normally suppresses the translation of target mRNAs involved in cell cycle, translation, proliferation and cell division [28]. Although FMRP is expressed in several tissues, it has an essential role in neuronal and intellectual development. FMRP regulates stability and translation of several genes involved in synaptic plasticity [29]. Mutation of FMRP normally results in the inability to inhibit translation and can lead to fragile X syndrome, mental retardation, premature ovarian failure, autism and Parkinson's disease. FMRP is found in RNA granules associated with ribosomal RNA (rRNA) in dendrites [30, 31]. TTP, a zinc finger protein, binds AU-rich sequences in mRNA transcripts to promote their decay. Target mRNAs are involved in cell cycle, inflammation, and carcinogenesis [32]. Nucleolin interacts with mRNAs bearing AU-rich or G-rich sequences to regulate mRNA stability and/or translation. Target transcripts are involved in several processes such as cell cycle, cell morphology, development, growth, proliferation, and carcinogenesis [3]. KH-type splicing regulatory protein (KSRP) RBP binds AU-rich sequences of target transcripts promoting mRNA decay. These targets encode cytokines, chemokines, transcription factors, proto-oncogenes, and cell-cycle regulators [33].

If the RBP functions to promote mRNA degradation such as AUF1 or TTP, then the mRNA half-life is shortened and therefore protein levels will be subsequently low. On the other hand, if the RBP functions to promote mRNA stability such as HuR, then the RBP will subsequently increase protein levels by extending the mRNA half-life. Similarly, if the RBP modulates mRNA translation, protein levels will be influenced accordingly. Figure 1 summarizes these general effects of RBPs as posttranscriptional gene regulators.

This chapter will focus on the effects of RBPs on mRNA stability and translation. It is believed that two or more RBPs may have a functional interplay among themselves and with small RNA molecules known as microRNAs, through binding to the same mRNA. Examples of stabilized and destabilized genes will be indicated, as well as translationally enhanced or suppressed mRNAs and the involvement of encoded proteins in the cellular process.

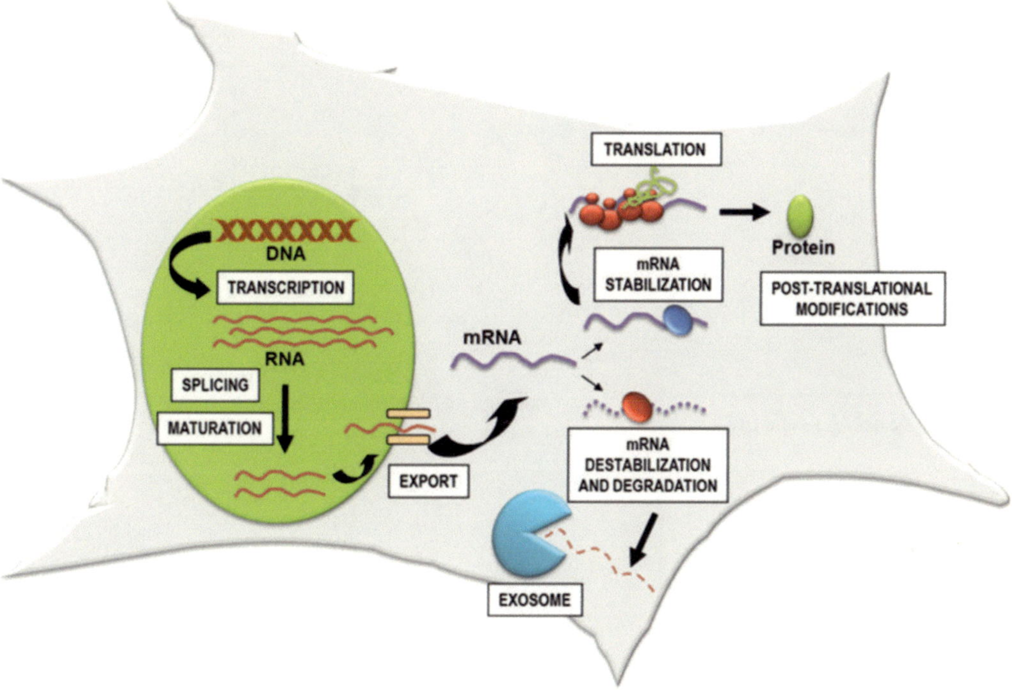

Figure 1. Regulation of mRNA stability and translation by RNA-binding proteins (RBPs). They mainly influence the fates of target mRNAs at the post-transcriptional levels. In the cytoplasm, stabilized mRNAs are protected from degradation leading to more protein levels. Destabilized mRNAs are driven to degradation machinery leading to lower protein levels. RBPs can also influence the abundance of mRNAs in the translation machinery (polysomes).

2. Methodology

In this section the methodology of investigating binding of RBPs to target mRNAs as well as the effects on mRNA stability and translation will be explained.

2.1. mRNA-ribonucleoprotein immunoprecipitation (mRNP-IP)

PAS beads from Sigma (P-3391) (or preswollen beads from Sigma) can be used to coat the IgG control antibody or the specific antibody recognizing the RBP. Mix 10 μg antibody, 60 μl volume beads and 200 μl of NT-2 buffer (50 mM Tris, pH 7.4, 150 mM NaCl, 1 mM MgCl2, 0.05% Nonidet P-40). Rotate overnight at 4°C.

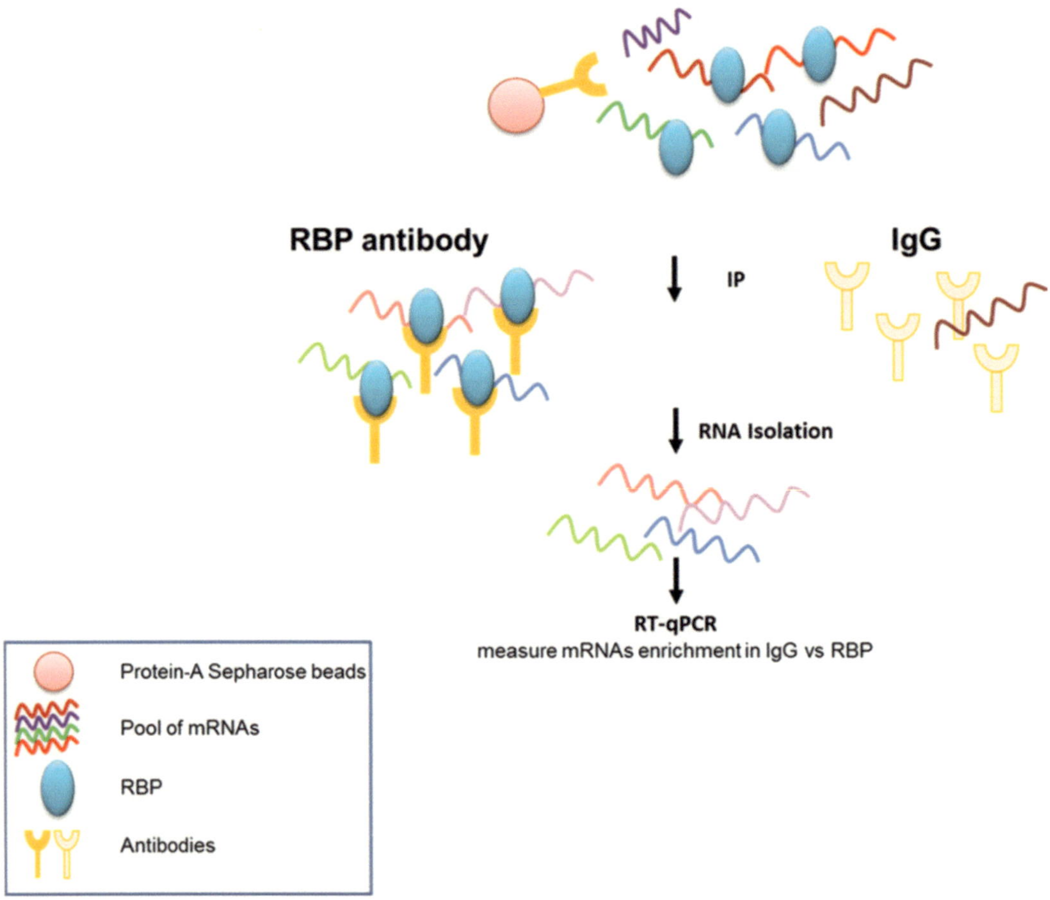

Figure 2. Schematic illustration of ribonucleoprotein immunoprecipitation (see text).

Harvest and lyse tissue culture cells in ice-cold lysis buffer supplemented with RNAse inhibitors and protease inhibitors for 10 minutes on ice. Lysis buffer is prepared by mixing 100 mM KCl, 5 mM MgCl2, 10 mM Hepes, pH 7.0, 0.5% Nonidet P-40, and 1 mM Dithiothrectol (DTT) added at the time of use. Spin 30 min at 14,000 rpm (20,000 x g) /4°C and transfer supernatant to the fresh tubes. Wash the pre-coated beads two times with NT2 buffer and add equal amounts of lysates to each antibody. Rotate at 4°C for one to two hours. Wash the beads Five times with 1 ml aliquots of ice-cold NT-2 buffer (5000 g, five minutes). Add 100 µl NT2 buffer having five µl DNase I (2 U/µl) and inculate at 37°C for 5-10 minutes. Add 1 ml NT2 buffer, spin at 5000 g for 5 minutes, and discard supernatant. Then, add the 5 µl of Proteinase K (10mg/ml), 1 µl 10% SDS and 100 µl NT-2 and incubate with shaking at 55°C for 15-30 minutes. Spin at 5000 g for 5 minutes to collect supernatant which contains the RNA. To the supernatants add 300 µl of the lower layer of acid phenol-$CHCl_3$ (Ambion) and vortex for one minute at room temperature. Spin at room temperature for one minute (14,000 rpm). Collect the upper layer, add 25 µl sodium acetate pH 5.2, 625 µl 100% ethanol and 5 µl glycoblue, mix well and store at 20°C overnight.

Spin at 14,000 rpm at 4°C for 30 minutes and discard supernatant. Wash the pellet with 1 ml 70% ethanol and spin at 14.000 rpm at 4°C for two minutes and then air dry pellet at room temperature for five minutes. Resuspend the pellet in 20-40 μl of RNAse-free water. This RNA can be used as any other RNA for real time PCR analysis or microarrays. If the gene of interest is enriched in RBP-IP which is twofold or higher compared to IgG-IP, then this gene and the RBP do interact. Figure 2 represents a schematic of mRNA-Ribonucleoprotein immunoprecipitation. For experimental examples see references [11, 34, 35].

2.2. Assessing the half-life ($t_{1/2}$) of target mRNAs

RBPs normally influence either mRNA stability or translation. Downregulation or overexpression of the RBP is helpful to determine whether the RBP affects mRNA stability. This can be achieved by transfection of either siRNA to downregulate, or a construct to overexpress, RBP of interest. Transfected cells are then treated with actinomycin D (2 μg/ml) to inhibit transcription. Cells can be harvested every hour for about six hours followed by isolation of RNA and real time PCR to measure the levels of genes of interest. The ribosomal RNA 18S is normally used for normalization. It is also recommended to measure the levels of a housekeeping gene or a gene that is not targeted by the RBP of interest. If the RBP influences mRNA stability, an increase or a decrease in the $t_{1/2}$ will be observed and can be calculated using this assay [11, 34, 35].

2.3. Evaluation of mRNA translation by polysome fractions

Prepare sucrose gradient solutions; 10-50% sucrose, 300 mM NaCl, 15mM $MgCl_2$, 15 mM Tris-Cl 7.5, 0.1 mg/ml cycloheximide and 1mg/ml Heparin. Layer the gradient with 2 ml of each solution starting with 10% (top) and ending with 50% (bottom). Be careful not to introduce any air bubbles into the gradient. Leave gradients at 4°C overnight to allow the step gradient to linearize. Lyse cells as described above (lysis buffer) and place cell lysates slowly at the top of the gradient. Use ultra-centrifugation spin for three hours at 35000 rpm at 4°C (SW41 rotor). Collect polysome fractions of 1ml each. An example of a polysome profile from HeLa cells is shown in Figure 3. It is important to note that the polysome profile might differ between cell lines and tissues. To analyze the distribution of a particular mRNA in the polysome profile, RNA is isolated from each fraction using Trizol followed by real time PCR and distribution can then be calculated. It is important to note that the sum of the mRNA distribution profile must be 100%. If the RBP affects mRNA translation, one or two observations can be found in the mRNA distribution profile. Significant changes in the amounts of mRNA in heavy translated fraction and a shift in the mRNA distribution profile either towards light or heavy fractions. These examples are illustrated in Figure 3 and reference [35].

3. Hu family

3.1. HuR

As mentioned above, the Hu family includes four RBPs, among them HuR which is ubiquitously expressed. HuR protein recognizes mRNAs through three RNA-recognition motifs [36]. It binds AU-rich sequences present in the 3'UTR or 5'UTR [11, 13]. The interaction of HuR with target mRNA is modulated by HuR phosphorylation through the checkpoint kinase Chk2 [34, 35]. This kinase also regulates HuR levels under heat shock conditions through ubiquitin-proteasome pathway [37]. Protein kinase C (PKC) and mitogen-activated protein kinase (MAPK) p38 also modulate the association of HuR with target mRNA [38-40]. Although HuR is predominantly nuclear, it is capable of shuttling to the cytoplasm through its nucleoyctoplasmic shuttling sequence (HNS) and transport machinery including chromosome region maintenance 1(CRM1), transportins 1 and 2, and importin-1α [41-44]. In addition, under stress conditions such as arsenite or heat shock, HuR aggregates in the cytoplasm with RNAs, known as RNA granules or stress granules, where mRNAs are stored or translationally suppressed [37, 45]. Levels of HuR are regulated by microRNA miR-519 which suppresses HuR mRNA translation [46]. Thus, these and other factors may influence the levels of HuR as a whole or its abundance in the cytoplasm and subsequently affect target mRNAs.

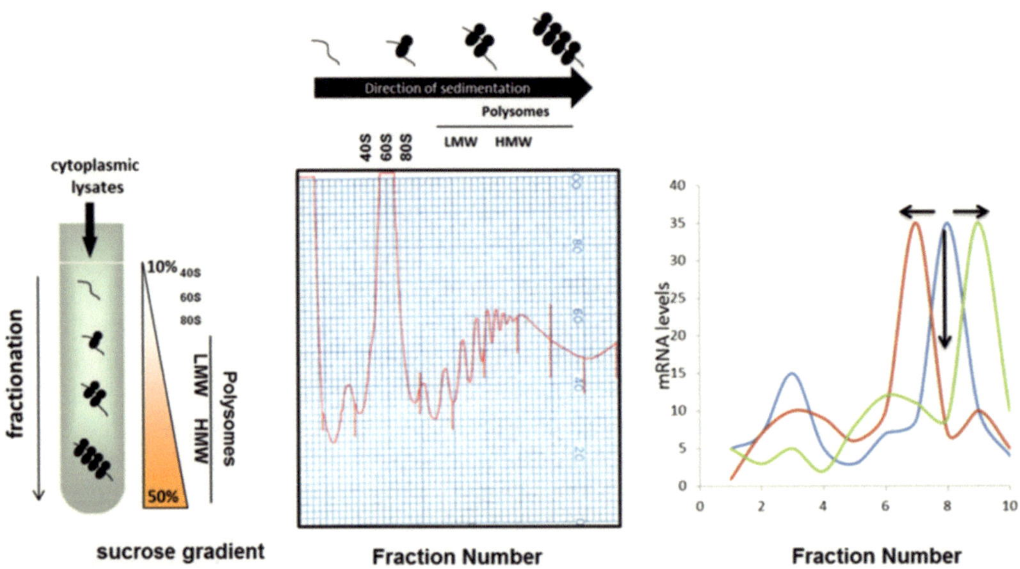

Figure 3. Schematic representations of translation assay (polysome profiling) to study the influence of RNA-binding proteins (RPBs) on mRNA translation (see text). Left; sucrose gradient, middle; example of a polysome profile using HeLa cells and right; examples of changes in mRNA distribution in polysome profile. Blue represents control, red represents an example of reduced mRNA translation and green represents an example of increased mRNA translation.

3.2. Stabilized HuR targets

Several target mRNAs are stabilized by HuR including cyclins A2, B1, E1, and D1 and p21. Proteins encoded by these mRNAs are involved in cell cycle, proliferation and cell survival. HuR also regulates the stability of genes such as silent mating type information regulation 2 homolog 1 (SIRT1), B-cell lymphoma 2 (BCL-2), epidermal growth factor (EGF), eukaryotic translation initiation factor 4E (eIF4E), and prothymosin α (ProTα) mRNAs.

These genes are involved in cell survival and proliferation. HuR promotes carcinogenesis by stabilizing mRNAs that encode for proteins such as Snail, matrix metallopeptidase 9 (MMP-9), urokinase (uPA) and urokinase receptor (uPAR), which enhance tumor invasion. Other genes such as vascular endothelial growth factor (VEGF) and cyclooxygenase-2 (COX-2) are also stabilized by HuR and involved in angiogenesis. Recent high-throughput analysis of HuR targets using photoactivatable ribonucleoside crosslinking and immunoprecipitation (PAR-CLIP) revealed the number of HuR binding sites per transcript, levels of binding, and degree of HuR-dependent RNA stabilization. Interestingly, HuR was found to bind pre-mRNAs and non-coding RNAs suggesting that HuR may integrate processing and stability [47].

These data suggest that HuR has a protective effect on its target mRNAs. While mRNAs can be recruited to the degradation machinery such as exosome and processing (P) bodies, HuR might be competing for binding to these labile mRNAs preventing or slowing down the degradation process. Since HuR is mostly present in the nucleus and PAR-CLIP identified pre-mRNAs bound to HuR, it is likely that HuR co-transcriptionally binds nuclear RNA substrates. This may also imply that HuR may play roles in splicing or maturation of these RNAs.

3.3. Translationally regulated HuR targets

HuR binds the 3'UTR of several mRNAs to enhance translation. For example, HuR enhances prothymosin α (ProTα), B-cell leukemia (BCL-2), and cyclin A2 mRNA translation. These genes are involved in cell cycle, proliferation, and cell survival [1]. While HuR binds the 3'UTR of wingless-type MMTV integration site family, member 5A (Wnt5a) mRNA to suppress translation, it binds the 3'UTR *of* thrombospondin 1 (TSP1) and vascular endothelial growth factor (VEGF) mRNAs to enhance its translation which are involved in carcinogenesis. In addition HuR binds 5'UTR of p27 and suppresses translation; p27 is involved in cell cycle, proliferation and cell survival. HuR also binds the 5' UTR of the hypoxia-inducible factor 1, alpha (HIF-1α) mRNA and promotes translation. This regulatory effect involves internal ribosome entry site (IRES) present in the 5'UTR of HIF-1α mRNA [48]. These data suggest that HuR can enhance mRNA translation through binding to the 3'UTR or 5'UTR. Future studies are required to investigate the roles of HuR coordinated with IRES located in the 5'UTRs to initiate mRNA translation.

3.4. HuD

Among Hu family proteins, HuD is also well studied. This RBP was initially described as neuronal specific [13]; however recent studies have shown HuD to be expressed in other cells such as pancreatic β cells [49, 50]. HuD is essential for neuronal development, identity, and differentiation through stabilization of mRNAs encoding proteins involved in these processes such as growth associated protein 43 (GAP-43), p21, acetylcholinesterase (AchE), and other targets [51-54]. In addition, HuD is involved in Parkinson's and Alzheimer's diseases and highly expressed in neuroblastomas [55-58]. Recent studies showed that HuD is regulated by the microRNA miR-375 which suppressed neuritis outgrowth [49]. In pancreatic β cells HuD was also found to bind the 5'UTR of preproinsulin mRNA and negatively regulate mRNA translation [50]. These findings suggest that HuD is expressed in other tissues than neuronal tissues and might have important regulatory functions yet to be investigated.

4. hnRNP family

These RBPs include several members such as hnRNP C, hnRNP D, and hnRNP K. hnRNP D, also known as AUF1, destabilizes mRNAs through binding to the 3'UTR. However some studies have indicated that AUF1 may also stabilize mRNAs and enhance mRNA translation. AUF1 post-transcriptionally regulate the expression of several genes involved in cancer and inflammation [21]. AUF1 is expressed as four isoforms due to alternative splicing of exons 2 and 7. The encoded isoforms are $p37^{AUF1}$, $p40^{AUF1}$, $p42^{AUF1}$, and $p45^{AUF1}$ according to their molecular masses. AUF1 isoforms contain two RNA recognition motifs (RRMs) that mediate binding to mRNA transcripts [21].

4.1. Influence of AUF1 on target mRNA

Unlike HuR, AUF1 promotes the degradation of the vast majority of its known targets through the recruitment of the mRNA to the exosome and the proteasome [23, 24], for example: cell cycle related genes such as cyclin D1, p21, p27 and p16INK4a [59-62], apoptosis regulators such as B cell leukemia (BCL-2) and growth arrest and DNA-damage-inducible protein alpha (GADD45α) [63, 64]; inflammatory related genes such as granulocyte-macrophage colony-stimulating factor (GM-CSF): and interleukin 6 (IL6) and human inducible nitric oxide synthase (NOS) [65-67] and DNA replication and repair related genes such as thymidylate synthase (TYMS), jun D proto-oncogene (JUND and c-fos (FOS) [68-70]. However, AUF1 can promote the stability and translation of some target transcripts. For example, AUF1 enhances c-MYC mRNA translation and stabilizes interleukin 1β (IL1B) mRNA in LPS stimulated cells [18, 71].

5. Other RBPs

In addition to the abovementioned RBPs, several others are known to post-transcriptionally regulate gene expression in similar fashions. For instance, TTP is known to promote the decay of mRNAs containing ARE sequences including several genes involved in cancer and inflammation such as IL-2, IL-3, IL-6, IL-10, and IL-12 [72-76].

Nucleolin post-transcriptionally modulates the fates of target mRNAs that bear AU-rich and/or G-rich sequences. Nucleolin targets include several genes involved in cellular processes such as proliferation, cell survival, and cell cycle as well as in diseases such as cancer and Alzheimer [3, 77]. For example, nucleolin binds the 3'UTR of BCL-2, GADD45A, gastrin (GAST) and β-globin enhancing mRNA stability. However, nucleolin binds the 3'UTR of APP mRNA, promoting its decay [78-83]. While nucleolin enhances the translation of mRNAs encoding for matrix metallopeptidase 9 (MMP9), AKT1 and cyclin I (CCNI) through binding to the 3′UTR, it suppresses translation of genes encoding for the tumor protein p53 (TP53) and prostaglandin endoperoxide H synthase-1 (PGHS-1) through binding to the 5′UTR [3, 84, 85].

Thus RBPs play an essential role in post-transcriptional gene regulation through binding to different regions of numerous mRNAs encoding for proteins involved in almost all cellular processes impacting cell fates in response to physiological and environmental stimuli.

6. RBPs interplay

Different RBPs are capable of binding to the same RNA inferring diverse effects on the fates of target transcripts. For instance HuR, AUF1, and nucleolin bind BCL-2 mRNA. While nucleolin and HuR promote the stability, AUF1 enhances the degradation of BCL-2 mRNA [63, 86-89]. This implies that HuR and nucleolin have a cooperative effect which is antagonized by AUF1.

Another example is illustrated in the case of GADD45A mRNA. While nucleolin stabilizes GADD45A mRNA, it seems that this effect might be antagonized by AUF1 which promotes its decay and TIAR which suppresses translation [64, 83].

These examples indicate that at least two or more RBPs can bind to the same mRNA molecule in a functional interplay to cooperatively or competitively regulate the fates of target mRNAs, translation and/or stability.

7. Interplay with microRNAs

MicroRNAs (miRNAs) are short RNA molecules, about 22 nt long, that regulate gene expression through RNA-induced silencing complex (RISC) [90, 91]. Targeted mRNAs are silenced either through degradation or translation suppression. RBPs RBPs jointly with miRNAs regulate the fates of mRNAs. While RBPs have diverse effects on target mRNAs, miRNAs only promote mRNA degradation or suppress its translation. In some cases miRNAs and RBPs cooperatively regulate the mRNA to a certain fate. For example, HuR was found to recruit let-7 to suppress c-MYC mRNA translation [92]. HuR competes with miR-494 and miR-548c-3p for the regulation of nucleolin and TOP2A mRNA respectively [93, 94]. These and several other examples indicate that RBPs are capable of competing or cooperating with other RNA binding factors such as miRNA to regulate the expression of target genes.

8. Concluding remarks

RBPs are involved in many cellular processes and pathological conditions such as cancer. Indeed, RBP such as HuR is highly expressed in cancer tissues and is believed to enhance tumorigenesis [2]. AUF1 is also involved in cancer progression through the modulation of neoplastic gene regulatory pathways [21]. Nucleolin is involved in cancer and Alzheimer's disease, while TTP is involved in cancer and inflammation [32].

Thus RBPs may influence not only gene expression but also diseases and disease-progression. Differential expression or subcellular localization of RBPs in diseases could be useful diagnostic markers and targeted for therapy. Indeed inhibitors of HuR and nucleolin have been reported to influence tumorigenesis in vitro, but their therapeutic usefulness in organisms remains untested [95-100].

In the past decade we have gained useful and specific knowledge about RBPs. We have advanced from <RNA binding> to <sequences specific binding> to <binding signatures/motifs> of RBPs. Nonetheless, it is important to identify the complete set of target RNAs which includes coding and non-coding RNAs in different cellular compartments. For example, the use of techniques such as photoactivatable-ribonucleoside-enhanced crosslinking and immunoprecipitation (PAR-CLIP) can provide a more global spectrum of RNA binding activities of RBPs [47, 101]. In addition, predominantly nuclear or nucleolar RBPs can be also studied by this technology to uncover their binding activities to other RNA species such as microRNAs, long non-coding RNAs, or even nuclear specific RNAs.

This will advance our knowledge in assessing other functions of RBPs in the regulation of gene expression.

Author details

Kotb Abdelmohsen
Laboratory of Molecular Biology and Immunology, NIA-IRP, NIH, Baltimore, MD, USA

Acknowledgement

K.A is supported by the Intramural Research Program of the National Institute on Aging, NIH. The author would like to thank Betty Landesman, MA/MLS/MS, National Institutes of Health (NIH) Library Writing Center, for her careful edits of this chapter.

9. References

[1] Srikantan, S. and M. Gorospe, HuR function in disease. Front Biosci, 2012. 17: p. 189-205.
[2] Abdelmohsen, K. and M. Gorospe, Posttranscriptional regulation of cancer traits by HuR. Wiley Interdiscip Rev RNA, 2010. 1(2): p. 214-29.
[3] Abdelmohsen, K., et al., Enhanced translation by Nucleolin via G-rich elements in coding and non-coding regions of target mRNAs. Nucleic Acids Res, 2011. 39(19): p. 8513-30.
[4] Kim, D.Y., et al., hnRNP Q mediates a phase-dependent translation-coupled mRNA decay of mouse Period3. Nucleic Acids Res, 2011. 39(20): p. 8901-14.
[5] Kwon, S., E. Barbarese, and J.H. Carson, The cis-acting RNA trafficking signal from myelin basic protein mRNA and its cognate trans-acting ligand hnRNP A2 enhance cap-dependent translation. J Cell Biol, 1999. 147(2): p. 247-56.

[6] Hitti, E., et al., Mitogen-activated protein kinase-activated protein kinase 2 regulates tumor necrosis factor mRNA stability and translation mainly by altering tristetraprolin expression, stability, and binding to adenine/uridine-rich element. Mol Cell Biol, 2006. 26(6): p. 2399-407.
[7] De Rubeis, S. and C. Bagni, Fragile X mental retardation protein control of neuronal mRNA metabolism: Insights into mRNA stability. Mol Cell Neurosci, 2010. 43(1): p. 43-50.
[8] Aroca, A., A. Diaz-Quintana, and I. Diaz-Moreno, A structural insight into the C-terminal RNA recognition motifs of T-cell intracellular antigen-1 protein. FEBS Lett, 2011. 585(19): p. 2958-64.
[9] Sawicka, K., et al., Polypyrimidine-tract-binding protein: a multifunctional RNA-binding protein. Biochem Soc Trans, 2008. 36(Pt 4): p. 641-7.
[10] Cuadrado, A., et al., Neuronal HuD gene encoding a mRNA stability regulator is transcriptionally repressed by thyroid hormone. J Neurochem, 2003. 86(3): p. 763-73.
[11] Lopez de Silanes, I., et al., Identification of a target RNA motif for RNA-binding protein HuR. Proc Natl Acad Sci U S A, 2004. 101(9): p. 2987-92.
[12] Abdelmohsen, K., et al., Posttranscriptional gene regulation by RNA-binding proteins during oxidative stress: implications for cellular senescence. Biol Chem, 2008. 389(3): p. 243-55.
[13] Hinman, M.N. and H. Lou, Diverse molecular functions of Hu proteins. Cell Mol Life Sci, 2008. 65(20): p. 3168-81.
[14] Lopez de Silanes, I., A. Lal, and M. Gorospe, HuR: post-transcriptional paths to malignancy. RNA Biol, 2005. 2(1): p. 11-3.
[15] Kuwano, Y. and M. Gorospe, Protecting the stress response, guarding the MKP-1 mRNA. Cell Cycle, 2008. 7(17): p. 2640-2.
[16] Abdelmohsen, K., et al., Posttranscriptional orchestration of an anti-apoptotic program by HuR. Cell Cycle, 2007. 6(11): p. 1288-92.
[17] Yi, J., et al., Reduced nuclear export of HuR mRNA by HuR is linked to the loss of HuR in replicative senescence. Nucleic Acids Res, 2010. 38(5): p. 1547-58.
[18] Liao, B., Y. Hu, and G. Brewer, Competitive binding of AUF1 and TIAR to MYC mRNA controls its translation. Nat Struct Mol Biol, 2007. 14(6): p. 511-8.
[19] Raineri, I., et al., Roles of AUF1 isoforms, HuR and BRF1 in ARE-dependent mRNA turnover studied by RNA interference. Nucleic Acids Res, 2004. 32(4): p. 1279-88.
[20] Vazquez-Chantada, M., et al., HuR/methyl-HuR and AUF1 regulate the MAT expressed during liver proliferation, differentiation, and carcinogenesis. Gastroenterology, 2010. 138(5): p. 1943-53.
[21] Zucconi, B.E. and G.M. Wilson, Modulation of neoplastic gene regulatory pathways by the RNA-binding factor AUF1. Front Biosci, 2012. 17: p. 2307-25.
[22] Gratacos, F.M. and G. Brewer, The role of AUF1 in regulated mRNA decay. Wiley Interdiscip Rev RNA, 2010. 1(3): p. 457-73.
[23] Chen, C.Y., et al., AU binding proteins recruit the exosome to degrade ARE-containing mRNAs. Cell, 2001. 107(4): p. 451-64.

[24] Laroia, G., et al., Control of mRNA decay by heat shock-ubiquitin-proteasome pathway. Science, 1999. 284(5413): p. 499-502.

[25] Kim, H.S., et al., Different modes of interaction by TIAR and HuR with target RNA and DNA. Nucleic Acids Res, 2011. 39(3): p. 1117-30.

[26] Damgaard, C.K. and J. Lykke-Andersen, Translational coregulation of 5'TOP mRNAs by TIA-1 and TIAR. Genes Dev, 2011. 25(19): p. 2057-68.

[27] Gilks, N., et al., Stress granule assembly is mediated by prion-like aggregation of TIA-1. Mol Biol Cell, 2004. 15(12): p. 5383-98.

[28] Kuwano, Y., et al., NF90 selectively represses the translation of target mRNAs bearing an AU-rich signature motif. Nucleic Acids Res, 2010. 38(1): p. 225-38.

[29] Bassell, G.J. and S.T. Warren, Fragile X syndrome: loss of local mRNA regulation alters synaptic development and function. Neuron, 2008. 60(2): p. 201-14.

[30] Antar, L.N., et al., Localization of FMRP-associated mRNA granules and requirement of microtubules for activity-dependent trafficking in hippocampal neurons. Genes Brain Behav, 2005. 4(6): p. 350-9.

[31] Rooms, L. and R.F. Kooy, Advances in understanding fragile X syndrome and related disorders. Curr Opin Pediatr, 2011. 23(6): p. 601-6.

[32] Sanduja, S., et al., The role of tristetraprolin in cancer and inflammation. Front Biosci, 2012. 17: p. 174-88.

[33] Briata, P., et al., KSRP, many functions for a single protein. Front Biosci, 2011. 16: p. 1787-96.

[34] Abdelmohsen, K., et al., Phosphorylation of HuR by Chk2 regulates SIRT1 expression. Mol Cell, 2007. 25(4): p. 543-57.

[35] Masuda, K., et al., Global dissociation of HuR-mRNA complexes promotes cell survival after ionizing radiation. EMBO J, 2011. 30(6): p. 1040-53.

[36] Burd, C.G. and G. Dreyfuss, Conserved structures and diversity of functions of RNA-binding proteins. Science, 1994. 265(5172): p. 615-21.

[37] Abdelmohsen, K., et al., Ubiquitin-mediated proteolysis of HuR by heat shock. EMBO J, 2009. 28(9): p. 1271-82.

[38] Doller, A., et al., Posttranslational modification of the AU-rich element binding protein HuR by protein kinase Cdelta elicits angiotensin II-induced stabilization and nuclear export of cyclooxygenase 2 mRNA. Mol Cell Biol, 2008. 28(8): p. 2608-25.

[39] Doller, A., et al., Protein kinase C alpha-dependent phosphorylation of the mRNA-stabilizing factor HuR: implications for posttranscriptional regulation of cyclooxygenase-2. Mol Biol Cell, 2007. 18(6): p. 2137-48.

[40] Lafarga, V., et al., p38 Mitogen-activated protein kinase- and HuR-dependent stabilization of p21(Cip1) mRNA mediates the G(1)/S checkpoint. Mol Cell Biol, 2009. 29(16): p. 4341-51.

[41] Gallouzi, I.E. and J.A. Steitz, Delineation of mRNA export pathways by the use of cell-permeable peptides. Science, 2001. 294(5548): p. 1895-901.

[42] Fan, X.C. and J.A. Steitz, HNS, a nuclear-cytoplasmic shuttling sequence in HuR. Proc Natl Acad Sci U S A, 1998. 95(26): p. 15293-8.

[43] von Roretz, C., A.M. Macri, and I.E. Gallouzi, Transportin 2 regulates apoptosis through the RNA-binding protein HuR. J Biol Chem, 2011. 286(29): p. 25983-91.
[44] Rebane, A., A. Aab, and J.A. Steitz, Transportins 1 and 2 are redundant nuclear import factors for hnRNP A1 and HuR. RNA, 2004. 10(4): p. 590-9.
[45] Kedersha, N., et al., Stress granules and processing bodies are dynamically linked sites of mRNP remodeling. J Cell Biol, 2005. 169(6): p. 871-84.
[46] Abdelmohsen, K., et al., miR-519 reduces cell proliferation by lowering RNA-binding protein HuR levels. Proc Natl Acad Sci U S A, 2008. 105(51): p. 20297-302.
[47] Mukherjee, N., et al., Integrative regulatory mapping indicates that the RNA-binding protein HuR couples pre-mRNA processing and mRNA stability. Mol Cell, 2011. 43(3): p. 327-39.
[48] Galban, S., et al., RNA-binding proteins HuR and PTB promote the translation of hypoxia-inducible factor 1alpha. Mol Cell Biol, 2008. 28(1): p. 93-107.
[49] Abdelmohsen, K., et al., miR-375 inhibits differentiation of neurites by lowering HuD levels. Mol Cell Biol, 2010. 30(17): p. 4197-210.
[50] Lee, E.K., et al., RNA-Binding Protein HuD Controls Insulin Translation. Mol Cell, 2012. 45(6): p. 826-35.
[51] Bolognani, F., T. Contente-Cuomo, and N.I. Perrone-Bizzozero, Novel recognition motifs and biological functions of the RNA-binding protein HuD revealed by genome-wide identification of its targets. Nucleic Acids Res, 2010. 38(1): p. 117-30.
[52] Chung, S., et al., The Elav-like proteins bind to a conserved regulatory element in the 3'-untranslated region of GAP-43 mRNA. J Biol Chem, 1997. 272(10): p. 6593-8.
[53] Deschenes-Furry, J., N. Perrone-Bizzozero, and B.J. Jasmin, The RNA-binding protein HuD: a regulator of neuronal differentiation, maintenance and plasticity. Bioessays, 2006. 28(8): p. 822-33.
[54] Pascale, A., M. Amadio, and A. Quattrone, Defining a neuron: neuronal ELAV proteins. Cell Mol Life Sci, 2008. 65(1): p. 128-40.
[55] Amadio, M., et al., nELAV proteins alteration in Alzheimer's disease brain: a novel putative target for amyloid-beta reverberating on AbetaPP processing. J Alzheimers Dis, 2009. 16(2): p. 409-19.
[56] Ball, N.S. and P.H. King, Neuron-specific hel-N1 and HuD as novel molecular markers of neuroblastoma: a correlation of HuD messenger RNA levels with favorable prognostic features. Clin Cancer Res, 1997. 3(10): p. 1859-65.
[57] DeStefano, A.L., et al., Replication of association between ELAVL4 and Parkinson disease: the GenePD study. Hum Genet, 2008. 124(1): p. 95-9.
[58] Noureddine, M.A., et al., Association between the neuron-specific RNA-binding protein ELAVL4 and Parkinson disease. Hum Genet, 2005. 117(1): p. 27-33.
[59] Lal, A., et al., Concurrent versus individual binding of HuR and AUF1 to common labile target mRNAs. EMBO J, 2004. 23(15): p. 3092-102.
[60] Trojanowicz, B., et al., The role of AUF1 in thyroid carcinoma progression. Endocr Relat Cancer, 2009. 16(3): p. 857-71.
[61] Chang, N., et al., HuR uses AUF1 as a cofactor to promote p16INK4 mRNA decay. Mol Cell Biol, 2010. 30(15): p. 3875-86.

[62] Wang, W., et al., Increased stability of the p16 mRNA with replicative senescence. EMBO Rep, 2005. 6(2): p. 158-64.

[63] Ishimaru, D., et al., Mechanism of regulation of BCL-2 mRNA by nucleolin and A+U-rich element-binding factor 1 (AUF1). J Biol Chem, 2010. 285(35): p. 27182-91.

[64] Lal, A., et al., Posttranscriptional derepression of GADD45alpha by genotoxic stress. Mol Cell, 2006. 22(1): p. 117-28.

[65] Sarkar, B., et al., Selective degradation of AU-rich mRNAs promoted by the p37 AUF1 protein isoform. Mol Cell Biol, 2003. 23(18): p. 6685-93.

[66] Paschoud, S., et al., Destabilization of interleukin-6 mRNA requires a putative RNA stem-loop structure, an AU-rich element, and the RNA-binding protein AUF1. Mol Cell Biol, 2006. 26(22): p. 8228-41.

[67] Pautz, A., et al., Similar regulation of human inducible nitric-oxide synthase expression by different isoforms of the RNA-binding protein AUF1. J Biol Chem, 2009. 284(5): p. 2755-66.

[68] Loflin, P., C.Y. Chen, and A.B. Shyu, Unraveling a cytoplasmic role for hnRNP D in the in vivo mRNA destabilization directed by the AU-rich element. Genes Dev, 1999. 13(14): p. 1884-97.

[69] Pullmann, R., Jr., et al., Differential stability of thymidylate synthase 3'-untranslated region polymorphic variants regulated by AUF1. J Biol Chem, 2006. 281(33): p. 23456-63.

[70] Zou, T., et al., Polyamines regulate the stability of JunD mRNA by modulating the competitive binding of its 3' untranslated region to HuR and AUF1. Mol Cell Biol, 2010. 30(21): p. 5021-32.

[71] Sarkar, S., et al., AUF1 isoform-specific regulation of anti-inflammatory IL10 expression in monocytes. J Interferon Cytokine Res, 2008. 28(11): p. 679-91.

[72] Ogilvie, R.L., et al., Tristetraprolin down-regulates IL-2 gene expression through AU-rich element-mediated mRNA decay. J Immunol, 2005. 174(2): p. 953-61.

[73] Stoecklin, G., et al., Somatic mRNA turnover mutants implicate tristetraprolin in the interleukin-3 mRNA degradation pathway. Mol Cell Biol, 2000. 20(11): p. 3753-63.

[74] Stoecklin, G., et al., Cellular mutants define a common mRNA degradation pathway targeting cytokine AU-rich elements. RNA, 2001. 7(11): p. 1578-88.

[75] Stoecklin, G., et al., Genome-wide analysis identifies interleukin-10 mRNA as target of tristetraprolin. J Biol Chem, 2008. 283(17): p. 11689-99.

[76] Jalonen, U., et al., Down-regulation of tristetraprolin expression results in enhanced IL-12 and MIP-2 production and reduced MIP-3alpha synthesis in activated macrophages. Mediators Inflamm, 2006. 2006(6): p. 40691.

[77] Dranovsky, A., et al., Cdc2 phosphorylation of nucleolin demarcates mitotic stages and Alzheimer's disease pathology. Neurobiol Aging, 2001. 22(4): p. 517-28.

[78] Chen, C.Y., et al., Nucleolin and YB-1 are required for JNK-mediated interleukin-2 mRNA stabilization during T-cell activation. Genes Dev, 2000. 14(10): p. 1236-48.

[79] Otake, Y., et al., Overexpression of nucleolin in chronic lymphocytic leukemia cells induces stabilization of BCL-2 mRNA. Blood, 2007. 109(7): p. 3069-75.

[80] Jiang, Y., X.S. Xu, and J.E. Russell, A nucleolin-binding 3' untranslated region element stabilizes beta-globin mRNA in vivo. Mol Cell Biol, 2006. 26(6): p. 2419-29.
[81] Rajagopalan, L.E., et al., hnRNP C increases amyloid precursor protein (APP) production by stabilizing APP mRNA. Nucleic Acids Res, 1998. 26(14): p. 3418-23.
[82] Lee, P.T., et al., Epidermal growth factor increases the interaction between nucleolin and heterogeneous nuclear ribonucleoprotein K/poly(C) binding protein 1 complex to regulate the gastrin mRNA turnover. Mol Biol Cell, 2007. 18(12): p. 5004-13.
[83] Zhang, Y., et al., Nucleolin links to arsenic-induced stabilization of GADD45alpha mRNA. Nucleic Acids Res, 2006. 34(2): p. 485-95.
[84] Takagi, M., et al., Regulation of p53 translation and induction after DNA damage by ribosomal protein L26 and nucleolin. Cell, 2005. 123(1): p. 49-63.
[85] Bunimov, N., et al., Translational regulation of PGHS-1 mRNA: 5' untranslated region and first two exons conferring negative regulation. Biochim Biophys Acta, 2007. 1769(2): p. 92-105.
[86] Sengupta, T.K., et al., Identification of nucleolin as an AU-rich element binding protein involved in BCL-2 mRNA stabilization. J Biol Chem, 2004. 279(12): p. 10855-63.
[87] Lossi, L., et al., Posttranslational regulation of BCL-2 levels in cerebellar granule cells: A mechanism of neuronal survival. Dev Neurobiol, 2009. 69(13): p. 855-70.
[88] Zhang, B., et al., Nucleolin/C23 is a negative regulator of hydrogen peroxide-induced apoptosis in HUVECs. Cell Stress Chaperones, 2010. 15(3): p. 249-57.
[89] Ishimaru, D., et al., Regulation of BCL-2 expression by HuR in HL60 leukemia cells and A431 carcinoma cells. Mol Cancer Res, 2009. 7(8): p. 1354-66.
[90] Shukla, G.C., J. Singh, and S. Barik, MicroRNAs: Processing, Maturation, Target Recognition and Regulatory Functions. Mol Cell Pharmacol, 2011. 3(3): p. 83-92.
[91] Bartel, D.P., MicroRNAs: target recognition and regulatory functions. Cell, 2009. 136(2): p. 215-33.
[92] Kim, H.H., et al., HuR recruits let-7/RISC to repress c-Myc expression. Genes Dev, 2009. 23(15): p. 1743-8.
[93] Tominaga, K., et al., Competitive regulation of nucleolin expression by HuR and miR-494. Mol Cell Biol, 2011. 31(20): p. 4219-31.
[94] Srikantan, S., et al., Translational control of TOP2A influences doxorubicin efficacy. Mol Cell Biol, 2011. 31(18): p. 3790-801.
[95] Meisner, N.C., et al., Identification and mechanistic characterization of low-molecular-weight inhibitors for HuR. Nat Chem Biol, 2007. 3(8): p. 508-15.
[96] Chae, M.J., et al., Chemical inhibitors destabilize HuR binding to the AU-rich element of TNF-alpha mRNA. Exp Mol Med, 2009. 41(11): p. 824-31.
[97] Soundararajan, S., et al., The nucleolin targeting aptamer AS1411 destabilizes BCL-2 messenger RNA in human breast cancer cells. Cancer Res, 2008. 68(7): p. 2358-65.
[98] Ireson, C.R. and L.R. Kelland, Discovery and development of anticancer aptamers. Mol Cancer Ther, 2006. 5(12): p. 2957-62.
[99] Destouches, D., et al., Suppression of tumor growth and angiogenesis by a specific antagonist of the cell-surface expressed nucleolin. PLoS One, 2008. 3(6): p. e2518.

[100] Krust, B., et al., Suppression of tumorigenicity of rhabdoid tumor derived G401 cells by the multivalent HB-19 pseudopeptide that targets surface nucleolin. Biochimie, 2011. 93(3): p. 426-33.

[101] Hafner, M., et al., PAR-CliP--a method to identify transcriptome-wide the binding sites of RNA binding proteins. J Vis Exp, 2010(41).

Chapter 6

Cationic Peptide Interactions with Biological Macromolecules

Monde Ntwasa

Additional information is available at the end of the chapter

http://dx.doi.org/10.5772/48492

1. Introduction

Cationic amphiphilic peptides (CAPs) are widely studied as effectors that are activated by microbial pathogens in immune signaling pathways of invertebrates and vertebrates. These peptides are non-specific effectors that can kill bacteria, fungi, viruses and protozoan parasites [1, 2]. They are a universal feature in all forms of life and are often found in all the major barriers such as the skin and epithelia that are naturally designed for protection against invading microorganisms. In the case of invertebrates, they play a pivotal role in innate immunity upon which these animals depend for defense against infection. The two immunes response strategies are interdependent and innate immunity has significant impact on the development of adaptive immunity [3-6]. In addition to innate immunity, vertebrates also rely on acquired immunity which is mediated by antibodies and cytotoxic T lymphocytes [7]. Identification of these antimicrobial peptides and the study of their structural features have led to the development of peptide drugs, sometimes through the design of synthetic peptides based on the known structures of the natural ones. A subset of cationic peptides has been found to have anti-tumour as well as wound-healing properties extending the prospects of these peptides as templates for drug design strategies against cancer and wound treatment [8]. The mechanisms by which these latter properties are manifested are not fully understood. Indeed, the mechanisms by which cationic peptides exert their wide biological activities are still under investigation and many theories have been proposed.

The mode of action of cationic peptides appears to be reliant heavily but not entirely, on their structural and biophysical features. As their name suggests, they are characterized by a net positive change which contrasts conveniently with the negative charge that is characteristic of microbial membranes and cancer cells.

Studies on the antibacterial peptide mode of action produced several models that suggest that the phospholipid bilayer forming membranes is the main target of peptide action. There is, however, evidence that shows that some cationic peptides can cross the plasma membrane and interact with intracellular macromolecules.

The mechanism by which cationic peptides inhibit viral infections is also not fully understood. They are understood to act primarily against enveloped RNA and DNA viruses but there are exceptions such as the non-enveloped adenovirus and a few others. Cationic peptides appear to target viral adsorption or the entry process, replication and gene expression [9] . It remains to be seen if the mode of action against viruses can be correlated to secondary structure features of the cationic peptides. Current knowledge points to interactions with the extracellular matrix and with membrane or viral envelope proteins. Intracellular targets whereby the host is stimulated to act against the virus are also suggested.

Antifungal peptides tend to be rich in polar and neutral amino acids suggesting a functional significance that is important for interfering with a unique fungal property. Furthermore, it has been shown that in peptides with activities against both fungi and bacteria different substitutions were required for optimizing the different types of activities. Overall, it seems that these peptides interact mainly with the phospholipid bilayer to effect lysis of certain microbes. However, mounting evidence that shows existence of intracellular targets that could be polypeptide or nucleic acid in nature, suggests a wider scope for investigation to establish how these peptides execute their biological functions.

CAPs are attractive candidates for therapeutic use but their development for commercialization is hampered by certain crucial obstacles. In this chapter, biochemical interactions of CAPs together with prospects for commercialization are discussed.

2. Classes of cationic peptides

Broadly, there are two major classes of cationic peptides with antimicrobial activities (Table 1). One group is produced by bacteria and fungi and consists of non-ribosomally synthesized peptides. These peptides are assembled by multifunctional peptide synthases in large and ordered multi-enzyme and co-factor systems following the "multiple carrier model" for peptide biosynthesis [10, 11]. Examples include Gramicidin, bacitracin, polymyxin B, streptogramins, vancomycin and others. This biosynthetic process results in an extensive chemical variety that includes peptides containing hydroxyl- L- D- and unusual amino acids which can be further modified by methylation, acylation, glycosylation or cyclic ring formation [11]. The major disadvantage of these peptides is that bacteria develop resistance to them e.g. vancomycin-resistant *Staphylococcus aureus* and enterococci [12, 13].

The second major class includes gene-encoded ribosomally synthesized peptides which are further subdivided into bacteriocins (produced by bacteria) and antimicrobial peptides (produced by eukaryotes). The latter are the main object of this chapter. A prominent group of bacteriocins, composed of rare and modified amino acids is also called lantibiotics. A good example is nisin, a peptide produced by *Lactococcus lactis* with rare amino acids such

Non-ribosomally synthetized	Gene-encoded
Contain a chemical variety of amino acid	Mainly D-amino acids
	Generally amphipathic with (12 – 20 amino acids)
	Have a high net positive charge and hydrophobic residues
Highly active at low concentrations	Active at higher concentrations
May be modified	Carry no unusual posttranslational modifications
Narrow spectrum	Broad spectrum

Table 1. Comparison between gene-encoded and non-ribosomally synthetized antimicrobial peptides

as lanthionine, 3-methyllanthionine, dehydroalanine and dehydrobutyrine [14]. Lantibiotics act by either pore formation leading to disruption of the bacterial cell wall or by interfering with biosynthesis of molecules such as the peptidoglycan component of the bacterial cell wall. This results in a thinner cell wall and eventual lysis of the bacterium [15].

Antimicrobial peptides are divided into four major structural groups namely; (a) peptides that form α-helical structures, (b) cysteine-rich peptides with intramolecular disulfide bonds, (c) peptides that form β-sheets connected by a single or two disulfide bridges, and (d) peptides rich in particular amino acids such as histidine, glycine, arginine and proline or tryptophan [16-20] (Table2 and Figure 1). They have considerable sequence diversity but share important physicochemical properties. They are 12 – 50 amino acids long, carry a positive (+2 to +9) charge and are composed of 40 – 50% hydrophobic residues. In their folded state, residues segregate into hydrophilic and hydrophobic clusters producing an amphipathic structure thus allowing them to be soluble in phospholipid membranes. The combination of these electrostatic and hydrophobic interactions results in membrane disruption and key structural features that contribute to their mode of action as described later in this chapter.

It is worth noting that the antimicrobial activity of cationic peptides is dependent upon physiological conditions [1]. They are regarded as antimicrobial peptides if they can kill pathogens at physiological concentrations of divalent cations such as Mg^{2+} and Ca^{2+} (1-2 mM), monovalent cations such as Na^{+} and K^{+} (100 mM) and polyanions and mucins.

Peptide type	Example	References
α-helical structures,	Cecropin A, magainins,dermaseptin, bombinin, mellitin, cathelicidin	[16, 115, 116]
Rich in cysteine residues,	HNP-1, 2 and 3 (human defensins)	[117]
β-sheets	Tachyplesins polyphemusin II (T22), lactoferricin	[18-20]
Rich in certain amino acids such as histidine, glycine, arginine and proline or tryptophan	Histatin (histidine), indolicidin (tryptophan), tritripticin, holotricin (glycine & histidine), coleoptericin (glycine), pyrrhocoricin (proline)	[69, 118-120]

Table 2. Classes of AMPs

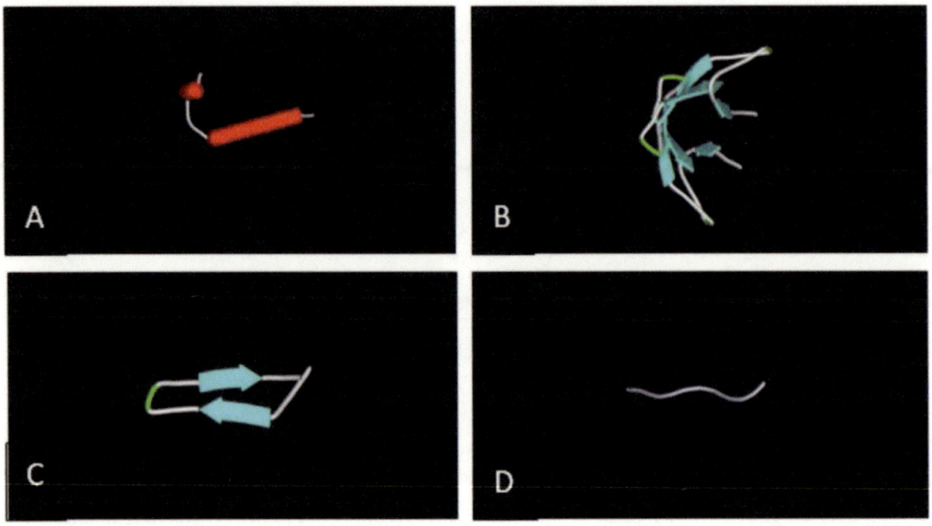

Figure 1. Structures and examples of cationic peptides representing different classes.. **A**. α-helical peptide - BMA-27 (PDB ID: 2KET). **B**. β-sheet peptide with disulfide bridges - human defensin (PDB ID: 3GNY) **C**. anti-parallel β-sheet - tachyplesin 1 (PDB ID: 1WO1), **D**. peptides with amino acid bias - Indolicidin (PDB ID: 1G89).

2. Modes of action of cationic peptides

The activity of antimicrobial peptides (AMPs) and their potential use as therapeutic agents rely on differences between mammalian and bacterial subcellular structures as well as between normal and abnormal (apoptotic and tumour) mammalian cells. The current dogma for microbial killing by cationic peptides is that they target the phospholipid bilayer and kill microorganisms by pore formation or membrane disruption leading to cell lysis. There is, however, growing evidence showing that some peptides act on intracellular macromolecular targets. In some cases it is debatable whether killing is due to intracellular targeting or a combination of this and membrane disruption. Nevertheless, good understanding of the mechanisms of action of AMPs should provide promising opportunities for drug design. Before reviewing their mode of action it is therefore necessary to consider the landscape of human and pathogen cell membranes. Generally, the cationic nature of antimicrobial peptides facilitates electrostatic attraction to the negatively charged microbial membrane phospholipids and their hydrophobicity facilitates cell membrane penetration. However, there are subtle differences in the mechanism of action of the various peptides.

Structural features of animal and bacterial cells

The distribution of phospholipids on the outer and inner leaflets of the plasma membrane in eukaryotic cells is asymmetric. Typically, the outer surface of normal mammalian cells is composed of neutral zwitterionic phospholipids and cholesterol [8]. It is largely composed of choline-containing phospholipids such as sphingolimyelin and phosphatidylcholine, while aminophospholipids such as phosphatidyliserine and phosphatidylyethanolamine dominate the inner leaflet [21]. In addition to the heterogeneity of headgroups and acyl chains, the presence of cholesterol in animal cells introduces more complexity to the membrane landscape by promoting the formation of lipid microdomains [22].

On the other hand, bacterial membranes are predominantly composed of acidic phospholipids (such as phosphatidylglycerol and cardiolipin) that confer a net negative charge to the surface of the membrane while phosphatidylethanolamine and phosphatidylserine are not detectable [23-25]. Since AMPs have to cross the negatively charged lipopolysaccharide layer before reaching the membrane, the possible impact of this barrier has been investigated. The negative charge on the lipopolysaccharide (LPS) rather than the size of the saccharide moiety is important for susceptibility of the bacterial cell to antimicrobial activity of the cationic peptides. This was demonstrated by experiments using bacterial LPS mutants with varying lengths of the polysaccharide moiety but an equal number of phosphate groups. In these mutants the phosphate groups would, however, be heterogeneous due to further modifications resulting in diverse phosphorylation patterns amongst mutants. It was found that the LPS mutants display differential susceptibility to cationic peptides in a manner that seems to be related to charge location and magnitude and to absence or presence of the O-antigen side chain [23, 26]. It is proposed that because of their greater affinity for LPS than divalent cations and their bulkiness, cationic peptides competitively displace these ions and create a passage through the outer bacterial membrane thus propelling themselves to the cytoplasmic membrane by a "self-promoted uptake" [27].

Loss of asymmetry with distinct bias in phospholipid types is observed in tumorigenic cells when compared to animal cells. Cancer cells are known to carry a predominantly negative charge due to high levels of the anionic phosphatidylserine, O-glycosylated mucins, sialylated gangliosides and heparin sulphates [28, 29]. The membranes of tumorigenic cells also contain a significantly higher number of microvilli compared to normal cells effectively increasing the surface area of cancer cells [21].

Cationic peptides interactions with the phospholipid bilayer of membranes

Cationic peptides are attracted to the negatively charged prokaryotic membranes and kill microbial pathogens by causing disintegration of their membranes and subsequent collapse of electrochemical gradients [23, 30, 31]. Various models of membranolytic activities of AMPs have been proposed. These include the (i) barrel stave (ii) Carpet (iii) toroidal model, and (iii) channel-forming models reviewed in [2, 32, 33] .

i. *The barrel stave model* – this model is based on the amphipathic α-helical peptides forming contacts with headgroups on the inner and outer surfaces of the membrane bilayer using their hydrophilic ends while their hydrophobic regions make contact with the acyl chains of the phospholipids. This results in transmembrane pore channels whose inner surface or lumen consists of the hydrophilic regions of the peptides. Binding to the membrane is probably driven by hydrophobic interactions with the membrane hydrophobic core and requires aggregation of several peptide monomers or oligomers in an α-helical form. This model proposes a stepwise sequence beginning with the peptides reaching the membrane and assembling at the surface. After recruitment of more monomers, they insert into the core of the membrane. Only a few pores are required to dissipate the transmembrane potential in cells [34]. The "barrel stave" model applies to certain peptides such as the non-ribosomally synthesized antibiotic, alamethicin [35] and the gene-encoded pardaxin, a polypetide *Purdachirus marmorutus* toxin with a helix-hinge-helix structure [36, 37].

ii. *The carpet model* – was first described for the action of dermaseptin and later for cecropin, the human cathelicidin LL-37 and others [33]. Binding of these peptides to the membrane is initially electrostatically driven and the peptides are not required to adopt a particular structural form. It is proposed that binding to bacterial membranes takes place in four defined steps [33, 34]. Initially, the peptides make contact with the LPS on Gram-negative bacteria or the teichoic acids on Gram-positive bacteria and traverse the membrane in a carpet-like fashion. The peptides then align themselves such that their hydrophobic regions face the lipids and their hydrophilic regions face the phospholipid headgroups. This is followed by the accumulation of peptides until a threshold concentration is reached. Finally, the peptides permeate the membrane and disrupt it causing the collapse of the bilayer. This model is sometimes referred as the *detergent model* and is characterized by the accumulation of the peptide which drives the eventual catastrophic collapse of the membrane.

iii. *The toroidal model* – was first proposed by [38, 39] to describe the action of the *Xenopus laevis* AMP, magainin 2. Later it was found that peptides such as mellitin and protegrins also induce transmembrane pores in the toroidal fashion [35]. In this model, the peptides aggregate such that both the phospholipid headgroups of the monolayers and the peptides line the lumen of the pore. This results in the formation of a dynamic core consisting of the lipid monolayers and peptides with a characteristic lipid flip-flop.

iv. *The aggregate or channel-forming model* – appears to be a subtle variation of the toroidal mechanism. It was first suggested after a study using short (10 – 14 amino acids) peptides and a membrane potential-sensitive cyanide dye. This model portrayed concentration- and voltage dependent peptide aggregation within the membrane without any fixed stoichiometry [40]. It was also described for sapecin, an antibacterial insect defensin isolated from the flesh fly, *Sarcophaga peregrina* [41]. In this study, the initial attraction to the membrane was found to be electrostatic with cardiolipin playing an important role. It had been shown previously that sapecin has a remarkable affinity for cardiolipin which is abundant in *Staphylococcus aureus*. Furthermore, *E. coli* mutants defective in cardiolipin synthesis were resistant to sapecin compared to wild type *E. coli* [42]. Using glucose leakage experiments it was shown that membrane permeabilization is dose-dependent and follows a sigmoidal curve. This cooperativity suggests that oligomerization is an important factor during permebilization [41]. A similar mechanism was noted in a previous study involving the wasp venom mastoparan which was found to exhibit pore formation dynamics that are concurrent with mellitin but with some differences [43, 44].

A recent review of these peptide modes of action introduces new models that have been proposed. Some of these are variations of the older ones described above [45]. They include the *detergent model,* the *sinking raft model,* the *lipid clustering mode,* the *interfacial activity models* and *molecular shape model*. These models have the common premise of non-pore formation.

Cationic peptide interaction with nucleic acids

There is considerable evidence that shows that some antimicrobial cationic peptides can pass the membrane with minimum disruption, suggesting that they may have intracellular targets. Furthermore several peptides have been shown to bind DNA *in vitro*. Others inhibit important cytosolic proteins thereby interfering with key cellular processes.

When, tachyplesin, a 17 residue arginine-rich peptide, was isolated it was shown to kill bacteria at low concentrations and to form complexes with bacterial lipopolysaccharide [46]. While evidence indicates that tachyplesin interacts with lipid membranes and kills bacteria by leakage, the exact mechanism of leakage and killing remains poorly defined [47]. Tachyplesin I is a cyclic broad-spectrum antimicrobial peptide with a rigid, antiparallel β-sheet and two intramolecular S-S linkages [46]. This structural motif is known to contribute to DNA binding [48]. Indeed, using DNase1 protection and other DNA footprinting-like techniques [49] showed that tachyplesin binds DNA. Furthermore, they showed that it probably binds to the minor groove as methylation of a guanine in the major groove was not affected by the presence of the peptide. However, the antiparallel β-sheet motif has been shown, by 3D solution structures of DNA complexes with proteins, to be involved in DNA binding by making contacts with the major groove [50, 51]. The chemical configuration in the major and minor groove is important as it indicates specificity and non-specificity or interactions respectively.

Another member of the tachyplesin family, polyphemusin I also accumulates in the cytoplasm fairly rapidly without causing membrane damage and shows subtle signs that it may interact with DNA [52]. In crossing the plasma membrane these peptides induce transient pore formation and membrane permeability [53-55]. Using unmodified and PEGylated versions tachyplesin I was shown to induce lipid flip-flops characteristic of the toroidal mode of pore formation. In these experiments, PEGylation did not alter the mode of interaction between the peptide and lipid membranes but lowered both DNA binding ability and antimicrobial activity. It may be reasonable therefore to assume that tachyplesin targets both the membrane and DNA but the main method of bacterial killing is still elusive.

Buforins represent another group of AMPs that translocate across the membrane via transient pores. The 21 amino acid peptide buforin 2 is a more potent derivative of buforin 1 and has broad spectrum antimicrobial activity [56]. It is translocated across the lipid bilayer in a manner similar to maganin2 but without inducing severe membrane permeabilization due to a proline (Pro^{11}) that distorts the helical form of the peptide, concentrating basic amino acids in a limited amphipathic region and thereby enhancing electrostatic repulsion within and efficient translocation through the pore. The rapid and transient nature of the translocation limits membrane permeabilization by buforin 2. DNA–binding studies show that buforin 2 binds DNA and RNA and that buforin influences cellular processes to do with nucleic acid metabolism [56, 57]. Buforin IIb, an anticancer synthetic analogue of buforin II, crosses the membrane without causing damage and accumulates in the nucleus. Furthermore, buforin IIb accumulates primarily in nuclei of Jurkat cells and induces mitochondria-dependent apoptosis in a mechanism that is not clearly understood [58]. Buforin 1 and II share complete sequence identity with the N-terminal region of histone H2A (H2A tail) that interacts directly with nucleic acids [59]. The H2A tails play a crucial role in maintaining the stability of the nucleosome by making specific interactions with DNA. In the nucleosome particle, they adopt a disordered conformation with many residues not making contact with DNA. The arginines, however, interact with the minor groove [60]. It is not clear whether the H2A tail interaction with chromatin can be taken as a model for buforin interactions. The helix–hinge-helix structure of buforin has been evaluated using phospholipid interactions but interactions with DNA have so far been demonstrated using techniques such as electrophoretic mobility shift assays. A 3D solution structure of a buforin- DNA complex may elucidate the exact nature of their interaction.

The actual contact between an AMP and DNA was demonstrated with indolicidin, a potent cationic peptide that enters bacterial cells without causing lysis and inhibits DNA replication [61]. These experiments showed that indolicidin assumes different environment-dependent conformations and prefers to bind certain sequences of double stranded DNA and that it binds poorly to single stranded DNA . This provides evidence that peptide-DNA interactions are not simple electrostatic attractions. Specific DNA-peptide interactions are often facilitated by the major groove environment which has richer chemical information than the minor groove [62, 63]. It may be expected then that the peptide makes specific contacts such as hydrogen bonds and hydrophobic interactions in the major groove and electrostatic contacts with the phosphate backbone. Other peptides may interact with nucleic acids. .

The DNA-binding property of cationic peptides together with subcellular localization into the nucleus may provide opportunities for development of delivery systems. Indeed a cationic amphipathic peptide called KALA was designed for delivery of DNA into cells [64]. Similarly the histidine-rich synthetic peptide known as LAH4 was also developed as a DNA carrier that can be used in a wide variety of applications including basic research, therapy and vaccination [65]. These prospects underline the importance of investigating the precise nature of the interaction between cationic peptides and nucleic acids.

Cationic peptide interaction with other subcellular targets

As stated earlier, some antimicrobial peptides have the ability to transiently permeabilize and translocate across the plasma membrane and cause death of the target pathogen without causing cell lysis. This indicates that these peptides may have intracellular targets. It is recorded that such cellular targets could include macromolecules in protein and lipid biosynthetic pathways and in nucleic acid metabolism (Table 3 and 4). It has not been established whether there are unique characteristics possessed by this class of peptides enabling them to target intracellular molecules.

Peptides	Mode of action	Reference
Buforin II and buforin IIb	Binds DNA	[56, 58, 70]
Tachyplesin	Binds DNA	[48, 121]
Mersadin	Inhibits cell wall synthesis	[122]
PR-39	Inhibits replication and protein synthesis	[123]
PR-26	Alters cytoplasmic membrane	[124]
Indolicidin	Replication, Alters cytoplasmic membrane	[61, 125]
Microcin 25	Alters cytoplasmic membrane	[126]
Pleurocidin	Inhibits nucleic acid metabolism	[127]
HNP-1	Inhibits nucleic acid metabolism	[128]
HNP-2	Inhibits nucleic acid metabolism	[128]
Dermaseptin	Inhibits nucleic acid metabolism	[127]
Histatins	Inhibits enzyme activity	[129]
Pyrrhocoricin	Inhibits enzyme activity	[129]
Drosocin	Inhibits enzyme activity	[129]
apidaecin	Inhibits enzyme activity	[129]
Pre-elafin/trappin-2	Binds DNA	[130, 131]
Lactoferricin	Regulation of transcription	[54] and references therein
Cecropin A	Gene expression	[132]

Table 3. Cationic peptides with intracellular killing activities

AMP	Interacting molecule	Reference
PR-39	Membrane receptor, multiple, SH3 domain-containing intracellular proteins and p85a (regulatory subunit of phosphatidylyinositol 3-kinase, (nucleic acids unconfirmed)	[123, 133]
Buforin II	Nucleic acids (both RNA and DNA), inhibits transcription or translation	[56]
Mellitin	Hyperactivation of phospholipase A_2	
Tachyplesin	C1q activating the classi complement pathway	[91]
Lactoferricin B	Heparin-like molecules preventing angiogenesis	[96]
Histatin 5	67 kDa fungal protein	[74]
Histatin 5	*B. gingivalis* trypsin-like protease	[78]
Pyrrhochoricin, drosocin, apidaecin	DnaK preventing chaperone-assisted protein folding	[66, 67]
Apidaecins	Probably a permease transporter and protein involved in protein synthesis	[85]
Cathelicidin LL-37/ hCAP-18	binds to formyl peptide receptor-like 1 (FPRL1), a G protein-coupled, seven-transmembrane cell receptor found on various cell types including macrophages, neutrophils and subsets of lymphocytes	[100]
Mouse Cathelin-related antimicrobial peptide (CRAMP)	binds to formyl peptide receptor-like 1 (FPRL1)	[101]

Table 4. Putative non-lipid molecular targets of CAPs

Peptides that belong to the proline-rich family, pyrrhocoricin, apidaecin and drosocin enter bacterial cells and macrophages and are distributed in all cellular compartments. These peptides bind specifically to the *E. coli* 70 kDa heat shock protein, DnaK preventing chaperone-assisted protein folding and death of the bacterium [66]. They appear to enter the cell in a LPS-mediated manner. Importantly, they do not bind to the equivalent human Hsp70 protein, pointing to a potential pharmaceutical benefit [67].

Proline is known to be a unique amino acid in facilitating macromolecular binding. Due to some unique biophysical reasons proline was found to facilitate macromolecular interactions by means of proline-rich motifs or even as a single proline residue [68]. Indeed it has been suggested that proline-rich modules may be a natural occurrence that facilitates membrane penetration [69]. Several examples have been recorded indicating that proline is important in AMP activity. The DNA-binding buforin II has a proline hinge which is crucial for membrane penetration [59, 70]. Cathelicidins have a α-helical N-terminus with antibacterial activity and a proline-containing C-terminus that is required for membrane penetration [69]. The endogenous proline-arginine (PR)-rich peptide, PR-39 inhibits NDPH oxidase by docking to the Src homology 3 (SH3) domain of this enzyme [71]. PR-39 is also implicated in blocking DNA replication [72]. This is consistent with established observations that proline-rich motifs are crucial for bind to signaling molecules with domains such as SH3 [68]. Detailed Structure-based analysis of the proline-rich motif and SH3 domain interaction shows how a crucial RXL motif in proline-rich ligands binds to the SH3 domain [73]. Systematic mutations of residues in the SH3 domain and the proline-rich ligand revealed that two crucial prolines interact directly with the domain while others form a molecular scaffold. Furthermore, arginine and lysine residues are involved in extensive interactions conferring specificity.

Some AMPs that are likely to have intracellular targets use unconventional mechanisms to enter the cell. These include the histatin family and apidaecins. Histatins, a family of histidine-rich AMPs found in human saliva enter the cell in a receptor-mediated manner and target the mitochondria [74]. The histatin family consists of AMPs that have potent activity against fungi and constitutes an important aspect of antifungal and wound healing activity in the oral cavity [74, 75]. It was found that histatin 5 kills intact *Candida albicans* without causing lysis and that spheroplasts (fragile with fragments of the cell wall) were 14-fold less susceptible compared to the intact cells. Binding studies showed that histatin 5 targets at least one specific protein that was detected in whole cell extracts and crude membrane fractions but not in the cell wall fraction and in spheroplasts [76]. Surprisingly, the human neutrophil defensin 1 (HNP-1) which differs structurally to histatins appeared to act in the same manner as histatin 5, probably sharing the same molecular target in *Candida albicans* [77]. Besides, histatin 5 was found to be an inhibitor of *B. gingivalis* trypsin-like protease probably accounting for natural protection against periodontitis [78]. They reduce the activity of a *Bacteroides gingivalis* trypsin-like protease by competitive inhibition [78]. This protease may be responsible for the periodontitis caused by *B. gingivalis* [79, 80], implying that histatins play an important role in combating oral pathogens. This was initially observed with lantibiotics such as nisin Z which uses Lipid II as a receptor [81] and mesentericin Y, a 37 amino acid peptide isolated from *Leuconostoc mesenteroides*. This peptide targets a specific receptor found only on the food-borne *listeria*. Generally, these peptides a have a characteristic structure with two domains; a recognition domain for binding to a receptor and an α-helical domain responsible for pore formation. Removal of the recognition domain results in loss of pathogen selectivity.

Some peptides exhibit anti-viral activity by mechanisms that albeit poorly understood, appear to be non-membrane dependent. The synthetic [Tyr5,12,Lys7]-polyphemusin II peptide (T22) inhibits HIV replication apparently by competition with cellular proteins required for viral attachment e.g. CD4 [82]. Mellitin and its inactive analogue can competitively inhibit the infectivity of the tobacco mosaic virus due to structural similarities with the virus capsid region required for RNA interaction [83].

Apidaecins are short proline-arginine-rich and highly antibacterial peptides that kill Gram-negative bacteria without forming pores [84, 85]. Their activity is limited to Gram-negative bacteria. Interestingly, they are distant relatives of the mammalian peptide PR-39. Apidaecin uptake was found to be actively driven by an energy-dependent mechanism, stereospecific and irreversible. The transporter-mediated model was demonstrated by the fact that pretreatment of cells with an oxidative phosphorylation uncoupler reduced uptake of apidaecin but did not prevent the uptake of a known pore-former, D-Mag (all D-magainin isomer). Furthermore, uptake of the apidaecin peptide was reduced by the presence of a proline-rich peptide (L-Pro) but not its enantiomer (D-Pro) indicating receptor dependence. Apidaecin may also act downstream on at least one indispensable cellular target as some peptide analogs entered the cell without killing it. Inhibition of protein synthesis by apidaecin suggests that it interferes with the translation machinery of the bacterium. The probable target is the 30S ribosomal subunit as cooperative inhibition by tetracycline (a known inhibitor of this subunit) and apidaecin was demonstrated [85]. Apidaecin is also implicated in interfering with protein folding by inhibiting the activity of DnaK [67, 86]. Since apidaecins are non-toxic to human cells better understanding of their mode of action is necessary. It seems probable that the intracellular targets of apidaecin are unique to Gram-negative bacteria. Nevertheless, the identification of intracellular targets of AMPs in general is important for the design of species- or strain-specific drugs.

Role of cationic peptides in anticancer therapy and wound healing

Current anticancer agents have limited success due to non-selective killing of cancer and normal cells and often result in the development of resistance. The discovery of new anticancer strategies is therefore urgent. Many studies have shown that cationic AMPs have anticancer properties. These peptides are divided into two classes; one that consists of peptides that are toxic to bacteria and cancer cells but not to human cells and another class with peptides that are toxic bacteria and to both cancer and normal human cells [87]. It is believed that they have membranolytic and non-membranolytic modes of action [8, 28]. The membranolytic activity is presumed to be based on the different compositions of cancer and normal membranes and includes the disruption of mitochondrial membrane. The disruption of the membrane probably occurs by some of the modes describes earlier; such as the "carpet" model. These peptides can also cause permeation of the mitochondrial membrane releasing cytochrome c followed by apoptosis. Such apoptosis would also cause caspase 9 activation and conversion of pro-caspase3 to caspase 3. Buforin IIb which displayed selective cytotoxicity against 62 cell lines provides a good example in this instance. It crosses cell membranes without causing damage and causes mitochondria-dependent apoptosis characterized by caspase 9 activation [58]. The exact mechanism of apoptotic killing is not clear as it is for many other cationic peptides. Mitochondria-dependent apoptosis can also occur by the death receptor associated pathway [88].

It seems that different Amps induce different apoptotic pathways and membranolytic mechanisms. A COOH-terminal fragment of the cathelicidin LL-37 pre-protein, hCAP-18 was found to selectively kill oral squamous carcinoma cells and not healthy human fibroblast or HaCaT cells by apoptosis that is characterized by mitochondrial depolarisation with no detectable caspase 3 or in a caspase-independent mechanism [89]. Tachyplesin that was conjugated to an integrin homing peptide killed both tumour and endothelial cells by a mitochondrial and death receptor -dependent pathways [90]. On the other hand, tachyplesin was shown to kill tumour cells by interacting with hyaluronan and C1q a key component of the complement pathway thus activating the classic complement pathway leading to loss of membrane integrity and cell lysis [91].

The non-membranolytic mechanism is probably facilitated by interaction with specific proteins or through processes that activate specific intracellular molecules. Mellitin is reported to selectively promote the destruction of ras oncogene-transformed cells by preferentially activating phospholipase A2 and causing calcium influx [92, 93]. Lactoferricin B (LfcinB), a cationic AMP that is cytotoxic to human and rodent cancer cells, kills human leukaemia and breast carcinoma cells by a sequential process involving generation of reactive oxygen species, mitochondrial membrane depolarization and activation of the caspase cascade leading to death by apoptosis [94]. However, LfcinB kills human B-lymphoma cells in a caspase-independent mechanism [95]. Furthermore, LfcinB was found to prevent angiogenesis by interacting with a heparin-like molecule on the surface of human umbilical vein endothelial cells (HUVECs) [96].

There is a growing number of AMPs that appear to promote wound healing. It is generally noticeable that wounds in the oral cavity heal faster than skin lesions for example but it has emerged recently that this may be attributable to the histatin family, at least in part. At least two histatins have been identified as the major wound healing factors in human saliva [75]. Moreover this property was associated with active uptake of histatin by epithelial cells and the activation of an extracellular signal-regulated kinases ½ signalling pathway suggesting a mechanism by which these peptides effect their non-AMP role. Wound healing is a localized process which involves inflammation, wound cell migration and mitosis, neovascularization, and regeneration of the extracellular matrix and is known to be mediated by peptide growth factors such as the epidermal growth factor (EGF) and transforming growth factor alpha (TGF-α) [97]. At least TGF-α has been shown to act by activating the expression of AMPs hCAP-18/LL-37 and human β-defensin 3 in addition to the larger proteins often found during injury, the neutrophil gelatinase-associated lipocalin, and secretory leukocyte protease inhibitor in human keratinocytes [98]. And cathelicidins are known to regulate cellular responses including cell proliferation, cell migration of inflammatory cells, release of cytokines and angiogenesis [99]. The cathelicidin hCAP-18 interacts with formyl peptide receptor-like 1 (FPRL1), a G protein-coupled, seven transmembrane cell receptor [100]. And the only known mouse cathelicidin-like protein the cathelin-related antimicrobial peptide (CRAMP) known to be angiogenic was further shown to be chemotactic for human monocytes, neutrophils, macrophages, and mouse peripheral blood leukocytes [101]. Clearly, as the multi-functional role of antimicrobial peptides unravels, the number of peptides involved in non-infection related processes and new molecular targets are set to increase.

3. Drug design strategies

Cationic antimicrobial peptides have key characteristics that make them attractive candidates for pharmaceutical development: (i) they are active against a broad spectrum of Gram-negative and Gram-positive bacteria (including the multiple drug resistant strains), fungi, viruses and protozoa – a single peptide can act against all these pathogens (ii) generally, they do not target specific pathogen molecules reducing development of resistance, and (iii) they are potent and kill pathogens rapidly [1, 102]. There are, however, obstacles that hinder the commercialization of AMPs. Commercialization of antimicrobial peptides is hindered by various pharmacokinetic obstacles that may require some engineering to resolve and are indeed the object of intensive research worldwide. Absorption, distribution, metabolism and excretion (ADME) are vital pharmacokinetic parameters that must be satisfied by successful drug candidates, and major challenges have emerged with respect to peptide drugs. Some of the key shortcomings that should be addressed to improve rational peptide-based drug design are:

i. Low bioavailability
ii. Toxicity
iii. High cost of production

There are several ideas about to overcome some of them (Table 5) and many researchers are investigating ways to remove these obstacles and move to commercialization.

Bioavailability and biodistribution

Peptide drugs have to overcome barriers that affect absorption, transport (systemic distribution) and translocation through membranes. These barriers are associated with the physicochemical properties of peptides such as aqueous solubility, lipophilicity, hydrogen bond formation and metabolic stability. Rapid degradation by proteolytic enzymes of the digestive tract, blood plasma and tissues is one of the major limitations attributed to peptide drugs as it limits oral availability and injection. These scenarios are further complicated by the fact that peptides are also subjected to rapid clearance by the liver and kidneys. Their physicochemical properties such as hydrophilicity and high conformation flexibility (no selectivity by specific receptors) also affect biodistribution.

Limitation	Cause	Solution	Reference
High cost	Regulatory and technological factors	Development of efficient and robust process of chemical synthesis Design short and compositionally simple peptides	[114, 134]
Low (especially oral) bioavailability	Peptides being substrates of digestive enzymes, blood plasma and tissues Rapid hepatic clearance Rapid renal clearance Poor biodistribution	Use of D-amino acids Peptide backbone alterations Protective delivery systems Chemical modification of protease cleavage sites	[1, 135]
Poor biodistribution	Hydrophilicity High conformational flexibility – non selective		
Toxicity	Immunogenicity Non-specific targets Some act on growth factors (wound healing) – may promote tumourigenesis	Pro-drug use e.g mellitin-biotin conjugates	[111]

Table 5. Challenges in drug design

There are several approaches to optimize lead peptides to circumvent bioavailability and biodistribution obstacles. These include (i) replacement of natural with unnatural or D- (rather than L-) amino acids, (ii) use of peptidometrics introducing non-peptidic backbones, (iii) adopting alternative formulations such as liposomes and (iv) modification to create protease resistant prodrugs [103]. The routes of drugs given systemically and orally are shown schematically in Figure 2 and Box 1 to indicate pharmacokinetic obstacles.

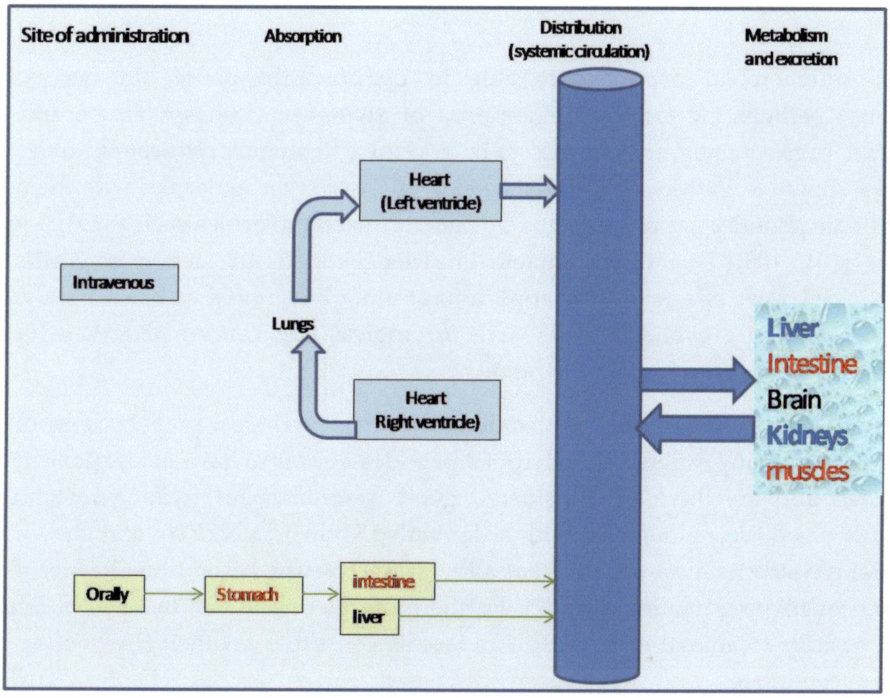

Figure 2. Distribution of drugs given intravenously and orally and obstacles that affect bioavailability. To be read together with Box 1.

BOX 1

When a drug is given intravenously it enters the systemic circulation via the right ventricle of the heart , flows past the lungs, into the left ventricle and finally into the rest of the circulatory system (Figure 2). Oral administration introduces the peptide into the strongly acidic environment of the stomach and later to high levels of proteolytic enzymes in the intestines. The main limitations to bioavailability of antimicrobial peptides are pre-systemic and systemic enzymatic degradation. When the peptide is given orally it could also undergo "first-pass" metabolism in the liver and the gastrointestinal tract. The major threat to the peptides lies in the small intestine where there are large quantities of peptidases [136]. Oral and intravenous delivery of peptides is therefore a major challenge for pharmaceutical science and demands innovative strategies. Biological barriers such as the Blood Brain Barrier (BBBB) and placenta are additional obstacles to delivery of AMPs.

Strategies that can be considered to circumvent these problems are:

i. Alternative routes of administration
- Subcutaneous injection
- Intramuscular
- Mucosal (nasal sprays)
- Sublingual delivery
- Transdermal routes (patches)

ii. Penetration enhancers
iii. Protease inhibitors

Toxicity

Broadly, antimicrobial peptides are able to disrupt prokaryotic but not eukaryotic membranes because the latter are composed of zwitterionic phospholipids and contain cholesterol. Consequently, they appear to be non-toxic to animals. However, some peptides have been shown to translocate into cells and even carry other molecules with them. Indeed some cationic peptides are proposed as carriers for macromolecules such as DNA in certain instances [104, 105]. Due to incomplete knowledge about the action of AMPs on the eukaryotic cell, toxic effects of their application cannot be ignored or taken lightly. Indeed, all the commercially available AMPs are for topical applications and there is lack of confidence in other forms of administration.

About 38% of drug candidates are abandoned in Phase I clinical trials because of toxicity [106]. However, many cationic antimicrobial peptides appear to have no cytotoxicity against mammalian and are therefore considered good candidates for treating infections. One example is plecstasin, a defensin with a derivative known as NZ2114 and shown to have additional physicochemical benefits that allow it to cross the blood brain barrier making it attractive for treating meningitis [107]. Furthermore plecstasin can be used at high doses without toxicity to animal cells [108]. Apidaecins constitute another group of apparently non-toxic candidates and have been discussed earlier in the chapter. Toxicity, of antimicrobial peptides is still a matter not rigorously investigated to date. Often their hemolytic activity is tested.

There are many unresolved issues about the mechanism of killing of AMPs compounded by the probable existence of intracellular targets. Fears are caused by the possibility that toxicity could emerge *in vivo* based on interaction between the AMPs and unknown subcellular targets. Currently, there is accumulating evidence showing that AMPs can kill eukaryotic cells by apoptosis. Two cathelicidins, BMAP-27 and BMAP-28 were shown to be toxic to transformed cell lines, fresh tumor cells and proliferating lymphocytes at microbicide concentrations. This cytotoxicity is associated with membrane disruption, calcium influx and subsequent apoptosis [109]. AMPs are apparently attracted to these cells because of an increase in negative charge introduced by sialylation of glycoproteins on transformed cells and activated lymphocytes as treatment of U937 cell by neuraminidase abrogated the toxic effect. Furthermore, the human cathelicidin LL-37 was shown to induce apoptosis *in vitro* in a human airway epithelial cell line and *in vivo* in a murine airway [110]. LL-37 induced dose-dependent and caspase 3 dependent apoptosis in human lung epithelial cell line A549 [110]. This cell death was inhibited by caspase 3 inhibitor and by human but not by bovine serum. Clearly, there is need to investigate the physiological impact of AMPs. Toxicity can be addressed by several means including the use of prodrug format whereby a drug conjugate is designed to be activated at specific tissues. For instance, the anticancer peptide mellitin was conjugated to a biotin moiety which could be selectively cleaved in ovarian carcinoma cells by matrix metalloproteinase-2 which are highly expressed in these cells [111].

Cost of production

Cost of peptide production tended to increase at an alarming rate in the past decade due to regulatory and technological factors [112]. Technically, the cost of producing a peptide is dependent on size. Size also determines the method of production. Peptides may be produced by chemical synthesis, recombinant DNA technology, cell free expression systems, enzymatic synthesis and by the use of transgenic animals and plants. Since these peptides can sometimes involve unnatural amino acids, chemical synthesis may provide a wide range of peptide derivatives. To this end the discovery of the solid phase peptide synthesis method was a major step boosting peptide drug production [113]. It is now possible to produce peptides as long as 50 amino acids by chemical synthesis and produce therapeutic peptides on a large scale [114]. Indeed, now the chemical synthesis of peptides provides cheaper manufacturing costs compared to recombinant production [103]. This obstacle is likely to be overcome in the near future.

4. Conclusion

Cationic peptides are attractive molecules for clinical use. They have multifunctional properties as anti-infective agents that are able to kill bacteria, fungi, viruses and parasites as well as cancer cells. Their activity depends largely on their structural features and unique features in the landscape of prokaryotic and eukaryotic cell membranes. Some of these peptides have gone through clinical trials and reached commercialization but only for topical application. There are many obstacles that hinder development of cationic peptides for administration by the oral route or by injection. These are bioavailability, biodistribution and potential toxicity. These obstacles can be overcome by better understanding of the mechanism of action and killing of these peptides. More research is required in this area. The high cost of production has been a major obstacle for a long time. New advances in the chemical synthesis technology have greatly reduced the cost of production and now large scale chemical synthesis is possible. This method is preferable because of the opportunities it provides for the inclusion of unnatural amino acids during production. Recombinant DNA synthesis is another method that can be perfected to manufacture peptides at low cost.

Author details

Monde Ntwasa
School of Molecular & Cell Biology, University of the Witwatersrand

5. References

[1] Hancock REW, Sahl H-G. Antimicrobial and host-defense peptides as new anti-infective therapeutic strategies. Nat Biotech. [10.1038/nbt1267]. 2006;24(12):1551-7.
[2] Wiesner J, Vilcinskas A. Antimicrobial peptides: The ancient arm of the human immune system. Virulence. 2010;1(5):440-64.

[3] Cederlund A, Gudmundsson GH, Agerberth B. Antimicrobial peptides important in innate immunity. FEBS Journal. 2011;278(20):3942-51.
[4] Medzhitov R, Janeway JCA. Innate immunity: The virtues of a nonclonal system of recognition. Cell. 1997;91:295-8.
[5] Akira S, Uematsu S, Takeuchi O. Pathogen recognition and innate immunity. Cell. 2006;124(4):783-801.
[6] Medzhitov R, Janeway Jr CA. Innate immunity: impact on the adaptive immune response. Current Opinion in Immunology. 1997;9(1):4-9.
[7] Salzet M. Vertebrate innate immunity resembles a mosaic of invertebrate immune responses. Trends in Immunology. 2001;22(6):285-8.
[8] Hoskin DW, Ramamoorthy A. Studies on anticancer activities of antimicrobial peptides. Biochimica et Biophysica Acta (BBA) - Biomembranes. 2008;1778(2):357-75.
[9] Wachinger M, Kleinschmidt A, Winder D, von Pechmann N, Ludvigsen A, Neumann M, et al. Antimicrobial peptides melittin and cecropin inhibit replication of human immunodeficiency virus 1 by suppressing viral gene expression. Journal of General Virology. 1998;79(4):731-40.
[10] Stein T, Vater J, Kruft V, Otto A, Wittmann-Liebold B, Franke P, et al. The multiple carrier model of nonribosomal peptide biosynthesis at modular multienzymatic templates. Journal of Biological Chemistry. 1996;271(26):15428-35.
[11] Hancock REW, Chapple DS. Peptide antibiotics. Antimicrobial Agents and Chemotherapy. 1999;43(6):1317-23.
[12] Hiramatsu K, Hanaki H, Ino T, Yabuta K, Oguri T, Tenover FC. Methicillin-resistant *Staphylococcus aureus* clinical strain with reduced vancomycin susceptibility. Journal of Antimicrobial Chemotherapy. 1997;40(1):135-6.
[13] Uttley A, Collins C, Naidoo J, George R. Vancomycin-resistant *enterococci*. Lancet. 1988;1(8575-76):57-8.
[14] deVos WM, Mulders JW, Siezen RJ, Hugenholtz J, Kuipers OP. Properties of nisin Z and distribution of its gene, nisZ, in Lactococcus lactis. Appl Environ Microbiol. 1993;59(1):213–8.
[15] Brötz H, Sahl H-G. New insights into the mechanism of action of lantibiotics—diverse biological effects by binding to the same molecular target. Journal of Antimicrobial Chemotherapy. 2000;46(1):1-6.
[16] Brogden KA. Antimicrobial peptides: Pore formers or metabolic inhibitors in bacteria? NATURE REVIEWS MICROBIOLOGY. 2005;3:238-50.
[17] Reddy KVR, Yedery RD, Aranha C. Antimicrobial peptides: premises and promises. International Journal of Antimicrobial Agents. 2004;24(6):536-47.
[18] Kawano K, Yoneya T, Miyata T, Yoshikawa K, Tokunaga F, Terada Y, et al. Antimicrobial peptide, tachyplesin I, isolated from hemocytes of the horseshoe crab (Tachypleus tridentatus). NMR determination of the beta-sheet structure. Journal of Biological Chemistry. 1990;265(26):15365-7.
[19] Tamamura H, Kuroda M, Masuda M, Otaka A, Funakoshi S, Nakashima H, et al. A comparative study of the solution structures of tachyplesin I and a novel anti-HIV synthetic peptide, T22 ([Tyr5,12, Lys7]-polyphemusin II), determined by nuclear

magnetic resonance. Biochim Biophys Acta (BBA) - General Subjects. 1993;1163(2):209-16.
[20] Hwang PM, Zhou N, Shan X, Arrowsmith CH, Vogel HJ. Three-dimensional solution structure of lactoferricin B, an antimicrobial peptide derived from bovine lactoferrin. Biochemistry. 1998 1998/03/01;37(12):4288-98.
[21] Zwaal RFA, Schroit AJ. Pathophysiologic Implications of Membrane Phospholipid Asymmetry in Blood Cells. Blood. 1997;89(4):1121-32.
[22] Brown DA, London E. Structure and origin of ordered lipid domains in biological membranes. Journal of Membrane Biology. 1998;164(2):103-14.
[23] Rana F, Macias E, Sultany C, Modzrakowski M, Blazyk J. Interactions between magainin 2 and Salmonella typhimurium outer membranes: effect of lipopolysaccharide structure. Biochemistry. 1991;30(24):5858-66.
[24] Contreras I, Shapiro L, Henry S. Membrane phospholipid composition of Caulobacter crescentus. Journal of Bacteriology. 1978;135(3):1130-6.
[25] Tucker AN, White DC. Heterogeneity of phospholipid composition in the bacterial membrane. Journal of Bacteriology. 1970;102(2):508-13.
[26] Rana FR, Blazyk J. Interactions between the antimicrobial peptide, magainin 2, and Salmonella typhimurium lipopolysaccharides. FEBS Letters. 1991;293(1–2):11-5.
[27] Hancock REW. Peptide antibiotics. The Lancet. 1997;349(9049):418-22.
[28] Schweizer F. Cationic amphiphilic peptides with cancer-selective toxicity. Eur J Pharmacol. 2009;625(1-3):190-4.
[29] Utsugi T, Schroit AJ, Connor J, Bucana CD, Fidler IJ. Elevated expression of phosphatidylserine in the outer membrane leaflet of human tumor cells and recognition by activated human blood monocytes. Cancer Research. 1991;51(11):3062-6.
[30] Matsuzaki K. Why and how are peptide–lipid interactions utilized for self defence? Biochemical Society Transactions. 2001;29:598-601.
[31] Matsuzaki K, Harada M, Handa T, Funakoshi S, Fujii N, Yajima H, et al. Magainin 1-induced leakage of entrapped calcein out of negatively-charged lipid vesicles. Biochimica et Biophysica Acta (BBA) - Biomembranes. 1989;981(1):130-4.
[32] Ntwasa M, Goto A, Kurata S. Coleopteran Antimicrobial Peptides: Prospects for Clinical Applications. International Journal of Microbiology. 2012;In press.
[33] Shai Y. Mechanism of the binding, insertion and destabilization of phospholipid bilayer membranes by α-helical antimicrobial and cell non-selective membrane-lytic peptides. Biochim et Biophys Acta 1999;1462 55-70.
[34] Shai Y. Mode of action of membrane active antimicrobial peptides. Peptide Science. 2002;66(4):236-48.
[35] Yang L, Harroun TA, Weiss TM, Ding L, Huang HW. Barrel-stave model or toroidal model? A case study on melittin pores. Biophysical Journal. 2001;81(3):1475-85.
[36] Oren Z, Shai Y. A class of highly potent antibacterial peptides derived from pardaxin, a pore-forming peptide isolated from Moses sole fish *Pardachirus marmoratus*. European Journal of Biochemistry. 1996;237(1):303-10.
[37] Zagorski MG, Norman DG, Barrow CJ, Iwashita T, Tachibana K, Patel DJ. Solution structure of pardaxin P-2. Biochemistry. 1991 1991/08/01;30(32):8009-17.

[38] Matsuzaki K, Murase O, Fujii N, Miyajima K. An antimicrobial peptide, magainin 2, induced rapid flip-flop of phospholipids coupled with pore formation and peptide translocation. Biochemistry. 1996 1996/01/01;35(35):11361-8.

[39] Ludtke SJ, He K, Heller WT, Harroun TA, Yang L, Huang HW. Membrane pores induced by magainin. Biochemistry. 1996 1996/01/01;35(43):13723-8.

[40] Wu M, Maier E, Benz R, Hancock REW. Mechanism of interaction of different classes of cationic antimicrobial peptides with planar bilayers and with the cytoplasmic membrane of *Escherichia coli*. Biochemistry. 1999 1999/06/01;38(22):7235-42.

[41] Takeuchi K, Takahashi H, Sugai M, Iwai H, Kohno T, Sekimizu K, et al. Channel-forming membrane permeabilization by an antibacterial protein, sapecin. Journal of Biological Chemistry. 2004;279(6):4981-7.

[42] Matsuyama K, Natori S. Mode of action of sapecin, a novel antibacterial protein of *Sarcophaga peregrina* (Flesh Fly). Journal of Biochemistry. 1990;108(1):128-32.

[43] Arbuzova A, Schwarz G. Pore-forming action of mastoparan peptides on liposomes: a quantitative analysis. Biochimica et Biophysica Acta (BBA) - Biomembranes. 1999;1420(1–2):139-52.

[44] Whiles JA, Brasseur R, Glover KJ, Melacini G, Komives EA, Vold RR. Orientation and effects of mastoparan X on phospholipid bicelles. Biophysical Journal. 2001;80(1):280-93.

[45] Wimley W, Hristova K. Antimicrobial peptides: Successes, challenges and unanswered questions. J Membrane Biol. 2011;239(1):27-34.

[46] Nakamura T, Furunaka H, Miyata T, Tokunaga F, Muta T, Iwanaga S, et al. Tachyplesin, a class of antimicrobial peptide from the hemocytes of the horseshoe crab (Tachypleus tridentatus). Isolation and chemical structure. Journal of Biological Chemistry. 1988;263(32):16709-13.

[47] Matsuzaki K, Fukui M, Fujii N, Miyajima K. Interactions of an antimicrobial peptide, tachyplesin I, with lipid membranes. Biochimica et Biophysica Acta (BBA) - Biomembranes. 1991;1070(1):259-64.

[48] Yonezawa A, Sugiura Y. Tachyplesin I as a model peptide for antiparallel beta-sheet DNA binding motif. Nucleic Acids Symp Ser 1992;27:161-2.

[49] Yonezawa A, Kuwahara J, Fujii N, Sugiura Y. Binding of tachyplesin I to DNA revealed by footprinting analysis: significant contribution of secondary structure to DNA binding and implication for biological action. Biochemistry. 1992 1992/03/01;31(11):2998-3004.

[50] Allen MD, Yamasaki K, Ohme-Takagi M, Tateno M, Suzuki M. A novel mode of DNA recognition by a [beta]-sheet revealed by the solution structure of the GCC-box binding domain in complex with DNA. EMBO J. [10.1093/emboj/17.18.5484]. 1998;17(18):5484-96.

[51] Raumann BE, Rould MA, Pabo CO, Sauer RT. DNA recognition by β-sheets in the Arc represser-operator crystal structure. Nature. [10.1038/367754a0]. 1994;367(6465):754-7.

[52] Powers J-PS, Martin MM, Goosney DL, Hancock REW. The antimicrobial peptide polyphemusin localizes to the cytoplasm of *Escherichia coli* following treatment. Antimicrobial Agents and Chemotherapy. 2006;50(4):1522-4.

[53] Hirakura Y, Kobayashi S, Matsuzaki K. Specific interactions of the antimicrobial peptide cyclic β-sheet tachyplesin I with lipopolysaccharides. Biochimica et Biophysica Acta (BBA) - Biomembranes. 2002;1562(1–2):32-6.

[54] Epand RM, Vogel HJ. Diversity of antimicrobial peptides and their mechanisms of action. Biochimica et Biophysica Acta (BBA) - Biomembranes. 1999;1462(1–2):11-28.

[55] Matsuzaki K, Yoneyama S, Fujii N, Miyajima K, Yamada K-i, Kirino Y, et al. Membrane permeabilization mechanisms of a cyclic antimicrobial peptide, tachyplesin I, and its linear analog. Biochemistry. 1997 1997/08/01;36(32):9799-806.

[56] Park CB, Kim HS, Kim SC. Mechanism of action of the antimicrobial peptide buforin II: Buforin II kills microorganisms by penetrating the cell membrane and inhibiting cellular functions. Biochem Biophys Res Commun 1998;244(1):253-7.

[57] Kobayashi S, Chikushi A, Tougu S, Imura Y, Nishida M, Yano Y, et al. Membrane translocation mechanism of the antimicrobial peptide buforin 2. Biochemistry. 2004 2004/12/01;43(49):15610-6.

[58] Lee HS, Park CB, Kim JM, Jang SA, Park IY, Kim MS, et al. Mechanism of anticancer activity of buforin IIb, a histone H2A-derived peptide. Cancer Letters. 2008;271(1):47-55.

[59] Cho JH, Sung BH, Kim SC. Buforins: Histone H2A-derived antimicrobial peptides from toad stomach. Biochimica et Biophysica Acta (BBA) - Biomembranes. 2009;1788(8):1564-9.

[60] Biswas M, Voltz K, Smith JC, Langowski J. Role of histone tails in structural stability of the nucleosome. PLoS Comput Biol. 2011;7(12):e1002279.

[61] Hsu C-H, Chen C, Jou M-L, Lee AY-L, Lin Y-C, Yu Y-P, et al. Structural and DNA-binding studies on the bovine antimicrobial peptide, indolicidin: evidence for multiple conformations involved in binding to membranes and DNA. Nucleic Acids Research. 2005;33(13):4053-64.

[62] White S, Szewczyk JW, Turner JM, Baird EE, Dervan PB. Recognition of the four Watson-Crick base pairs in the DNA minor groove by synthetic ligands. Nature. [10.1038/35106]. 1998;391(6666):468-71.

[63] Kielkopf CL, White S, Szewczyk JW, Turner JM, Baird EE, Dervan PB, et al. A structural basis for recognition of A·T and T·A base pairs in the minor groove of B-DNA. Science. 1998;282(5386):111-5.

[64] Wyman TB, Nicol F, Zelphati O, Scaria PV, Plank C, Szoka FC. Design, synthesis, and characterization of a cationic peptide that binds to nucleic acids and permeabilizes bilayers. Biochemistry. 1997 1997/03/01;36(10):3008-17.

[65] Kichler A, Mason AJ, Bechinger B. Cationic amphipathic histidine-rich peptides for gene delivery. Biochimica et Biophysica Acta (BBA) - Biomembranes. 2006;1758(3):301-7.

[66] Kragol G, Lovas S, Varadi G, Condie BA, Hoffmann R, Otvos L. The antibacterial peptide pyrrhocoricin inhibits the ATPase actions of DnaK and prevents chaperone-assisted protein folding. Biochemistry. 2001 2001/03/01;40(10):3016-26.

[67] Otvos L, O I, Rogers ME, Consolvo PJ, Condie BA, Lovas S, et al. Interaction between heat shock proteins and antimicrobial peptides. Biochemistry. 2000 2000/11/01;39(46):14150-9.

[68] Kay BK, Williamson MP, Sudol M. The importance of being proline: the interaction of proline-rich motifs in signaling proteins with their cognate domains. The FASEB Journal. 2000;14(2):231-41.

[69] Kragol G, Hoffmann R, Chattergoon MA, Lovas S, Cudic M, Bulet P, et al. Identification of crucial residues for the antibacterial activity of the proline-rich peptide, pyrrhocoricin. European Journal of Biochemistry. 2002;269(17):4226-37.

[70] Jang SA, Kim H, Lee JY, Shin JR, Kim DJ, Cho JH, et al. Mechanism of action and specificity of antimicrobial peptides designed based on buforin IIb. Peptides. 2012(0).

[71] Shi J, Ross CR, Leto TL, Blecha F. PR-39, a proline-rich antibacterial peptide that inhibits phagocyte NADPH oxidase activity by binding to Src homology 3 domains of p47 phox. Proceedings of the National Academy of Sciences. 1996;93(12):6014-8.

[72] Lehrer RI, Ganz T. Cathelicidins: a family of endogenous antimicrobial peptides. Current Opinion in Hematology. 2002;9(1):18-22.

[73] Yu H, Chen JK, Feng S, Dalgarno DC, Brauer AW, Schrelber SL. Structural basis for the binding of proline-rich peptides to SH3 domains. Cell. 1994;76(5):933-45.

[74] Kavanagh K, Dowd S. Histatins: antimicrobial peptides with therapeutic potential. Journal of Pharmacy and Pharmacology. 2004;56(3):285-9.

[75] Oudhoff MJ, Bolscher JGM, Nazmi K, Kalay H, van 't Hof W, Amerongen AVN, et al. Histatins are the major wound-closure stimulating factors in human saliva as identified in a cell culture assay. The FASEB Journal. 2008;22(11):3805-12.

[76] Edgerton M, Koshlukova SE, Lo TE, Chrzan BG, Straubinger RM, Raj PA. Candidacidal activity of salivary histatins. Journal of Biological Chemistry. 1998;273(32):20438-47.

[77] Edgerton M, Koshlukova SE, Araujo MWB, Patel RC, Dong J, Bruenn JA. Salivary histatin 5 and human neutrophil defensin 1 kill *Candida albicans* via shared pathways. Antimicrob Agents Chemother. 2000;44(12):3310-6.

[78] Nishikata M, Kanehira T, Oh H, Tani H, Tazaki M, Kuboki Y. Salivary histatin as an inhibitor of a protease produced by the oral bacterium Bacteroides gingivalis. Biochemical and Biophysical Research Communications. 1991;174(2):625-30.

[79] Slots J, Bragd L, Wikström M, Dahlén G. The occurrence of *Actinobacillus actinomycetemcomitans, Bacteroides gingivalis* and *Bacteroides intermedius* in destructive periodontal disease in adults. Journal of Clinical Periodontology. 1986;13(6):570-7.

[80] Slots J, Listgarten MA. *Bacteroides gingivalis, Bacteroides intermedius* and *Actinobacillus actinomycetemcomitans* in human periodontal diseases. Journal of Clinical Periodontology. 1988;15(2):85-93.

[81] Breukink E, Wiedemann I, Kraaij Cv, Kuipers OP, Sahl H-G, Kruijff Bd. Use of the cell wall precursor lipid II by a pore-forming peptide antibiotic. Science. 1999;286:2361-4.

[82] Weeks BS, Nomizu M, Otaka A, Weston CA, Okusu A, Tamamura H, et al. The synthetic (Tyr5,12,Lys7)-polyphemusin II peptide (T22) binds to the CD4 cell surface molecule. Biochemical and Biophysical Research Communications. 1995;215(2):626-31.

[83] Marcos JF, Beachy RN, Houghten RA, Blondelle SE, Pérez-Payá E. Inhibition of a plant virus infection by analogs of melittin. Proceedings of the National Academy of Sciences. 1995;92(26):12466-9.

[84] Piantavigna S, Czihal P, Mechler A, Richter M, Hoffmann R, Martin L. Cell penetrating apidaecin peptide interactions with biomimetic phospholipid membranes. International Journal of Peptide Research and Therapeutics. 2009;15(2):139-46.
[85] Castle M, Nazarian A, Yi SS, Tempst P. Lethal effects of apidaecin on *Escherichia coli* involve sequential molecular interactions with diverse targets. Journal of Biological Chemistry. 1999;274(46):32555-64.
[86] Li W-F, Ma G-X, Zhou X-X. Apidaecin-type peptides: Biodiversity, structure–function relationships and mode of action. Peptides. 2006;27(9):2350-9.
[87] Papo N, Shai Y. Host defense peptides as new weapons in cancer treatment. Cellular and Molecular Life Sciences. 2005;62(7):784-90.
[88] Thorburn A. Death receptor-induced cell killing. Cellular Signalling. 2004;16(2):139-44.
[89] Okumura K, Itoh A, Isogai E, Hirose K, Hosokawa Y, Abiko Y, et al. C-terminal domain of human CAP18 antimicrobial peptide induces apoptosis in oral squamous cell carcinoma SAS-H1 cells. Cancer Lett 2004;212(2):185-94.
[90] Chen Y, Xu X, Hong S, Chen J, Liu N, Underhill CB, et al. RGD-tachyplesin inhibits tumor growth. Cancer Research. 2001;61(6):2434-8.
[91] Chen J, Xu X-M, Underhill CB, Yang S, Wang L, Chen Y, et al. Tachyplesin activates the classic complement pathway to kill tumor cells. Cancer Research. 2005;65(11):4614-22.
[92] Sharma S. Melittin resistance: a counterselection for ras transformation. Oncogene. 1992;7(2):193-201.
[93] Sharma S. Melittin-induced hyperactivation of phospholipase A2 activity and calcium influx in ras-transformed cells. Oncogene. 1993;8(4):939-47.
[94] Mader JS, Salsman J, Conrad DM, Hoskin DW. Bovine lactoferricin selectively induces apoptosis in human leukemia and carcinoma cell lines. Molecular Cancer Therapeutics. 2005;4(4):612-24.
[95] Furlong SJ, Mader JS, Hoskin DW. Bovine lactoferricin induces caspase-independent apoptosis in human B-lymphoma cells and extends the survival of immune-deficient mice bearing B-lymphoma xenografts. Experimental and Molecular Pathology. 2010;88(3):371-5.
[96] Mader JS, Smyth D, Marshall J, Hoskin DW. Bovine lactoferricin inhibits basic fibroblast growth factor- and vascular endothelial growth factor165-induced angiogenesis by competing for heparin-like binding sites on endothelial cells. The American Journal of Pathology. 2006;169(5):1753-66.
[97] Schultz G, Clark W, Rotatori DS. EGF and TGF-α in wound healing and repair. Journal of Cellular Biochemistry. 1991;45(4):346-52.
[98] Sørensen OE, Cowland JB, Theilgaard-Mönch K, Liu L, Ganz T, Borregaard N. Wound healing and expression of antimicrobial peptides/polypeptides in human keratinocytes, a consequence of common growth factors. The Journal of Immunology. 2003;170(11):5583-9.
[99] Bals R, Wilson JM. Cathelicidins- a family of multifunctional antimicrobial peptides. Cell Mol Life Sci. 2003;60:711-20.

[100] Yang D, Chertov O, Oppenheim JJ. Participation of mammalian defensins and cathelicidins in anti-microbial immunity: receptors and activities of human defensins and cathelicidin (LL-37). Journal of Leukocyte Biology. 2001;69(5):691-7.

[101] Kurosaka K, Chen Q, Yarovinsky F, Oppenheim JJ, Yang D. Mouse cathelin-related antimicrobial peptide chemoattracts leukocytes using formyl peptide receptor-like 1/mouse formyl peptide receptor-like 2 as the receptor and acts as an immune adjuvant. The Journal of Immunology. 2005;174(10):6257-65.

[102] Marr AK, Gooderham WJ, Hancock REW. Antibacterial peptides for therapeutic use: obstacles and realistic outlook. Current Opinion in Pharmacology. 2006;6(5):468-72.

[103] Vlieghe P, Lisowski V, Martinez J, Khrestchatisky M. Synthetic therapeutic peptides: science and market. Drug Discovery Today. 2010;15(1–2):40-56.

[104] Lau YE, Rozek A, Scott MG, Goosney DL, Davidson DJ, Hancock REW. Interaction and cellular localization of the human host defense peptide LL-37 with lung epithelial cells. INFECTION AND IMMUNITY. 2005;73(1):583-91.

[105] Sandgren S, Wittrup A, Cheng F, Jönsson M, Eklund E, Busch S, et al. The human antimicrobial peptide LL-37 transfers extracellular DNA plasmid to the nuclear compartment of mammalian cells via lipid rafts and proteoglycan-dependent endocytosis. Journal of Biological Chemistry. 2004;279(17):17951-6.

[106] Kola I, Landis J. Can the pharmaceutical industry reduce attrition rates? Nat Rev Drug Discov. [10.1038/nrd1470]. 2004;3(8):711-6.

[107] Østergaard C, Sandvang D, Frimodt-Møller N, Kristensen H-H. High cerebrospinal fluid (CSF) penetration and potent bactericidal activity in CSF of NZ2114, a novel plectasin variant, during experimental pneumococcal meningitis. Antimicrobial Agents and Chemotherapy. 2009;53(4):1581-5.

[108] Hara S, Mukae H, Sakamoto N, Ishimoto H, Amenomori M, Fujita H, et al. Plectasin has antibacterial activity and no affect on cell viability or IL-8 production. Biochemical and Biophysical Research Communications. 2008;374(4):709-13.

[109] Risso A, Zanetti M, Gennaro R. Cytotoxicity and apoptosis mediated by two peptides of innate immunity. Cellular Immunology. 1998;189(2):107-15.

[110] Lau YE, Bowdish DME, Cosseau C, Hancock REW, Davidson DJ. Apoptosis of airway epithelial cells. American Journal of Respiratory Cell and Molecular Biology. 2006;34(4):399-409.

[111] Holle L, Song W, Holle E, Wei Y, Wagner T, Yu X. A matrix metalloproteinase 2 cleavable melittin/avidin conjugate specifically targets tumor cells in vitro and in vivo. Int J Oncol. 2003;22(1):93-8.

[112] Rawlins MD. Cutting the cost of drug development? Nat Rev Drug Discov. [10.1038/nrd1347]. 2004;3(4):360-4.

[113] Merrifield R. Solid phase peptide synthesis. I. The synthesis of a tetrapeptide. J Am Chem Soc. 1963;85:2149-54.

[114] Bray BL. Large-scale manufacture of peptide therapeutics by chemical synthesis. Nat Rev Drug Discov. [10.1038/nrd1133]. 2003;2(7):587-93.

[115] Gesell J, Zasloff M, Opella SJ. Two-dimensional 1H NMR experiments show that the 23-residue magainin antibiotic peptide is an α-helix in dodecylphosphocholine micelles,

sodium dodecylsulfate micelles, and trifluoroethanol/water solution. Journal of Biomolecular NMR. 1997;9(2):127-35.
[116] Bechinger B. Structure and functions of channel-forming peptides: Magainins, cecropins, melittin and alamethicin. Journal of Membrane Biology. 1997;156(3):197-211.
[117] Ouellette A. Paneth cell α-defensins in enteric innate immunity. Cellular and Molecular Life Sciences. 2011;68(13):2215-29.
[118] Sagisaka A, Miyanoshita A, Ishibashi J, Yamakawa M. Purification, characterization and gene expression of a glycine and proline-rich antibacterial protein family from larvae of a beetle, Allomyrina dichotoma. Insect Molecular Biology. 2001;10(4):293-302.
[119] Lee S, Moon H, Kurata S, Natori S, Lee B. Purification and cDNA cloning of an antifungal protein from the hemolymph of Holotrichia diomphalia larvae. Biol Pharm Bull 1995;18(8):1049-52.
[120] Rozek A, Friedrich CL, Hancock REW. Structure of the bovine antimicrobial peptide indolicidin bound to dodecylphosphocholine and sodium dodecyl sulfate micelles. Biochemistry. 2000 2000/12/01;39(51):15765-74.
[121] Bruckdorfer T, Marder O, Albericio F. From production of peptides in milligram amounts for research to multi-tons quantities for drugs of the future. Curr Pharm Biotechnol. 2004;5(1):29-43.
[122] Yeung A, Gellatly S, Hancock R. Multifunctional cationic host defence peptides and their clinical applications. Cell Mol Life Sci. 2011;68(13):2161-76.
[123] Imura Y, Nishida M, Ogawa Y, Takakura Y, Matsuzaki K. Action mechanism of tachyplesin I and effects of PEGylation. Biochimica et Biophysica Acta (BBA) - Biomembranes. 2007;1768(5):1160-9.
[124] Brötz H, Bierbaum G, Leopold K, Reynolds PE, Sahl H-G. The lantibiotic mersacidin inhibits peptidoglycan synthesis by targeting lipid II. Antimicrobial Agents and Chemotherapy. 1998;42(1):154-60.
[125] Boman HG, Agerberth B, Boman A. Mechanisms of action on *Escherichia coli* of cecropin P1 and PR-39, two antibacterial peptides from pig intestine. Infection and Immunity. 1993;61(7):2978-84.
[126] Shi J, Ross CR, Chengappa MM, Sylte MJ, McVey DS, Blecha F. Antibacterial activity of a synthetic peptide (PR-26) derived from PR-39, a proline-arginine-rich neutrophil antimicrobial peptide. Antimicrobial Agents and Chemotherapy. 1996;40(1):115-21.
[127] Subbalakshmi C, Sitaram N. Mechanism of antimicrobial action of indolicidin. FEMS Microbiol Lett. 1998;160(1):91-6.
[128] Salomón RA, Farías RN. Microcin 25, a novel antimicrobial peptide produced by *Escherichia coli*. Journal of Bacteriology. 1992;174(22):7428-35.
[129] Patrzykat A, Friedrich CL, Zhang L, Mendoza V, Hancock REW. Sublethal concentrations of pleurocidin-derived antimicrobial peptides inhibit macromolecular synthesis in *Escherichia coli*. Antimicrobial Agents and Chemotherapy. 2002;46(3):605-14.
[130] Lehrer RI, Barton A, Daher KA, Harwig SS, Ganz T, Selsted ME. Interaction of human defensins with *Escherichia coli*. Mechanism of bactericidal activity. The Journal of Clinical Investigation. 1989;84(2):553-61.

[131] Andreu D, Rivas L. Animal antimicrobial peptides: An overview. Peptide Science. 1998;47(6):415-33.

[132] Bellemare A, Vernoux N, Morin S, Gagne S, Bourbonnais Y. Structural and antimicrobial properties of human pre-elafin/trappin-2 and derived peptides against *Pseudomonas aeruginosa*. BMC Microbiol. 2010;10(1):253.

[133] Baranger K, Zani M-L, Chandenier J, Dallet-Choisy S, Moreau T. The antibacterial and antifungal properties of trappin-2 (pre-elafin) do not depend on its protease inhibitory function. FEBS Journal. 2008;275(9):2008-20.

[134] Hong RW, Shchepetov M, Weiser JN, Axelsen PH. Transcriptional profile of the *Escherichia coli* response to the antimicrobial insect peptide cecropin A. Antimicrobial Agents and Chemotherapy. 2003;47(1):1-6.

[135] Chan YR, Gallo RL. PR-39, a syndecan-inducing antimicrobial peptide, binds and affects p130^{Cas}. Journal of Biological Chemistry. 1998;273(44):28978-85.

[136] Woodley J. Enzymatic barriers for GI peptide and protein delivery. Crit Rev Ther Drug Carrier Syst. 1994;11(2-3):61-95.

Chapter 7

The Study of MASPs Knockout Mice

Minoru Takahashi, Daisuke Iwaki, Yuichi Endo and Teizo Fujita

Additional information is available at the end of the chapter

http://dx.doi.org/10.5772/50500

1. Introduction

Plasma proteases, e.g. thrombin, factor X, complement factor D and C1s are responsible for the physiological activities, such as coagulation and complement system. These proteases circulate as their zymogen in blood and are activated by various stimulations. In this chapter, we focus on a family of plasma serine proteases, called MASP (MBL/ficolin-associated serine protease) that can activate the complement. Three distinct MASP, MASP-1, MASP-2 and MASP-3 have been identified in many species of vertebrates. Although the contribution of MASP-2 in activation of complement was well defined, the substrates for MASP-1 and MASP-3 were still obscure. We have generated MASP-1- and MASP-3-deficient mice (*Masp1/3*$^{-/-}$) to verify roles of MASP-1 and MASP-3 proteases *in vivo*. One major finding is that MASP-1, considered being a lectin pathway component—also acts as a pro-factor D (Df) convertase, the initiator of the alternative pathway. Our results emphasize a unique feature of MASP-1, participating two complement pathways. We also generated MASP-2 deficient mice. In here, we would like to summarize the results obtained from these knockout mice.

2. Complement system

The complement system is an important part of the innate immune system, mediating several major effector functions, such as directly killing pathogens, promoting phagocytosis, and clearance of immune complexes and apoptotic cells and modulating adaptive immune responses, as describing in some excellent reviews (Ricklin, et al., 2010) (Fujita, et al., 2004) (Carroll, 2004). On the other hand, inappropriate activation of complement affects the pathogenesis of inflammatory diseases (Holers, 2003). Therefore, well-understanding of the mechanisms of its activation is very important. More than 30 proteins in plasma consist of the complement system. The most abundant protein among them is the third component (C3). Once the complement system is activated, a chain of reactions involving restricted proteolysis and assembly occurs, resulting in cleavage of C3 into C3b and C3a. The cascade up to C3 cleavage is called the activation pathway. There are three distinct activation pathways of the complement cascade; the classical, alternative, and lectin pathways, that all converge on factor C3 and lead to activation of complement effector functions as above (Walport, 2001a)(Fig. 1).

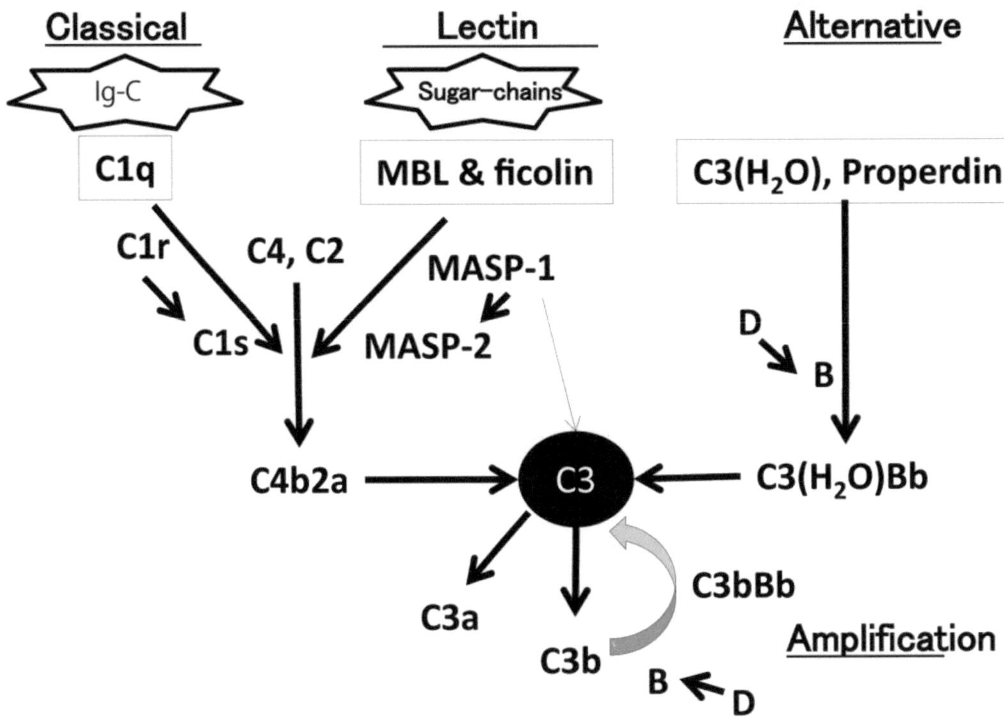

Figure 1. Activation pathways for complement system.

In the mammalian complement system, the pivotal molecule circulating C3 is cleaved into C3a and C3b by two different C3 convertases, C4b2a and C3bBb. C4b2a is generated by the classical and lectin pathway and C3bBb is generated by the alternative pathway.

2.1. The classical pathway

The classic pathway is initiated by recognition of the first C1 binding to a variety of targets, most prominently immune complexes (Walport, 2001a) (Walport, 2001b). C1 consists of a single C1q molecule associated with dimers of C1r and C1s(Lepow, et al., 1963). C1r and C1s are plasma serine proteases, normally existing in an inactive pro-enzyme form. The conformational exchange of C1q by binding to immune complexes results in the activation of C1r. C1r is thought to be cleaved in some autocatalytic manner and once C1r molecule is activated, it activate C1s, which in turn cleaves C4 and then C2(Arlaud, et al., 2002). The C4 cleavage products are C4a and C4b. The latter molecule may be bound to non-self surfaces on pathogens and is bound to C2 to form the classical pathway C3 convertase.

2.2. The alternative pathway

In the alternative pathway, spontaneous hydrolysis of C3, designated C3(H_2O) results in triggering complement activation with complement factor B, making another C3 convertase, C3(H_2O)Bb on foreign cells (Muller-Eberhard and Gotze, 1972, Pangburn, et al., 1981). This leads to the cleavage of factor B by factor D, giving rise to an active enzyme complex with the fragment Bb as the enzyme. The alternative pathway does not involve specific recognition molecules and also functions to amplify C3 activation (amplification loop) (Brouwer, et al., 2006).

2.3. The lectin pathway

Activation of the lectin pathway is similar with that of the classical pathway (Degn, et al., 2010). The lectin pathway is initiated by some serum lectins binding to pathogen-associated molecular patterns, mainly carbohydrate structures present on bacterial, fungal, or viral pathogens. In 1978, a serum lectin, designated mannose-binding lectin (MBL), which recognizes carbohydrates such as mannose and N-acetylglucosamine was first isolated from rabbit liver (Kawasaki, et al., 1978). MBL acts as the pattern recognition molecule, which recognizes sugar chains on some foreign pathogens. MBL is also found to have an avidity of complement activation (Ikeda, et al., 1987) (Holmskov, et al., 2003) (Turner, 1996). It has been thought that MBL activates complement by $C1r_2C1s_2$ protease complex that consists of classical pathway (Ohta, et al., 1990). However, in 1992, Matsushita and Fujita found a new plasma serum protease designated MBL-associated serine protease (MASP) that binds MBL (Matsushita and Fujita, 1992) (Matsushita, et al., 1998). Recent studies identified ficolins that are also plasma proteins with binding activity for carbohydrates to associate with MASP and to activate complement (Matsushita, et al., 2000, Matsushita, et al., 2001) (Cseh, et al., 2002). Ficolins has a collagen-like domain and a fibrinogen-like domain. Furthermore, CL-K1 (Keshi, et al., 2006) was also identified as a collectin that associates with MASP(Hansen, et al., 2010).

3. MBL-associated serine proteases

3.1. Three MASP proteins were associated with MBL and ficolins

MASP is homologue of C1r and C1s of the classical pathway, sharing the well-described domains structure in the order from N-terminus, CUB-I, EGF, CUB-II, CCP-I, CCP-II and SP (Sato, et al., 1994). The CUB (C1r/C1s, embryonic sea Urchin protein [Uefg], and Bone-morphogenetic protein 1 [Bmp1]) domain is approximately 110 aa, predicting a molecular structure of an antiparallel beta-barrel similar to those in immunoglobulins (Bork and Beckmann, 1993). The EGF (epidermal growth factor-like) domain of approximately 50 aa is also found in many proteins and is known to mediate protein-protein interactions via calcium ion. The N-terminal three domains consisting of CUB-I, EGF and CUB-II of the MASP are responsible for dimerization and for the calcium-dependent binding to MBL and ficolins(Feinberg, et al., 2003). The two contiguous CCPs (complement control protein) of

MASP, especially the second CCP domain, have been implicated in the binding of macromolecular substrates. The CCP domains of around 60 aa are found in a number of complement factors and other proteins(Chou and Heinrikson, 1997). The SP (serine protease) domain is the catalytically active unit of the proteases and defines them as part of the S1A family of chymotrypsin-like proteases (Yousef, et al., 2004). MASP is able to cleave C4 and C2 to generate a C3 convertase, C4b2a. Recent studies isolated two additional MASPs in human MBL complex (Thiel, et al., 1997) (Dahl, et al., 2001). These newly identified MASPs are called as MASP-2 and MASP-3 and the former one is MASP-1(Schwaeble, et al., 2002).

3.2. Substrates for MASP

It is apparently defined that MASP-2 cleaves C4 that is similar with C1s in the classical pathway (Vorup-Jensen, et al., 1998) (Ambrus, et al., 2003). However, substrates for MASP-1 and MASP-3 are still obscure. Several candidates were demonstrated by recent studies as shown in Table 1.

MASP	Substrates (reference)
MASP-1	C3 (Matsushita and Fujita, 1995), C2, fibrinogen, Factor XIII(Hajela, et al., 2002), PAR4 (Megyeri, et al., 2009), Df(Takahashi, et al., 2010)
MASP-2	C4, C2(Ambrus, et al., 2003), prothrombin
MASP-3	IGFBP-5 (Cortesio and Jiang, 2006), Df(Iwaki, et al., 2011)
C1r	C1s
C1s	C4, C2

Table 1. Substrates for MASPs

3.3. *MASP* genes

3.3.1. *MASP1*

MASP1 is located on chromosome 3q27-q28 in human and chromosome 16 (B2-B3) in mouse (Takada, et al., 1995). Three gene products, MASP-1, MASP-3 and MAP44 are encoded from this gene by alternative splicing. MAP44 is a truncated protein of MASP-1/3 and lacks serine protease domain (Degn, et al., 2009) (Skjoedt, et al., 2010). MAP44 is thought to be a regulatory factor, attenuating activation of the lectin pathway. *MASP1* gene has a unique structure. A single exon, encoding whole MASP-3 light-chain and the six sprit exons, encoding MASP-1 are tandem located (Dahl, et al., 2001). Therefore, MASP-1 and MASP-3 consist of a common heavy-chain and the distinct light-chain.

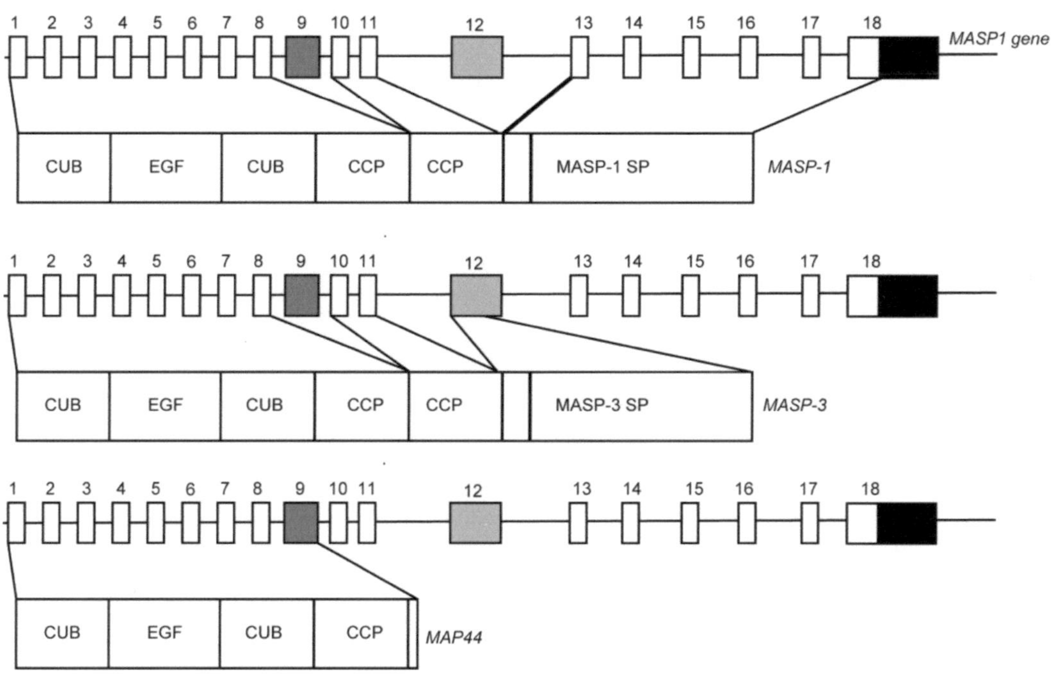

Figure 2. Schematic representation of *MASP1* gene

MASP1 gene consists of 18 exons, encoding three gene products, MASP-1, MASP-3 and MAP44 by alternative splicing.

3.3.2. MASP2

MASP2 gene is located on human chromosome 1p36.3-p36.2(Stover, et al., 1999a). And mouse Masp2 gene is located on chromosome 4(Lawson and Reid, 2000). It was shown that the MASP2 gene encodes two gene products, the 76 kDa MASP-2 serine protease and a plasma protein of 19 kDa, termed sMAP/MAp19 by alternative splicing (Takahashi, et al., 1999) (Stover, et al., 1999b). sMAP/MAp19 consist of only CUB-I and EGF-like domain of MASP-2, lacking catalytic domain.

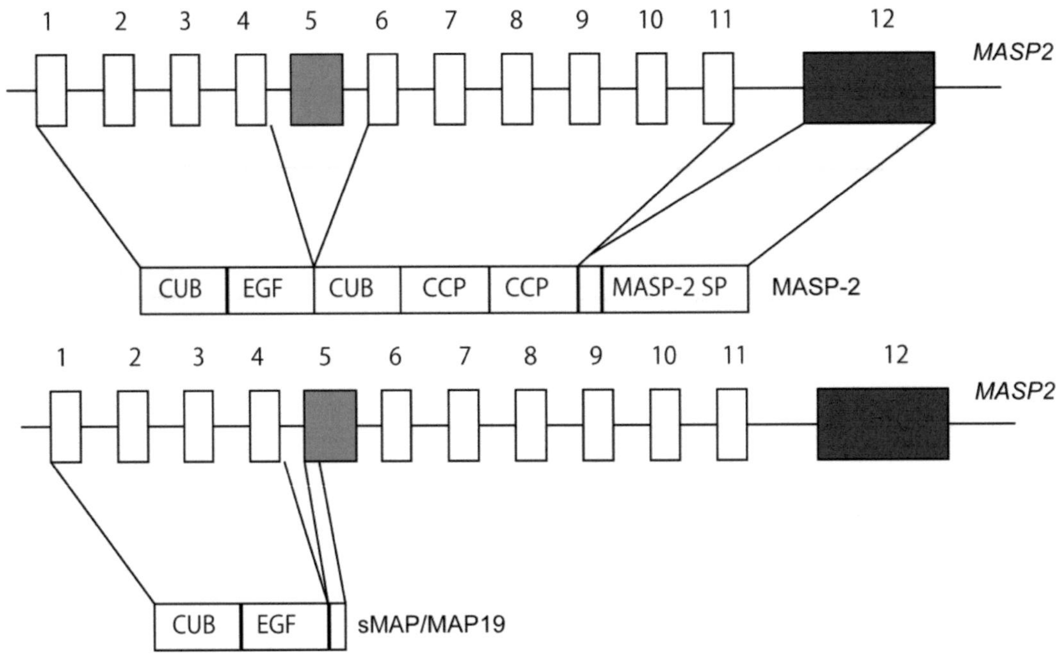

Figure 3. Schematic representation of *MASP2* gene

MASP2 gene consists of 12 exons, encoding two gene products, MASP-2 and sMAP/Map19 by alternative splicing.

4. Studies for the Masp-knockout mice

Knockout mice	Mutant allele	chromosome	Targeted exon
Masp1/3$^{-/-}$	Masp1^{tm1Tefu}	16	2
sMAP/Masp2$^{-/-}$	Masp2^{tm1Tefu}	4	5
Masp2$^{-/-}$	Masp2^{tm1Wjsc}	4	11 &12

Table 2. Masps knockout mice

4.1. MASP-1 and MASP-3-deficient mice (*Masp1/3*$^{-/-}$)

To investigate the role of MASP-1 in complement activation, we planned to disrupt the second exon of Masp1 gene by a conventional gene targeting (Takahashi, et al., 2008). When this project was proceeding, MASP-3 was identified (Dahl, et al., 2001). Surprisingly, both gene products were produced from *MASP1* gene. Since the targeted second exon is at upstream of both transcripts, it was predicted that MASP-3 is also absent in this knockout mice. It was confirmed that not only MASP-1, but also MASP-3, is absent in *MASP1/3*$^{-/-}$ mice (Takahashi, et al., 2008).

4.1.1. *Masp1/3$^{-/-}$* shows the abnormality of the lectin pathway activation

Serum from *Masp1/3$^{-/-}$* shows the abnormality of both C4 and C3 activation on mannan and it is restored by adding recombinant MASP-1. This result supported that MASP-1 contributes the lectin pathway through C4 activation. Furthermore, MASP-2 activation is delayed in *Masp1/3$^{-/-}$* to be compared with that of wild type. This result reveals that MASP-1 and/or MASP-3 may involve in the lectin pathway activation through the acceleration of MASP-2 activation (Takahashi, et al., 2008).

4.1.2. *Masp1/3$^{-/-}$* shows the abnormality of the alternative pathway activation

Further study noticed us that not only lectin pathway but also alternative pathway is abnormal in *Masp1/3$^{-/-}$*. We found that complement factor D (Df) circulates as a zymogen in *Masp1/3$^{-/-}$* (Takahashi, et al., 2010). Df was known to be active-form, but not a zymogen in circulation (Lesavre and Muller-Eberhard, 1978). However, it has become evident that most proteases in blood are secreted as zymogen. Df was thought to be an exception. We also found that Df is synthesized as zymogen from adipocytes (Takahashi, et al., 2010) (Fig. 4). This result supports the general consensus for Df. Interestingly, increasing evidence suggests that the alternative pathway is involved in human disease, such as inflammatory arthritis and ischemia/reperfusion injury (Thurman and Holers, 2006).

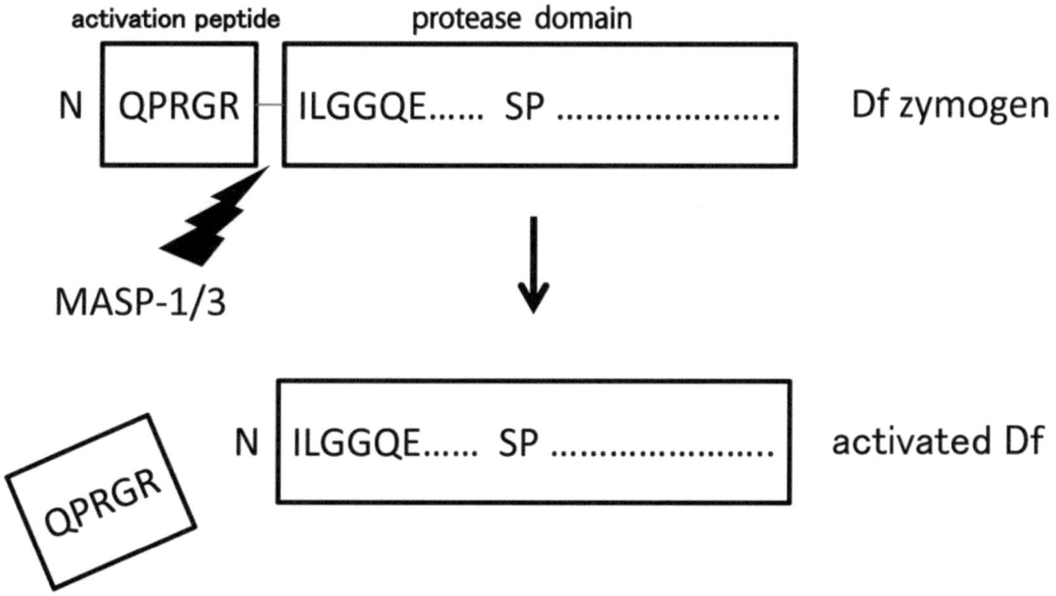

Figure 4. MASP-1 and/or MASP-3 involve in activating a zymogen of complement factor D

Complement factor D (Df) is synthesized as a zymogen (Pro-Df) from adipocytes. In serum of *Masp1/3$^{-/-}$*, Pro-Df that has an activation peptide (QPRGR) at N-terminal of Df was observed.

4.1.3. MASP-1 and/or MASP-3 involve the fat metabolism through Df activation

It was also reported that the alternative pathway is involved in fat metabolism in adipose tissue (Paglialunga, et al., 2008). Recent studies have indicated that acylation-stimulating protein (ASP), which is identical to C3adesArg, stimulates fat storage in adipocytes (Yasruel, et al., 1991) (Maslowska, et al., 1997). ASP is a derivative of complement C3; thus, $C3^{-/-}$ mice are lean owing to ASP deficiency. Furthermore, plasma ASP levels are decreased in Bf-deficient and Df-deficient mice, indicating that the alternative pathway stimulates production of ASP. We found that $Masp1/3^{-/-}$ mice are also apparently lean (Takahashi, et al., 2008), strongly indicating a contribution of MASP-1 to fat metabolism via alternative pathway. We measured the plasma concentration of leptin and TNF-alpha (Fig. 5). Leptin plays a critical role in the regulation of body weight by inhibiting food intake and stimulating energy expenditure. Leptin appears to be a hormone secreted by adipocyte (Zhang, et al., 1994). It was shown that level of leptin in $Masp1/3^{-/-}$ significantly decrease. Furthermore, we determined that one of inflammatory factor, TNF-alpha increases in $Masp1/3^{-/-}$. As shown in Fig. 4, adipose tissues in Masp1/3-/- apparently show atrophy. Therefore, fat metabolisms in Masp1/3-/- adipose tissue might be reduced.

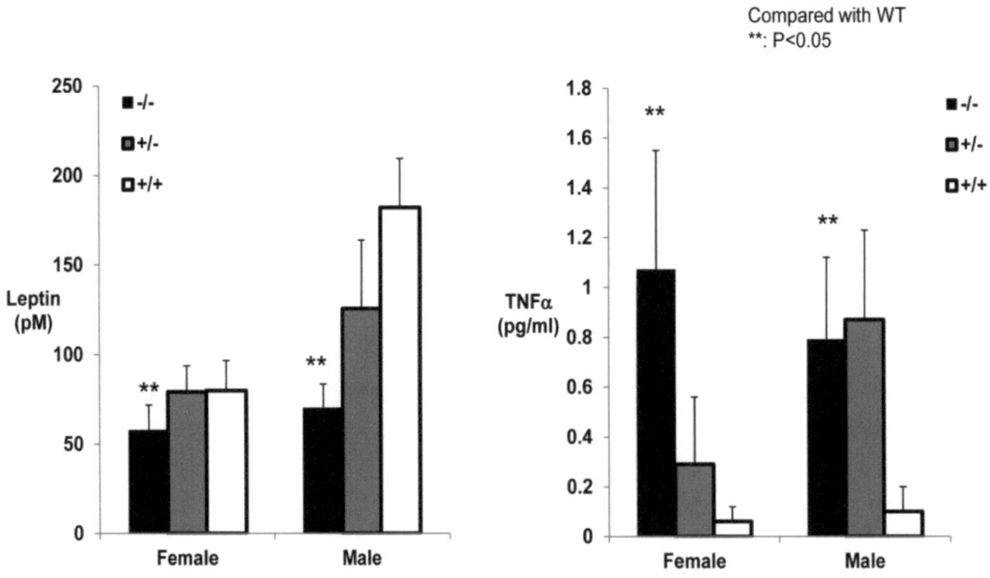

Figure 5. Serum leptin and TNF-alpha level in $Masp1/3^{-/-}$

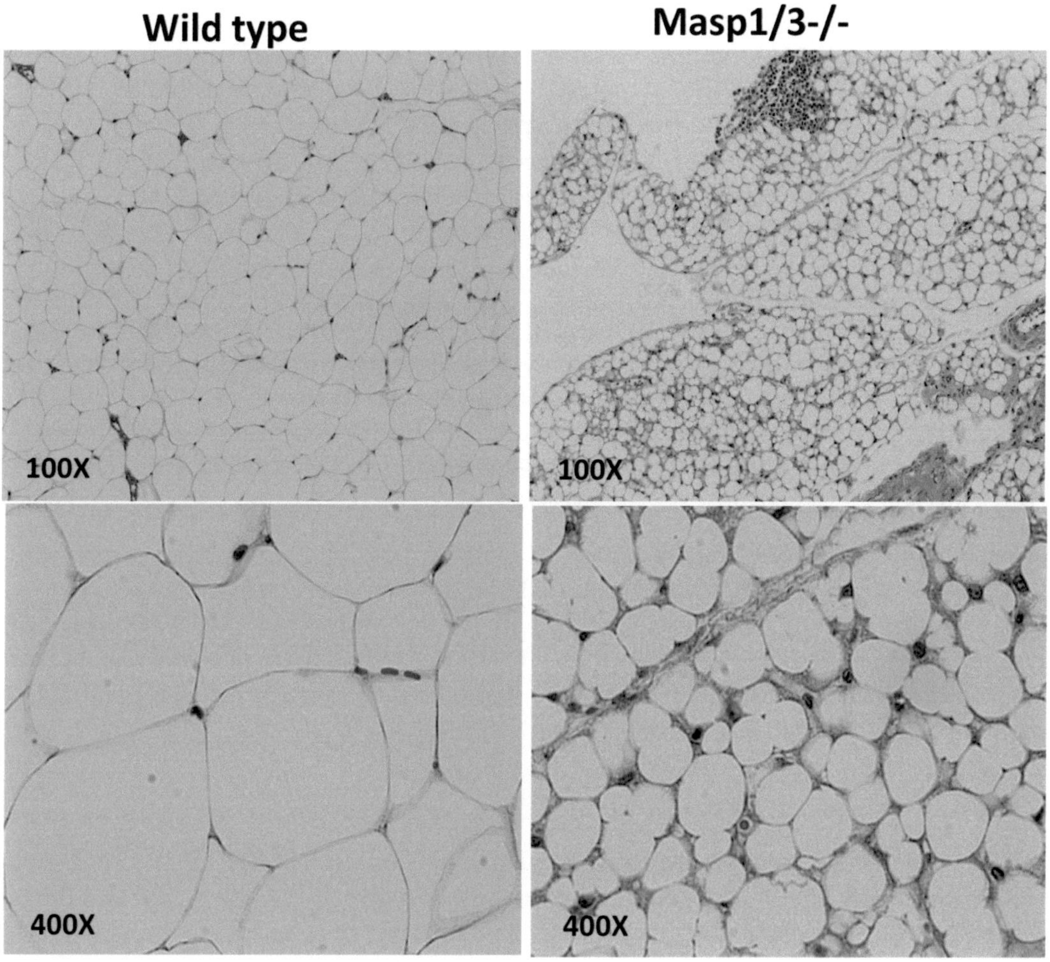

Figure 6. H&E staining of mouse adipose tissue

4.1.4. Masp1/3$^{-/-}$ is resistant to AP-mediated joint damage

Banda et al. demonstrated that *Masp1/3$^{-/-}$* mice are highly resistant to CAIA as evidenced by a significant decrease in the histological scores as compared with WT mice (Banda, et al., 2010). Recent studies supported that the alternative pathway is both necessary and sufficient to induce disease in murine collagen Ab-induced arthritis (CAIA) (Banda, et al., 2006) (Banda, et al., 2007). This model mouse confirmed that *Masp1/3$^{-/-}$* shows the abnormality of the alternative pathway.

4.1.5. MASP3 mutation causes 3MC syndrome

3MC syndrome (Malpuech-Michels-Mingarelli-Carnevale syndrome) are four rare autosomal recessive disorders (Carnevale, et al., 1989) (Mingarelli, et al., 1996) (Malpuech, et al., 1983) (Michels, et al., 1978). This syndrome shows facial dysmorphic traits. Recent observations for families, including patients who suffer from 3MC syndrome found the genetic mutations in *CL-K1* and *MASP1* genes (Rooryck, et al., 2011). This result was very interesting, since a possibility was raised that MASP-3 may be responsible to not only complement system, but also development system with a recognition molecule, CL-K1. In 2010, Sirmaci, et al. also found the mutations of *MASP1* gene in two Turkish familes (Sirmaci, et al., 2010). Preliminary results was obtained that *Masp1/3* knockout mice have some developmental disorders (publication preparing).

4.2. sMAP and MASP-2-deficient mice (*sMAP/Masp2*$^{-/-}$)

To clarify the role of sMAP/Map19, we also generated another mutant mice, disrupting the fifth exon of *MASP2* gene by replacement with *neo*^{r}-gene (Iwaki, et al., 2006). Since this targeted region is the sMAP/Map19-specific exon, it was predicted that MASP-2 might be intact in this knockout mice. However, MASP-2 was not detected in their serum. Therefore, these mutant mice were named as *sMAP/Masp2*$^{-/-}$.

When recombinant sMAP and recombinant MASP-2 (rMASP-2) reconstituted the MBL-MASP-sMAP complex in deficient serum, the binding of these recombinant proteins to MBL was competitive, and the C4 cleavage activity of the MBL-MASP-sMAP complex was restored by the addition of rMASP-2. On the other hand, the addition of recombinant sMAP attenuated the activity. Therefore, MASP-2 is essential for the activation of C4 and sMAP plays a regulatory role in the activation of the lectin pathway(Iwaki, et al., 2006).

4.3. MASP-2-deficient mice (*Masp2*$^{-/-}$)

An England group generated MASP-2-deficient mice(Schwaeble, et al., 2011). This strain lacks exon 11 and 12 of *Masp2* gene, encoding the C-terminal part of the CCPII and the SP domains. In their knockout mice, sMAP/Map19 is predicted to be intact. In vitro analysis of *MASP2*$^{-/-}$ plasma showed a total absence of lectin pathway-dependent C4 cleavage on mannan- and zymosan-coated surfaces. They investigated whether MASP-2 affect the inflammatory process using a model of myocardial ischemia reperfusion injury (MIRI). It was observed that *MASP2*$^{-/-}$ was protected from MIRI.

5. Conclusion

Here, we focus on analyses of three strains for *Masps* knockout mice, *Masp1/3*$^{-/-}$, *sMAP/Masp2*$^{-/-}$ and *Masp2*$^{-/-}$. All strains show that activation of lectin pathway is deficient. We also detected the abnormality of the alternative pathway in *Masp1/3*$^{-/-}$. But *Masp2*-deficient phenotype does not affect the activity. MASPs are associated with MBL, ficolins and CL-K1. MBL-deficient mice were generated and analysed (Takahashi, et al., 2002, Shi, et al., 2004). Surprisingly, MBL-null mice show the comparable level of the alternative pathway with that of wild type. If MASP-1 and/or MASP-3 involve the activation of alternative pathway with MBL, MBL-null mice must be affected. Other recognition molecules, ficolin or CL-K1 might be involved in this phenomenon. This problem should be resolved in future study.

Recently MASP1 mutants were identified in human patients, suffering from 3MC syndrome. However, the mechanisms how MASP-1 and/or MASP-3 contribute the facial development are still unclear. Further study using Masp1/3-/- would provide a powerful tool to resolve this problem.

Author details

Minoru Takahashi, Daisuke Iwaki, Yuichi Endo and Teizo Fujita
Department of Immunology, Fukushima Medical University School of Medicine, Japan

6. References

Ambrus, G., Gal, P., Kojima, M., Szilagyi, K., Balczer, J., Antal, J., Graf, L., Laich, A., Moffatt, B. E., Schwaeble, W., Sim, R. B. and Zavodszky, P. (2003). Natural substrates and inhibitors of mannan-binding lectin-associated serine protease-1 and -2: a study on recombinant catalytic fragments. *J Immunol,* Vol. 170, No. 3, pp. 1374-1382

Arlaud, G. J., Gaboriaud, C., Thielens, N. M., Budayova-Spano, M., Rossi, V. and Fontecilla-Camps, J. C. (2002). Structural biology of the C1 complex of complement unveils the mechanisms of its activation and proteolytic activity. *Molecular Immunology,* Vol. 39, No. 7-8, pp. 383-394

Banda, N. K., Takahashi, K., Wood, A. K., Holers, V. M. and Arend, W. P. (2007). Pathogenic complement activation in collagen antibody-induced arthritis in mice requires amplification by the alternative pathway. *J Immunol,* Vol. 179, No. 6, pp. 4101-4109

Banda, N. K., Takahashi, M., Levitt, B., Glogowska, M., Nicholas, J., Takahashi, K., Stahl, G. L., Fujita, T., Arend, W. P. and Holers, V. M. (2010). Essential role of complement mannose-binding lectin-associated serine proteases-1/3 in the murine collagen antibody-induced model of inflammatory arthritis. *J Immunol,* Vol. 185, No. 9, pp. 5598-5606

Banda, Nirmal K., Thurman, Joshua M., Kraus, Damian, Wood, Allyson, Carroll, Michael C., Arend, William P. and Holers, V. Michael. (2006). Alternative Complement Pathway Activation Is Essential for Inflammation and Joint Destruction in the Passive Transfer Model of Collagen-Induced Arthritis. *The Journal of Immunology,* Vol. 177, No. 3, pp. 1904-1912

Bork, P. and Beckmann, G. (1993). The CUB domain. A widespread module in developmentally regulated proteins. *Journal of molecular biology,* Vol. 231, No. 2, pp. 539-545

Brouwer, N., Dolman, K. M., van Zwieten, R., Nieuwenhuys, E., Hart, M., Aarden, L. A., Roos, D. and Kuijpers, T. W. (2006). Mannan-binding lectin (MBL)-mediated opsonization is enhanced by the alternative pathway amplification loop. *Mol Immunol,* Vol. 43, No. 13, pp. 2051-2060

Carnevale, F., Krajewska, G., Fischetto, R., Greco, M. G. and Bonvino, A. (1989). Ptosis of eyelids, strabismus, diastasis recti, hip defect, cryptorchidism, and developmental delay in two sibs. *Am J Med Genet,* Vol. 33, No. 2, pp. 186-189

Carroll, M. C. (2004). The complement system in regulation of adaptive immunity. *Nature immunology,* Vol. 5, No. 10, pp. 981-986

Chou, K. C. and Heinrikson, R. L. (1997). Prediction of the tertiary structure of the complement control protein module. *Journal of protein chemistry,* Vol. 16, No. 8, pp. 765-773

Cortesio, C. L. and Jiang, W. (2006). Mannan-binding lectin-associated serine protease 3 cleaves synthetic peptides and insulin-like growth factor-binding protein 5. *Arch Biochem Biophys,* Vol. 449, No. 1-2, pp. 164-170

Cseh, S., Vera, L., Matsushita, M., Fujita, T., Arlaud, G. J. and Thielens, N. M. (2002). Characterization of the interaction between L-ficolin/p35 and mannan-binding lectin-associated serine proteases-1 and -2. *J Immunol,* Vol. 169, No. 10, pp. 5735-5743

Dahl, M. R., Thiel, S., Matsushita, M., Fujita, T., Willis, A. C., Christensen, T., Vorup-Jensen, T. and Jensenius, J. C. (2001). MASP-3 and its association with distinct complexes of the mannan-binding lectin complement activation pathway. *Immunity,* Vol. 15, No. 1, pp. 127-135

Degn, S. E., Hansen, A. G., Steffensen, R., Jacobsen, C., Jensenius, J. C. and Thiel, S. (2009). MAp44, a human protein associated with pattern recognition molecules of the complement system and regulating the lectin pathway of complement activation. *J Immunol,* Vol. 183, No. 11, pp. 7371-7378

Degn, S. E., Jensenius, J. C. and Bjerre, M. (2010). The lectin pathway and its implications in coagulation, infections and auto-immunity. *Current opinion in organ transplantation,* Vol. No. pp.

Feinberg, H., Uitdehaag, J. C., Davies, J. M., Wallis, R., Drickamer, K. and Weis, W. I. (2003). Crystal structure of the CUB1-EGF-CUB2 region of mannose-binding protein associated serine protease-2. *The EMBO journal,* Vol. 22, No. 10, pp. 2348-2359

Fujita, T., Matsushita, M. and Endo, Y. (2004). The lectin-complement pathway--its role in innate immunity and evolution. *Immunol Rev,* Vol. 198, No. pp. 185-202

Hajela, K., Kojima, M., Ambrus, G., Wong, K. H., Moffatt, B. E., Ferluga, J., Hajela, S., Gal, P. and Sim, R. B. (2002). The biological functions of MBL-associated serine proteases (MASPs). *Immunobiology,* Vol. 205, No. 4-5, pp. 467-475

Hansen, S., Selman, L., Palaniyar, N., Ziegler, K., Brandt, J., Kliem, A., Jonasson, M., Skjoedt, M. O., Nielsen, O., Hartshorn, K., Jorgensen, T. J., Skjodt, K. and Holmskov, U. (2010). Collectin 11 (CL-11, CL-K1) is a MASP-1/3-associated plasma collectin with microbial-binding activity. *Journal of immunology (Baltimore, Md. : 1950),* Vol. 185, No. 10, pp. 6096-6104

Holers, V. M. (2003). The complement system as a therapeutic target in autoimmunity. *Clin Immunol,* Vol. 107, No. 3, pp. 140-151

Holmskov, U., Thiel, S. and Jensenius, J. C. (2003). Collections and ficolins: humoral lectins of the innate immune defense. *Annu Rev Immunol,* Vol. 21, No. pp. 547-578

Ikeda, K., Sannoh, T., Kawasaki, N., Kawasaki, T. and Yamashina, I. (1987). Serum lectin with known structure activates complement through the classical pathway. *J Biol Chem,* Vol. 262, No. 16, pp. 7451-7454

Iwaki, D., Kanno, K., Takahashi, M., Endo, Y., Lynch, N. J., Schwaeble, W. J., Matsushita, M., Okabe, M. and Fujita, T. (2006). Small mannose-binding lectin-associated protein plays a regulatory role in the lectin complement pathway. *J Immunol,* Vol. 177, No. 12, pp. 8626-8632

Iwaki, Daisuke, Kanno, Kazuko, Takahashi, Minoru, Endo, Yuichi, Matsushita, Misao and Fujita, Teizo. (2011). The Role of Mannose-Binding Lectin-Associated Serine Protease-3 in Activation of the Alternative Complement Pathway. *The Journal of Immunology,* Vol. 187, No. 7, pp. 3751-3758

Kawasaki, T., Etoh, R. and Yamashina, I. (1978). Isolation and characterization of a mannan-binding protein from rabbit liver. *Biochem Biophys Res Commun,* Vol. 81, No. 3, pp. 1018-1024

Keshi, H., Sakamoto, T., Kawai, T., Ohtani, K., Katoh, T., Jang, S. J., Motomura, W., Yoshizaki, T., Fukuda, M., Koyama, S., Fukuzawa, J., Fukuoh, A., Yoshida, I., Suzuki, Y. and Wakamiya, N. (2006). Identification and characterization of a novel human collectin CL-K1. *Microbiol Immunol,* Vol. 50, No. 12, pp. 1001-1013

Lawson, P. R. and Reid, K. B. (2000). A novel PCR-based technique using expressed sequence tags and gene homology for murine genetic mapping: localization of the complement genes. *International immunology,* Vol. 12, No. 3, pp. 231-240

Lepow, I. H., Naff, G. B., Todd, E. W., Pensky, J. and Hinz, C. F. (1963). Chromatographic resolution of the first component of human complement into three activities. *The Journal of experimental medicine,* Vol. 117, No. pp. 983-1008

Lesavre, P. H. and Muller-Eberhard, H. J. (1978). Mechanism of action of factor D of the alternative complement pathway. *J Exp Med,* Vol. 148, No. 6, pp. 1498-1509

Malpuech, G., Demeocq, F., Palcoux, J. B. and Vanlieferinghen, P. (1983). A previously undescribed autosomal recessive multiple congenital anomalies/mental retardation (MCA/MR) syndrome with growth failure, lip/palate cleft(s), and urogenital anomalies. *Am J Med Genet,* Vol. 16, No. 4, pp. 475-480

Maslowska, M., Sniderman, A. D., Germinario, R. and Cianflone, K. (1997). ASP stimulates glucose transport in cultured human adipocytes. *Int J Obes Relat Metab Disord,* Vol. 21, No. 4, pp. 261-266

Matsushita, M., Endo, Y. and Fujita, T. (1998). MASP1 (MBL-associated serine protease 1). *Immunobiology,* Vol. 199, No. 2, pp. 340-347

Matsushita, M., Endo, Y. and Fujita, T. (2000). Cutting edge: complement-activating complex of ficolin and mannose-binding lectin-associated serine protease. *J Immunol,* Vol. 164, No. 5, pp. 2281-2284

Matsushita, M., Endo, Y., Hamasaki, N. and Fujita, T. (2001). Activation of the lectin complement pathway by ficolins. *Int Immunopharmacol,* Vol. 1, No. 3, pp. 359-363

Matsushita, M. and Fujita, T. (1992). Activation of the classical complement pathway by mannose-binding protein in association with a novel C1s-like serine protease. *J Exp Med,* Vol. 176, No. 6, pp. 1497-1502

Matsushita, M. and Fujita, T. (1995). Cleavage of the third component of complement (C3) by mannose-binding protein-associated serine protease (MASP) with subsequent complement activation. *Immunobiology,* Vol. 194, No. 4-5, pp. 443-448

Megyeri, M., Mako, V., Beinrohr, L., Doleschall, Z., Prohaszka, Z., Cervenak, L., Zavodszky, P. and Gal, P. (2009). Complement protease MASP-1 activates human endothelial cells: PAR4 activation is a link between complement and endothelial function. *J Immunol,* Vol. 183, No. 5, pp. 3409-3416

Michels, V. V., Hittner, H. M. and Beaudet, A. L. (1978). A clefting syndrome with ocular anterior chamber defect and lid anomalies. *J Pediatr,* Vol. 93, No. 3, pp. 444-446

Mingarelli, R., Castriota Scanderbeg, A. and Dallapiccola, B. (1996). Two sisters with a syndrome of ocular, skeletal, and abdominal abnormalities (OSA syndrome). *J Med Genet,* Vol. 33, No. 10, pp. 884-886

Muller-Eberhard, H. J. and Gotze, O. (1972). C3 proactivator convertase and its mode of action. *J Exp Med,* Vol. 135, No. 4, pp. 1003-1008

Ohta, M., Okada, M., Yamashina, I. and Kawasaki, T. (1990). The mechanism of carbohydrate-mediated complement activation by the serum mannan-binding protein. *J Biol Chem,* Vol. 265, No. 4, pp. 1980-1984

Paglialunga, S., Fisette, A., Yan, Y., Deshaies, Y., Brouillette, J. F., Pekna, M. and Cianflone, K. (2008). Acylation-stimulating protein deficiency and altered adipose tissue in alternative complement pathway knockout mice. *Am J Physiol Endocrinol Metab,* Vol. 294, No. 3, pp. E521-529

Pangburn, M. K., Schreiber, R. D. and Muller-Eberhard, H. J. (1981). Formation of the initial C3 convertase of the alternative complement pathway. Acquisition of C3b-like activities by spontaneous hydrolysis of the putative thioester in native C3. *J Exp Med,* Vol. 154, No. 3, pp. 856-867

Ricklin, D., Hajishengallis, G., Yang, K. and Lambris, J. D. (2010). Complement: a key system for immune surveillance and homeostasis. *Nature immunology,* Vol. 11, No. 9, pp. 785-797

Rooryck, C., Diaz-Font, A., Osborn, D. P., Chabchoub, E., Hernandez-Hernandez, V., Shamseldin, H., Kenny, J., Waters, A., Jenkins, D., Kaissi, A. A., Leal, G. F., Dallapiccola, B., Carnevale, F., Bitner-Glindzicz, M., Lees, M., Hennekam, R., Stanier, P., Burns, A. J., Peeters, H., Alkuraya, F. S. and Beales, P. L. (2011). Mutations in lectin complement pathway genes COLEC11 and MASP1 cause 3MC syndrome. *Nat Genet,* Vol. 43, No. 3, pp. 197-203

Sato, T., Endo, Y., Matsushita, M. and Fujita, T. (1994). Molecular characterization of a novel serine protease involved in activation of the complement system by mannose-binding protein. *Int Immunol,* Vol. 6, No. 4, pp. 665-669

Schwaeble, W., Dahl, M. R., Thiel, S., Stover, C. and Jensenius, J. C. (2002). The mannan-binding lectin-associated serine proteases (MASPs) and MAp19: four components of the lectin pathway activation complex encoded by two genes. *Immunobiology,* Vol. 205, No. 4-5, pp. 455-466

Schwaeble, W. J., Lynch, N. J., Clark, J. E., Marber, M., Samani, N. J., Ali, Y. M., Dudler, T., Parent, B., Lhotta, K., Wallis, R., Farrar, C. A., Sacks, S., Lee, H., Zhang, M., Iwaki, D., Takahashi, M., Fujita, T., Tedford, C. E. and Stover, C. M. (2011). Targeting of mannan-binding lectin-associated serine protease-2 confers protection from myocardial and gastrointestinal ischemia/reperfusion injury. *Proc Natl Acad Sci U S A,* Vol. 108, No. 18, pp. 7523-7528

Shi, L., Takahashi, K., Dundee, J., Shahroor-Karni, S., Thiel, S., Jensenius, J. C., Gad, F., Hamblin, M. R., Sastry, K. N. and Ezekowitz, R. A. (2004). Mannose-binding lectin-deficient mice are susceptible to infection with Staphylococcus aureus. *J Exp Med,* Vol. 199, No. 10, pp. 1379-1390

Sirmaci, A., Walsh, T., Akay, H., Spiliopoulos, M., Sakalar, Y. B., Hasanefendioglu-Bayrak, A., Duman, D., Farooq, A., King, M. C. and Tekin, M. (2010). MASP1 mutations in patients with facial, umbilical, coccygeal, and auditory findings of Carnevale, Malpuech, OSA, and Michels syndromes. *Am J Hum Genet,* Vol. 87, No. 5, pp. 679-686

Skjoedt, M. O., Hummelshoj, T., Palarasah, Y., Honore, C., Koch, C., Skjodt, K. and Garred, P. (2010). A novel mannose-binding lectin/ficolin-associated protein is highly expressed in heart and skeletal muscle tissues and inhibits complement activation. *The Journal of biological chemistry,* Vol. 285, No. 11, pp. 8234-8243

Stover, C. M., Schwaeble, W. J., Lynch, N. J., Thiel, S. and Speicher, M. R. (1999a). Assignment of the gene encoding mannan-binding lectin-associated serine protease 2 (MASP2) to human chromosome 1p36.3-->p36.2 by in situ hybridization and somatic cell hybrid analysis. *Cytogenet Cell Genet,* Vol. 84, No. 3-4, pp. 148-149

Stover, C. M., Thiel, S., Thelen, M., Lynch, N. J., Vorup-Jensen, T., Jensenius, J. C. and Schwaeble, W. J. (1999b). Two constituents of the initiation complex of the mannan-binding lectin activation pathway of complement are encoded by a single structural gene. *J Immunol,* Vol. 162, No. 6, pp. 3481-3490

Takada, F., Seki, N., Matsuda, Y., Takayama, Y. and Kawakami, M. (1995). Localization of the genes for the 100-kDa complement-activating components of Ra-reactive factor (CRARF and Crarf) to human 3q27-q28 and mouse 16B2-B3. *Genomics,* Vol. 25, No. 3, pp. 757-759

Takahashi, K., Gordon, J., Liu, H., Sastry, K. N., Epstein, J. E., Motwani, M., Laursen, I., Thiel, S., Jensenius, J. C., Carroll, M. and Ezekowitz, R. A. (2002). Lack of mannose-binding lectin-A enhances survival in a mouse model of acute septic peritonitis. *Microbes Infect,* Vol. 4, No. 8, pp. 773-784

Takahashi, M., Endo, Y., Fujita, T. and Matsushita, M. (1999). A truncated form of mannose-binding lectin-associated serine protease (MASP)-2 expressed by alternative polyadenylation is a component of the lectin complement pathway. *Int Immunol,* Vol. 11, No. 5, pp. 859-863

Takahashi, M., Ishida, Y., Iwaki, D., Kanno, K., Suzuki, T., Endo, Y., Homma, Y. and Fujita, T. (2010). Essential role of mannose-binding lectin-associated serine protease-1 in activation of the complement factor D. *J Exp Med,* Vol. 207, No. 1, pp. 29-37

Takahashi, M., Iwaki, D., Kanno, K., Ishida, Y., Xiong, J., Matsushita, M., Endo, Y., Miura, S., Ishii, N., Sugamura, K. and Fujita, T. (2008). Mannose-binding lectin (MBL)-associated serine protease (MASP)-1 contributes to activation of the lectin complement pathway. *J Immunol,* Vol. 180, No. 9, pp. 6132-6138

Thiel, S., Vorup-Jensen, T., Stover, C. M., Schwaeble, W., Laursen, S. B., Poulsen, K., Willis, A. C., Eggleton, P., Hansen, S., Holmskov, U., Reid, K. B. and Jensenius, J. C. (1997). A second serine protease associated with mannan-binding lectin that activates complement. *Nature,* Vol. 386, No. 6624, pp. 506-510

Thurman, J. M. and Holers, V. M. (2006). The central role of the alternative complement pathway in human disease. *J Immunol,* Vol. 176, No. 3, pp. 1305-1310

Turner, M. W. (1996). Mannose-binding lectin: the pluripotent molecule of the innate immune system. *Immunology today,* Vol. 17, No. 11, pp. 532-540

Vorup-Jensen, T., Jensenius, J. C. and Thiel, S. (1998). MASP-2, the C3 convertase generating protease of the MBLectin complement activating pathway. *Immunobiology,* Vol. 199, No. 2, pp. 348-357

Walport, M. J. (2001a). Complement. First of two parts. *N Engl J Med,* Vol. 344, No. 14, pp. 1058-1066

Walport, M. J. (2001b). Complement. Second of two parts. *N Engl J Med,* Vol. 344, No. 15, pp. 1140-1144

Yasruel, Z., Cianflone, K., Sniderman, A. D., Rosenbloom, M., Walsh, M. and Rodriguez, M. A. (1991). Effect of acylation stimulating protein on the triacylglycerol synthetic pathway of human adipose tissue. *Lipids,* Vol. 26, No. 7, pp. 495-499

Yousef, G. M., Elliott, M. B., Kopolovic, A. D., Serry, E. and Diamandis, E. P. (2004). Sequence and evolutionary analysis of the human trypsin subfamily of serine peptidases. *Biochimica et biophysica acta,* Vol. 1698, No. 1, pp. 77-86

Zhang, Y., Proenca, R., Maffei, M., Barone, M., Leopold, L. and Friedman, J. M. (1994). Positional cloning of the mouse obese gene and its human homologue. *Nature,* Vol. 372, No. 6505, pp. 425-432

Chapter 8

CELF1, a Multifunctional Regulator of Posttranscriptional Networks

Daniel Beisang, Paul R. Bohjanen and Irina A. Vlasova-St. Louis

Additional information is available at the end of the chapter

http://dx.doi.org/10.5772/48780

1. Introduction

In order to assure the precise utilization of genetic information, gene expression is regulated at the level of transcription as well as multiple post-transcriptional levels including splicing, transport, localization, mRNA stability, and translation [1],[2],[3],[4],[5],[6],[7]. During evolution, cells developed precise mechanisms to ensure that each transcript is appropriately stored, modified, translated or degraded, depending on the need for the mRNA or encoded protein by the cell. Steady-state protein levels within a cell correlate poorly with steady-state levels of mRNA, leading scientists to hypothesize that the gene expression is regulated at post-transcriptional levels [8]. Work over the past quarter century has resulted in the identification of unifying concepts in post-transcriptional regulation. One unifying concept states is that post-transcriptional regulation is mediated by two major molecular components: *cis*-acting regulatory sequence elements and *trans*-acting factors. *Cis*-acting regulatory sequence elements are sub-sequences contained in the 5′ untranslated region (UTR), coding region, and 3′UTR of mRNA that are selectively recognized by a complementary set of one or more *trans*-acting factors to regulate post-transcriptional gene expression. *Trans*-acting factors include RNA-binding proteins (RBPs) and microRNAs (miRNAs) which are able to influence the fate of mRNA by controlling processes such as translation and mRNA degradation (reviewed in references [9],[10],[11],[12]). The combinatorial interplay between various miRNAs and RBPs binding to a given mRNA allows for the transcript specific regulation critical to many cellular decisions during development [13],[14],[15],[16] and in response to environmental stimuli (reviewed in references [17],[18],[19],[20],[21],[22]).

Various experimental approaches have been developed to understand the interaction between RBPs and the network of transcripts that they regulate. One of the most widely used techniques involves immunopurification of specific RNA-binding proteins from cellular extracts followed by high-throughput analysis of the co-purified RNA species [23]. The coupling of this technique to powerful bioinformatic analysis methods has lead researchers to understand the binding specificity of a wide-variety of RBPs. The advent of new technology such as next generation sequencing and chemical cross-linking procedures have improved these methodologies and allowed for the fine-scale mapping of RBP binding sites, as well as the refinement of RBP binding motifs. Microarray-based studies that evaluated mRNA decay rates on a global basis have also provided valuable information about the role of post-transcriptional regulation of a wide variety of transcripts that have important physiological functions [24],[25],[26],[27],[28],[29].

This chapter focuses on the role of CELF1 (CUGBP and embryonically lethal abnormal vision-type RNA binding protein 3-like factor 1) in the regulation of posttranscriptional gene expression. CELF1 functions to regulate posttranscriptional gene expression by binding to RNA sequences known as GU-rich elements (GREs). Genome-wide measurements of mRNA decay and bioinformatic sequence motif discovery methods were used to identify the GRE as a highly conserved sequence that was enriched in the 3'UTR of mRNA transcripts with short half lives in primary human T lymphocytes [30]. This sequence resembled previously characterized binding sites for CELF1 [31],[32], and CELF1 was found to bind with high affinity to GRE sequences and mediate mRNA degradation [30]. This chapter reviews how CELF1 and its target transcripts function as an evolutionarily conserved posttranscriptional regulatory network which plays important roles in health and disease.

2. Evolutionary conservation of CELF proteins

The CELF protein family is an evolutionarily conserved family of RNA-binding proteins that play essential roles in post-transcriptional gene regulation [28],[33]. These proteins contain three highly conserved RNA-Recognition Motifs (RRM) with the 2 N-terminal RRMs and the C-terminal RRM being separated by a highly divergent linker domain [34]. The RRMs confer RNA binding activity, and it is postulated that the divergent linker domain is an important site for functional regulation. Six members of the CELF family have been identified in humans and mice: CELF1 (CUGBP1) and CELF2 (CUGBP2) proteins are expressed ubiquitously and play vital role in embryogenesis [35],[36],[37],[38],[39], whereas CELF proteins 3-6 are restricted to adult tissues and found almost exclusively in the nervous system [40],[41]. CELF proteins often serve multiple functions in both the cytoplasm and the nucleus [42],[43]. Human CELF1 and its orthologs in *Gallus gallus, Zebrafish, Xenopus, Drosophila* and *C. elegans* have been known for many years to regulate gene expression at posttranscriptional levels and to control important developmental processes [31],[44],[45],[46],[47],[48],[49].

CELF1 function is conserved across evolution at the level of biochemical mechanism as well as its function in regulating development. Transcript deadenylation is often the first step in the mRNA degradation process, and CELF1 has been shown to promote transcript deadenylation in diverse species [28],[50]. In *Xenopus* embryos the CELF1 homologue

Embryo Deadenylation Element Binding Protein (EDEN-BP), which is 88% identical to CELF1, regulates transcript deadenylation, and human CELF1 was able to functionally replace the deadenylation function of EDEN-BP in *Xenopus* extracts [51]. In HeLa cell extracts CELF1 also promotes transcript deadenylation and was shown to recruit PolyA Ribonuclease (PARN) [52]. In addition to the evolutionary conservation of the biochemical function of CELF1, the developmental programs regulated by CELF1 may also be conserved. For example, CELF1 appears to be an important factor in muscle development in diverse species. Studies investigating the function of CELF1 in *Drosophila, Xenopus* and mice have shown that CELF1 is critical for regulating the muscle developmental program [45], [53], [54]. More recent work suggests that CELF1 is a crucial factor in the regulation of mRNA degradation in mouse myoblasts [55]. Thus, in addition to the conservation of its biochemical function as a regulator of deadenylation, the role of CELF1 in muscle development may also be conserved.

As described below, CELF proteins from diverse species bind to RNA preferentially at GU-rich sequences and thereby regulate post-transcriptional processes such as mRNA splicing, translation, deadenylation and mRNA degradation. The structure and biochemical properties of CELF family members suggest functional redundancy [56], yet each CELF protein targets specific sub-populations of RNA transcripts and appears to have distinct functions [57]. We are starting to understand the mechanisms by which an individual CELF protein can serve multiple biochemical functions to coordinately regulate gene expression at posttranscriptional levels [30].

3. Biochemistry of binding by CELF proteins to target mRNA

CELF 1 and 2 proteins were first isolated and characterized as novel heterogeneous nuclear ribonucleoproteins (hnRNPs). Timchenko et.al. demonstrated that these proteins bound to RNA containing the sequence $(CUG)_8$ within the 3'UTR of myotonin protein kinase mRNA *in vitro* [58],[59]. Subsequent searches for the RNA-binding specificities of CELF1 and CELF2 used systemic evolution of ligands exponential enrichment (SELEX), revealing that CELF1 and CELF2 both bound preferentially to GU-rich RNA sequences [60]. Binding by CELF1 to GU-rich sequences *in vitro* and *in vivo* was abrogated by mutation of G nucleotides to C [30],[61]. Takanashi et. al. used a yeast three hybrid system for evaluating RNA-protein interactions, and found CELF1 bound preferentially to UG repeats rather than to CUG repeats [32]. CELF1 bound with high specificity to $(UG)_{15}$ based on a surface plasmon resonance (SPR) quantitative binding assay [62]. Orthologues of CELF1 in other species also appear to have preferences for binding to GU-rich sequences. In *Xenopus,* the CELF1 orthologue EDEN-BP (embryo deadenylation element binding protein) binds to the GU-rich EDEN element, which contains the sequence $(UGUA)_{12}$, and functions as a deadenylation signal in *Xenopus* embryos after fertilization [31],[51]. In *Drosophila,* the CELF1 orthologue Bru-3 was found to bind specifically to $(UG)_{15}$ repeats and also was able to bind to the *Xenopus* EDEN element [46]. The *Zebrafish* protein Brul, a homologue of EDEN-BP with 81% identity, was also shown to preferentially bind to GU-rich RNAs [63]. EDEN-BP and Bru-3 can bind to GRE-RNA as dimers [64],[65] and may require GU-rich sequences of sufficient length to allow dimer formation [66]. In addition to the primary GU-rich sequence, adjacent sequence elements may also be important for assembly of CELF proteins on RNA by allowing optimal secondary structure to facilitate the formation of RNA-protein complexes [67],[68].

Structural studies have provided valuable insight into the mechanisms underlying the RNA-binding activity of CELF1. CELF proteins all contain two N-terminal and one C-terminal RNA recognition motifs (RRMs), separated by a 160-230 residue divergent domain [69],[70]. The highly conserved RRMs bind to RNA in a sequence-specific manner [69],[71]. Nuclear Magnetic Resonance spectroscopic (NMR)-based solution studies demonstrated that both RRM1 and RRM2 each contribute to binding to a 12-nt target RNA containing two UUGUU motifs. The tandem RRM1/2 domains together show increased affinity compared to the binding by each domain separately to an RNA sequence with two sequential UUGU(U) motifs, thus indicating binding cooperativity between the two RRMs [34],[72]. Crystallographic studies showed that both RRM2 and RRM1 bind to GRE-RNA, and RRM1 is important for crystal-packing interactions [73].

In addition to RRM1 and RRM2, RRM3 also has RNA-binding activity. According to NMR analysis, RRM3 specifically recognizes the UGU trinucleotide segment of bound $(UG)_3$ RNA through extensive stacking and hydrogen-bonding interactions within the pocket formed by the beta-sheet and the conserved N-terminal extension [71]. Experiments investigating CELF1 function through a yeast three hybrid system suggested that deletion/mutation of RRM1 or RRM2 does not abrogate binding to GU-rich RNA, suggesting that RRM3 may recognize GU-repeats more avidly than RRM1 or RRM2 [62]. Additionally, it has been reported that RRM3 is able to recognize a poorly defined G/C-rich sequence from the 5'UTR of Cyclin D1 when combined with the divergent domain [65]. The divergent domain also appears to be important for RNA-binding since the presence of divergent domain within recombinant CELF1/CELF4 chimeric proteins increased RNA-binding affinity, perhaps by conveying important conformational changes necessary for RNA-binding [32],[62],[70]. The divergent domain may also facilitate CELF:CELF homotypic interactions [64] which may influence its activity. For example, CELF:CELF interactions appear to activate RNA deadenylation in *Xenopus* extracts [66].

3.1. Regulation of CELF1 function through phosphorylation

CELF1 is a known phosphoprotein with multiple predicted phosphorylation sites, and CELF1 phosphorylation appears to regulate its function as a mediator of alternative splicing, mRNA decay, and translational regulation [74],[75],[76],[77]. One of the pathologic events which occurs in the disease Myotonic Dystrophy type 1 (DM1) is an increase in the protein abundance of CELF1 and an associated increase in CELF1 mediated alternative splicing activity. This increase in CELF1 protein abundance is a result of increased CELF1 protein stability secondary to hyperphosphorylation [75]. In DM1, the (CUG)n expansion of the DMPK 3'UTR leads to protein kinase C (PKC) activation through an unknown mechanism. PKC, in turn, hyperphosphorylates CELF1, resulting in increased protein stability and abundance as well as increased splicing activity [78]. Additionally, in transgenic mouse models of DM1, mice treated with specific inhibitors of the PKC pathway showed amelioration of cardiac abnormalities associated with the disease phenotype [79]. Phosphorylation of CELF1 also influences its ability to regulate muscle development (reviewed in [80]). CELF1 phosphorylation by Akt kinase at Ser 28 in normal muscle myoblasts influences its ability to affect the translation of its target transcripts during differentiation [65]. Phosphorylation of CELF1 also directly influences its RNA-binding activity. For example, cyclin D3-Cdk4/6 phosphorylates CELF1 at Ser 302, altering the binding specificity of CELF1 to RNA and translation initiation proteins, such as eIF2α [81]. During the process of T cell activation, phosphorylation of CELF1 alters binding by CELF1 to target transcripts. Shortly following T cell activation, CELF1 becomes phosphorylated, dramatically decreasing its affinity for mRNA and leading to stabilization of CELF1 target transcripts [77]. Overall, these studies show that phosphorylation regulates the many functions of CELF1 in posttranscriptional gene regulation.

3.2. Identification of CELF1 target transcripts

Insight into the biological significance of CELF1 function as a coordinate regulator of post-transcriptional network was revealed through the experimental determination of CELF1 target transcripts. A technique involving RNA-immunoprecipitation followed by microarray analysis of associate transcripts (RIP-Chip) has allowed for the unbiased, genome-wide experimental identification of RNA-binding protein target transcripts. This technique involves immunoprecipitating an RNA-binding protein of interest from cell lysates under conditions that preserve RNA:Protein interactions. The co-purified RNA found associated with the immunoprecipitated RNA-binding protein is then isolated and interrogated using high throughput methods such as microarrays. Using this methodology, CELF1 targets have been identified in HeLa cells, resting and activated human T cells, and mouse myoblasts [55],[77],[82]. CELF1 targets, identified in cytoplasmic extracts from HeLa cells using an anti-CELF1 antibody, were analyzed to identify the CELF1 target sequence, which is known as the GRE. The sequence profile of CELF1 target transcripts was analyzed for enriched sequences using a Markov Chain Monte Carlo based gibbs sampler algorithm (BioProspector) as well as an overrepresentation algorithm, and the previously described GRE sequence, UGUUUGUUUGU, and a GU-repeat sequence, UGUGUGUGUGU, were found to be highly overrepresented in the 3′UTRs of the CELF1 target transcripts [83]. Both sequences were validated as CELF1-binding targets and were shown to function as mRNA decay elements by accelerating the decay of reporter transcripts. While GU-repeat sequences had previously been identified as a CELF1 recognition motif through *in vitro* SELEX protocol [60]. These and other experiments identified putative binding targets of CELF1 in cells [32],[62]. Because (as described later in this chapter) the UGUUUGUUUGU sequence and the GU-repeat sequence both bound to CELF1 and functioned as decay elements, the GRE was redefined to contain both of these sequences [83],[84]. The RIP-Chip approach was also used to immunoprecipitate endogenous RNA binding complexes from mouse myoblasts, using an anti-CELF1 antibody and similar G and U rich target sequences were identified [55]. In *Xenopus* extracts, target transcripts identified by RIP-Chip using an antibody against the CELF1 sequence homolog, EDEN-BP, were enriched in GU-rich sequences very similar to GREs [85]. These GU-rich containing target transcripts represented approximately 5% of the tested transcripts on the microarray [85]. In this work, the authors proposed a 15-nucleotide consensus motif $(UGU/UG)_3$ to be the target motif of EDEN-BP [85],[86]. The RIP-Chip approach was also used to investigate the cytoplasmic target transcripts of CELF1 in resting and activated primary human T cells, and target transcripts were highly enriched for the presence of the GRE in their 3'UTRs, but the number of CELF1 target transcripts decreased dramatically following T cell activation [77]. Overall, numerous CELF1 target transcripts have been identified in several different systems indicating the CELF1 functions to regulate an important posttranscriptional network of gene expression.

Another approach to identify targets of RNA-binding proteins utilizes a cross-linking step prior to immunoprecipitation (CLIP) and subsequent high throughput methods to identify protein binding sequences. Using this method, 315 CELF1 RNA targets were identified in whole cell extracts from mouse hindbrain [87]. These RNA-binding targets for CELF1 were enriched in UG repeat sequences, with 64% of target sequences found in introns and 25% found in 3' UTR sequences [87]. Similar analysis of CELF1 in the C2C12 mouse myoblast cell line [88] extensively characterized RNA-binding sites of CELF1 and found that CELF1 bound predominantly in 3'UTRs and caused mRNA decay. The authors found significant enrichment of CELF1 binding sites in intronic regions flanking exons, supporting a role for CELF1 in alternative splicing [88]. Overall, these studies suggest that GU-rich sequences serve as genuine binding sites for CELF1 in a manner that has been conserved through evolution. In the next sections, we review the data supporting the model that CELF1 recognizes GU-rich sequences and thereby regulates pre-mRNA splicing, translation, and/or mRNA deadenylation/decay depending on the cellular and environmental context.

4. CELF1 as a regulator of splicing

Pre-mRNA alternative splicing is a common mechanism for generating transcript and protein diversity. An estimated 90% of human genes produce alternatively spliced transcripts [89],[90]. Alignment of the genomic regions adjacent to mammalian intron-exon splice sites, identified TG-rich motifs (TTCTG and TGTT) as conserved *cis*-elements found at splicing acceptor sites associated with alternative splicing [91],[92]. These C/UG-rich sequences serve as binding sites for CELF proteins which activate or repress the splicing of pre-mRNA targets, depending on the context [93]. Recent evidence has re-confirmed the position-dependence of CELF1-binding sites in regulating exon inclusion or skipping (Figure 1) [88]. Although alternative splicing regulation was initially considered the primary function of CELF1 proteins in the nucleus, CELF members have also been implicated in nuclear C to U RNA editing in mammalian cells [94],[95].

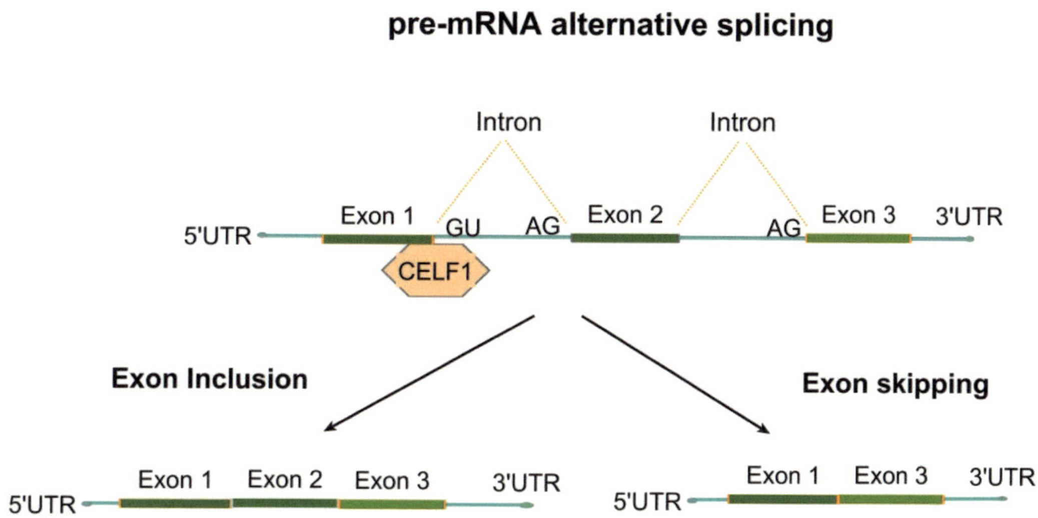

Figure 1. Alternative pre-mRNA splicing by CELF1 protein modulates the temporal and spatial diversity of genes during development. CELF1 binds to GU-rich intronic sequences in precursor mRNA and regulates exon inclusion or exon skipping during stage-specific alternative splicing transitions.

CELF1-mediated regulation of alternative splicing is critical for maintenance of normal muscle structure and function [43],[96],[97]. Much of what we know about the role of CELF1 in alternative splicing comes from studies investigating the role of CELF1 in the pathogenesis of the neuromuscular disease myotonic dystrophy type 1 (DM1). In this disease, aberrant gain of CELF1 function is combined with a corresponding loss of function of the splicing factor MBNL1, resulting in the mis-splicing of a number of crucial genes (reviewed in [11]). Minigene reporter systems that contain alternative splice sites proved to be a useful tools for the identification of pre-mRNA targets for CELF1, including genes for cardiac troponin T (TNNT2) [98], insulin receptor (INSR) [99], and chloride channel1 (CLCN1) [100],[101]. Interestingly, these genes were all shown to be mis-regulated in tissues from patients who suffered from DM1. Minigene systems have been particularly useful in demonstrating that individual pre-mRNA splicing events are affected by loss or gain of activities of specific regulatory proteins. Studies performed in cultured cells with transiently transfected minigenes have identified a number of alternative gene regions regulated by CELF1 and other family members [43], [69], [98], [99], [100], [101], [102], [103], [104], [105], [106],[107],[108]. However, as in other chimeric systems, the results of minigene overexpression experiments may not necessarily reflect the full-length pre-mRNA splicing patterns observed *in vivo*, especially during certain stages of organism development [109]. CELF proteins have been found to regulate the switch from fetal to adult splicing patterns of several skeletal muscle transcripts through the use of transgenic mouse models [101],[100],[110]. In mice, splicing microarray studies found that nearly half of transcripts that undergo fetal-to-adult alternative splicing transitions in heart respond to over-expression of CELF1, suggesting that the level of CELF1 activity directly regulates the alternative splicing pattern of endogenous transcripts [111]. The development of dominant negative (DN) and tissue specific transgenic mice was advantageous for studying CELF-specific alternative splicing *in vivo* [96],[104],[109],[110]. For example, dominant negative CELF (DNΔCELF) expressed under the control of a cardiac muscle-specific promoter, promoted the development of dilatated cardiomyopathy and cardiac dysfunction over time [96]. In contrast, when DNΔCELF was expressed under the control of a skeletal muscle-specific promoter, mice exhibit reduction in muscle intersticia and an increase in slow twitch fibers [110]. In near future, we will see more phenotypic studies using a nucleus-restricted form of the dominant negative CELF protein which would specifically block only the CELF1 nuclear function, leaving the cytoplasmic function intact [112], [113], [114].

5. CELF proteins as regulators of deadenylation, translation, and mRNA decay

5.1. Deadenylation

CELF1 plays important roles in mRNA stability and translation in diverse species. In eukaryotic organisms, the length of a transcript's polyA tail influences the translational state of a transcript, and deadenylation is regulated by GU-rich sequences and CELF1 proteins across evolution. Regulation of translation through deadenylation in *Xenopus* embryos is the best characterized model of posttranscriptional gene regulation by CELF proteins. In this model, the shortening or lengthening of the polyA tail causes activation or repression of translation of a number of transcripts [115]. However, as we describe below, deadenylation can also be the first step leading to mRNA degradation in mammalian cells, and the deadenylation machinery seems to be conserved although the consequences of deadenylation (translation or degradation) is regulated differently in diverse species.

In *Xenopus,* maternal transcripts are stored in the cytoplasm of oocytes in a translationally silent form (reviewed in [116]). After fertilization of *Xenopus* oocytes, the CELF1 homologue EDEN-BP binds to the EDEN element which activates transcript deadenylation and leads to the translation of EDEN-containing mRNA transcripts, including transcripts that encode important cell cycle regulators [31],[33],[50],[117],[118],[119]. Furthermore, human CELF1, which has 88% identity with EDEN-BP, was able to functionally substitute for EDEN-BP to mediate transcript deadenylation in *Xenopus* extracts [51], suggesting that the deadenylation function of GU-rich sequences and CELF proteins were conserved in diverse species.

Removal of the polyA tail is the rate-limiting step in the degradation of the majority of mammalian mRNAs [120],[121]. In human cell lines, CELF1 has been shown to associate with the deadenylase enzyme polyA ribonuclease (PARN) and to stimulate polyA tail shortening in a cell-free assay using S100 extracts from human cells [52]. It is not known if CELF1 activates other deadenylases in mammalian cells or how deadenylated transcripts are subsequently degraded. PARN, EDEN-BP and cytoplasmic polyadenylation element-binding proteins (CPEB) are present in *Xenopus* oocyte extracts [122], [123]. Theoretically, the balance between the rate of deadenylation versus polyadenylation depends upon the ability of EDEN-BP to recruit PARN and bind to polyA tail with higher affinity than CPEB

[122]. Since EDEN-BP in *Xenopus* is a regulator of deadenylation, it is likely that CELF1 also regulates deadenylation in mammalian cells, leading to transcript degradation through unknown mechanisms.

5.2. Translation

Translation is a critical layer of post-transcriptional control of gene expression that is regulated in response to environmental and developmental changes. CELF proteins have been shown to be involved in the activation of translation of several mRNA species at various stages of development [124]. Additionally, CELF proteins have been shown to function as inhibitors of translation under conditions of stress, where they act as translational silencers in conjunction with other protein binding partners. The involvement of CELF1 in translational regulation is evolutionarily conserved, with several CELF1 homologues having been shown to regulate translation. For example, in the *Drosophila* oocyte, translational repression is mediated by the protein Bruno (CELF1 orthologue), that binds specifically to bruno response elements (BREs) within the oskar mRNA 3'UTR. Binding by the CELF1 orthologue Bru-3 to GU-rich sequences in 3′UTR of gurken, cyclin A and oskar mRNA leads to their translational repression [44]. The suggested mechanism underlying Bru-3 mediated translational regulation is through the formation of a Bru-3/eIF4E/5′-cap translational silencing complex during specific stages of embryo development [125]. CELF1 has also been shown to play a role in translational regulation in mammalian cells. In human cell lines, tethering of CELF1 to the 3′UTR of mRNA through an interaction with the MS2 coat protein led to decreased steady state levels of reporter transcripts that contained a MS2 RNA-binding site, while reporter protein levels increased [126]. CELF1 increases the translation of p21 (CDKN1A28) protein [127], and Mef2a29 [128] during normal muscle cell differentiation via direct interaction with (GC)n repeats located within the 5′UTR of those mRNAs. The data suggests that CELF1 mediates translational regulation through interaction with a G- and C-rich motif in the 5′UTR, whereas CELF1 mediates its splicing and degradation effects through interaction with a G- and U-rich motif in introns and 3′UTRs, respectively. Our experiments determining CELF1 binding targets through high-throughput means have failed to identify enrichment of GC-rich motifs or 5′UTR binding by CELF1 [82]. It may be that CELF1 mediated translational regulation is rare, and only occurs in the context of very specific mRNA species and cellular contexts. Recently, an additional mechanism for CELF1 mediated translational regulation through interaction with the 3′UTR was discovered. Binding of CELF1 to the 3′UTR of Serine hydroxymethyltransferase (SHMT) RNA [129],[130] and cyclin dependent kinase inhibitor p27 (Kip1) RNA [131], was found to regulate internal ribosome entry site (IRES) mediated translation activation. This implicated CELF1 in participating in an IRES mode of initiation of mRNA translation. In addition, IRES translation is achieved through CELF1/hnRNPH complex formation, which promotes circularization of RNA transcripts by mediating 5′/3′ ends interactions [129]. Whether CELF1 recruits the translation machinery to the 5′UTR via additional interaction with eIF2 (Eukaryotic Initiation Factor 2) or another initiation factor remains to be determined (Figure 2).

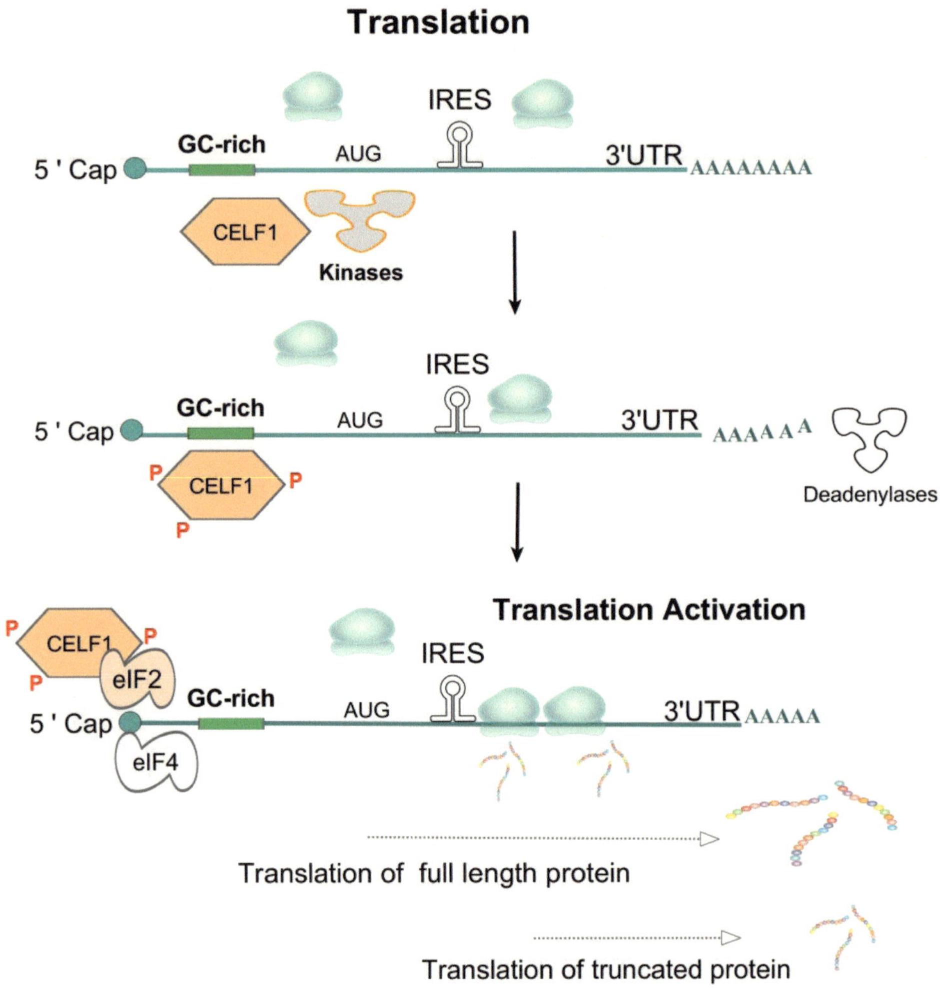

Figure 2. Simplified representation of the role of CELF1 in mRNA translation. Several mechanisms have been proposed for CELF1 mediated regulation of translation. Many of these mechanisms involve CELF1 interacting with mRNA through sequences in the 5'UTR and subsequent translation via an internal ribosomal entry site. If (hyper)/phosphorylated, CELF1 interacts with eIF2 and other translation initiation factors, this serves to promote the production of truncated protein products.

One well studied instance of CELF1 mediated translational control involves the translation of alternative isoforms of the transcription factor CCAAT/enhancer-binding protein (CEBPbeta) [132],[133],[134]. In a rat model, CELF1 phosphorylation was activated by partial hepatectomy, which promoted the formation of a complex between CELF1 and eIF2a. This subsequently led to selective translation of the liver enriched inhibitory protein (LIP) isoform of CCAAT/enhancer-binding protein [76]. It was later shown that in liver, CELF1 undergoes hyper-phosphorylation through a GSK3beta-cyclin D3-cdk4 kinase pathway, and the activity of this pathway seemed to increase with age [135]. Similar to the partial hepatectomy model, the cdk4-mediated hyper-phosphorylation of CELF1 was involved in the age-associated induction of the CELF1-eIF2 complex [136]. In the rat aging model, the CELF1-eIF2 complex binds to the 5′UTR of HDAC1 mRNA and increases histone deacetylase 1 protein levels in aging liver [136],[137]. It was further shown that during rat aging, CELF1 phosphorylation promotes its interaction with a GC-rich sequence in 5′UTR of p21 mRNA causing p21 translational arrest and senescence in fibroblasts [138]. In myocytes, p21 mRNA is stabilized in discrete cytoplasmic structures called stress granules, which serve as reversible storage sites for mRNA under conditions of stress. Interestingly, only during late senescence did p21s localization in stress granules interfere with its translation [138],[139]. One important component of stress granules is the RNA-binding protein T cell internal antigen 1 (TIA1). Consistent with CELF1's recruitment to stress granules, CELF1 has been shown to function as a translational silencer through interaction with the TIA1 protein [140]. Further support for this model comes from experiments utilizing DM1 cell harboring CUG repeat RNA. The presence of a CUG repeat expansion was found to cause stress and activation of the PKR-phospho-eIF2α–CELF1 pathway leading to stress granule formation and inhibition of mRNA translation [81]. This disruption to physiologic mRNA translation pathways by cellular stress signals might contribute to the progressive muscle loss in DM1 patients. Taken together, this data suggests that CELF proteins may function as activators or repressors of translation, depending on the context.

5.3. mRNA Decay

Bioinformatic analysis of short lived-transcripts in primary human T cells led to the identification of the conserved, GU-rich element (GRE) enriched in transcript's 3′UTRs. CELF1 was subsequently identified as a protein that specifically bound to the GRE *in vitro* and then to regulate the decay of exogenously expressed GRE-containing transcripts within cells [30],[141]. Further verification of the role of CELF1 in GRE-mediated mRNA decay came from the observation that in HeLa cells, siRNA-mediated knockdown of CELF1 led to stabilization of GRE-containing beta-globin reporter transcripts, as well as endogenous GRE-containing transcripts [30],[83],[142]. These results implicated CELF1 as a mediator of GRE-dependent mRNA decay. In primary human T cells, GREs and CELF1 appear to be involved in the rapid changes in gene expression patterns observed following T cell receptor-mediated activation. Identification the cytoplasmic binding targets of CELF1 before and after T cell activation led to the discovery that CELF1 dissociated from GRE-containing transcripts following T cell activation in a manner correlated with a transient upregulation of CELF1 target mRNAs [77]. The dissociation of CELF1 from its target transcripts upon T cell activation was the result of an activation-dependent phosphorylation of CELF1 and a resultant decrease in the ability of CELF1 to bind to GRE-containing RNAs [77]. Many of the transiently up-regulated CELF1 target transcripts encoded proteins necessary for the transition from a quiescent state to a state of cellular activation and proliferation. This supported a model whereby CELF1 suppresses a network of transcripts involved in activation and proliferation in resting T cells, and subsequent activation-induced phosphorylation of CELF1 allows for de-repression and accumulation of these transcripts within activated cells.

In mouse myoblasts, cytoplasmic CELF1 bound hundreds of target transcripts that contained GU-rich sequences, including networks of transcripts that regulated cell cycle, intracellular transport and cell survival [55]. Knockdown of CELF1 in this myoblast cell line led to the stabilization of many endogenous GRE-containing targets, as well as luciferase reporter RNAs [88]. Many CELF1 target transcripts were found to be significantly stabilized in CELF1 knockout myoblasts, suggesting that CELF1 mediates the decay of a network of transcripts during myoblast growth and differentiation [55]. In the DM1 disease model, there is aberrant activation of the protein kinase C pathway as a result of the CTG expansion, and this results in CELF1 phosphorylation. Mouse myoblasts (C2C12 cells) made to express CTG expanded RNA were shown to experience stabilization of tumor necrosis factor alpha (TNF-alpha) mRNA [143]. This result suggested that the over-expression of TNF-alpha observed in DM1 could be coming from muscle, and this TNF-alpha overexpression may contribute to the muscle wasting and insulin resistance that are characteristic of this disease [143]. In summary, CELF1 and its GRE-containing target transcripts define posttranscriptional regulatory networks that function to control cellular growth, activation, and differentiation (Figure 3).

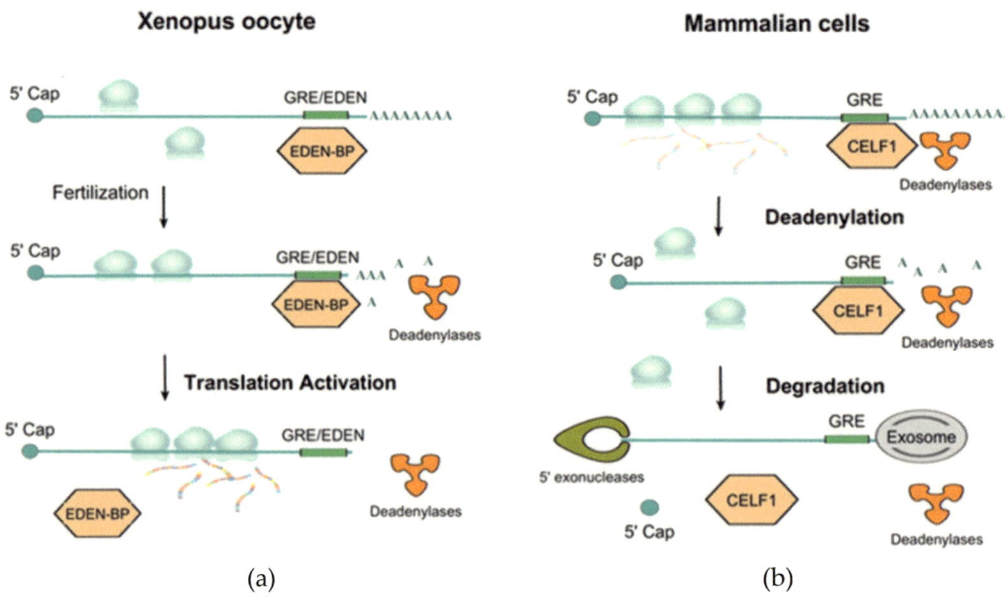

Figure 3. Evolutionary conservation of deadenylation by CELF1 protein and GU-rich sequences. (a). In *Xenopus* and *Drosophila* eggs, after fertilization, EDEN-BP (CELF1 homologue) bound to EDEN-containing maternal mRNAs, causing deadenylation and subsequent translational activation. (b). In mammalian cells, CELF1 binds to GREs within the 3' UTR of specific transcripts and promotes their deadenylation (by deadenylases) and subsequent decay by the exosome.

6. The GRE/CELF1 posttranscriptional network in human diseases

The CELF family is an evolutionarily conserved family of RNA-binding proteins that plays an essential role in several aspects of post-transcriptional gene regulation and participates in the control of important developmental processes. Disruption of CELF1/GRE-mediated mRNA regulation may play a role in the pathophysiology of developmental defects [87],[113],[144], or cancer [145],[146]. In *Xenopus*, injecting "masking" oligonucleotides into embryos to specifically inhibit the binding of CELF1 to mRNA causes developmental defects, such as the loss of somatic segmentation [147]. Genetic deletion of CELF1 in *Caenorhabditis elegans* and transgenic mice caused severe developmental abnormalities and death [38],[45]. CELF1 knockout mice were mostly non-viable, but the few surviving pups displayed severe muscular and fertility defects [38]. The finding that CELF1 knockout mice displayed muscle pathophysiology was not surprising since CELF1 was first described as a protein that bound to the abnormally expanded CUG mRNA repeats occurring in patients with the neuromuscular disease: type I myotonic dystrophy [58],[59]. It has since been shown that the molecular pathogenesis of DM1 involves an increase in both nuclear and cytoplasmic CELF1 levels [148],[149] due to hyper-phosphorylation of the protein [74]. Kuyumcu-Martinez and colleagues reported that CELF1 hyper-phosphorylation was triggered by the presence of abnormal CUG repeats in DMPK RNA, which caused cellular stress and a resultant activation of the Protein kinase C stress response pathway. This stress response and CELF1 hyper-phosphorylation was shown to trigger stabilization of the CELF1 protein and thus upregulation in DM1 myoblasts [75]. The importance of CELF1 upregulation is highlighted by the finding that over-expression of CELF1 in mouse heart and skeletal muscle recapitulated many of the aberrant splicing patterns observed in DM1 patient tissues [54],[78],[97],[128],[148],[150]. Interestingly, the repression of CELF1 activity can restore normal alternative splicing events in transgenic mouse model of DM1 [114]. It has become increasingly clear that abnormal splicing underlies the molecular pathogenesis of muscular degenerative disorders, and in addition to occurring in muscle tissue, these splicing changes have been reported in brain tissues [151] which correlated with the presence of neurologic impairment [152] and abnormal Ca(2+) metabolism in DM1 patients [153]. DM1-like alternative splicing dysregulation and altered expression of CELF1 also occurs in mouse models of other muscular dystrophies and muscle injury, most likely due to recapitulation of neonatal splicing patterns in regenerating fibers [113]. CELF1 function is altered in other neuromuscular diseases due to its sequestration to nuclear inclusions in oculopharyngeal muscular dystrophy (OPMD) [154], fragile-X-associated tremor/ataxia syndrome [152], and in spinal bulbar muscular atrophy [155], suggesting a key role for this protein in muscle pathophysiology. It will be interesting to investigate whether altered CELF1 regulation in muscle diseases could also have deleterious effects through altering the stability of GU-rich mRNA targets, given the role of CELF1 in mRNA decay. The discovery of disease-causing splicing patterns in muscle disease has yielded a wealth of information about both physiologic and dysregulated RNA biology and this information is currently being leveraged to develop novel therapies for DM1 and other RNA based neuromuscular disorders [156].

Despite the fact that the field of CELF1 biology is relatively young, there is some data supporting a potential link between dysregulated CELF1 mediated RNA metabolism and a cancerous phenotype. One recent study found CELF1 to be one to the top ten candidates in a transposon-based genetic screen in mice to identify potential drivers of colorectal tumorigenesis [157]. Additionally, CELF1 expression has been shown to be lost through a t(1;11)(q21;q23) translocation in certain forms of pediatric acute leukemia [158]. One way in which disruption of CELF1 may contribute to a malignant phenotype is through disregulation of C/EBPbeta expression. In HER2-overexpressing breast cancer cells CELF1 is activated favoring the production of the C/EBPbeta transcription-inhibitory isoform LIP over that of the active isoform LAP, and this contributed to evasion of TGFbeta and oncogene-induced senescence [146]. Treatment of HER2-transformed metastatic breast cancer cells with the anti-HER2/neu monoclonal antibody trastuzumab reduced CELF1 protein level and it's activity, suggesting that the targeting of CELF1 may be a viable adjunct therapy in the treatment of breast cancer [159]. Expressions of C/EBPbeta and C/EBPalfa are translationally repressed in BCR/ABL cells (chronic myelogenous leukemia) and it can be re-induced by imatinib via a mechanism that appears to depend on the activity of CELF1 and the integrity of the CUG-rich intercistronic region of C/EBPbeta mRNA [160],[161].

Another potential mechanism of CELF1 mediated tumor promotion comes from our lab's results of RIP-Chip experiments investigating CELF1's targets in normal and malignant cells. In primary human T cells, we observed that CELF1 bound to a large number of transcripts involved in cell cycle and apoptosis regulation pathways, and that upon activation and proliferation of these cells, CELF1 bound to a drastically reduced mRNA population [77]. This result suggests that CELF1 inhibition is correlated with a cellular state of proliferation and altered apoptotic response. We also identified hundreds of CELF1 target transcripts in human HeLa cells (carcinoma cell line) and many of these transcripts were different than those in normal T cells suggesting again that altered CELF1's RNA binding specificity may correlate with malignancy [82].

CELF1-HDAC1-C/EBPbeta pathway is activated in young rat liver cells and in human tumor liver samples suggesting that CELF1-HDAC1-C/EBPbeta complexes are involved in the development of liver tumors [162],[163]. The inhibition of the ubiquitin-dependent proteasome system (UPS) via specific drugs (such as Bortezomib) is one type of approach used to combat cancer [164]. Gareau et. al. showed that CELF1 is required for p21 mRNA stabilization and localization in stress granules induced upon treatment with Bortezomib. The authors postulated that this may allow cancer cells survive stress and escape apoptosis [165]. This mechanism may explain why some tumors are refractory to Bortezomib treatment.

Thus, the dysregulation of CELF1 and GREs appears to contribute to malignant phenotype, perhaps by abrogating its ability to mediate the rapid and timely degradation of GRE-containing growth-regulatory transcripts and promote translation of some cell cycle regulators and oncogenes.

7. Conclusion

In summary, we have learned a wealth of information about CELF1-mRNA complexes and their importance in development, regeneration, aging and disease. CELF1 binds preferentially to GRE-containing transcripts, and affects expression of transcripts encoding other transcription factors and RNA-binding proteins that regulate cell growth, apoptosis, and development/differentiation (reviewed in [28],[166]). Thus, CELF1 may be functioning as a posttranscriptional "regulator of regulators", whereby CELF1 influences the expression of a network of target transcripts encoding RNA/DNA binding proteins. This, in turn regulates individual subnetworks of transcripts necessary for development or environmental responses, such as immune activation, requiring transition from a quiescent state to a state of cellular activation and proliferation.

Understanding gene regulatory networks and the integration of transcriptional and posttranscriptional events are the next important tasks in translational medicine. It will require innovations in computational methods, experimental techniques and new animal models. It is also important to further investigate *in vivo* biochemical interactions between CELF proteins and RNA, to discover unknown components of CELF protein-containing complexes bound to RNA that may be involved in splicing, deadenylation, decay, and/or translation regulation. The lists of conserved RNA-binding proteins and mRNA cis-elements has been expanding over the past decade, but the mechanisms of the precise assembly of RNA-binding complexes in an orchestrated temporal and spatial manner have not been comprehensively described. Furthermore, little work has been done on how the expression and function of CELF1 is regulated, specifically by microRNAs (such as mir-222 [167], mir-503 [168], and miR-23a/b [169]). The more details we learn about intracellular signaling, cross-talk, molecular assembly and localization of RNA-protein complexes, the more unifying principles we may find. Understanding the biochemistry of posttranscriptional regulation will lead to elucidation of posttranscriptional regulatory pathways and networks and lead to a better understanding of normal cellular function and disease states.

Authors details

Daniel Beisang, Paul R. Bohjanen and Irina A. Vlasova-St. Louis
Department of Microbiology, Center for Infectious Diseases and Microbiology Translational Research, University of Minnesota, Minneapolis, MN, USA

Paul R. Bohjanen
Department of Medicine, University of Minnesota, Minneapolis, MN, USA

Acknowledgment

This work was supported by NIH grants AIO57484 and AIO72068 to P.R.B. D.B. was supported by MSTP grant T32 GM008244 from the NIH. I.A.V-S. was funded through a fellowship from the Lymphoma Research Foundation.

8. References

[1] Antic D, Keene JD (1997) Embryonic lethal abnormal visual RNA-binding proteins involved in growth, differentiation, and posttranscriptional gene expression. Am J Hum Genet 61: 273-278.

[2] Jans DA, Xiao CY, Lam MH (2000) Nuclear targeting signal recognition: a key control point in nuclear transport? Bioessays 22: 532-544.

[3] Jansen RP (2001) mRNA localization: message on the move. Nat Rev Mol Cell Biol 2: 247-256.

[4] Faustino NA, Cooper TA (2003) Pre-mRNA splicing and human disease. Genes Dev 17: 419-437.

[5] Mata J, Marguerat S, Bahler J (2005) Post-transcriptional control of gene expression: a genome-wide perspective. Trends Biochem Sci 30: 506-514.

[6] Moore MJ (2005) From birth to death: the complex lives of eukaryotic mRNAs. Science 309: 1514-1518.

[7] Keene JD (2007) RNA regulons: coordination of post-transcriptional events. Nat Rev Genet 8: 533-543.

[8] Mansfield KD, Keene JD (2009) The ribonome: a dominant force in co-ordinating gene expression. Biol Cell 101: 169-181.

[9] Keene JD (2007) Biological clocks and the coordination theory of RNA operons and regulons. Cold Spring Harb Symp Quant Biol 72: 157-165.

[10] Moroy T, Heyd F (2007) The impact of alternative splicing in vivo: mouse models show the way. RNA 13: 1155-1171.

[11] Lee JE, Cooper TA (2009) Pathogenic mechanisms of myotonic dystrophy. Biochem Soc Trans 37: 1281-1286.

[12] Fabian MR, Sonenberg N, Filipowicz W (2010) Regulation of mRNA translation and stability by microRNAs. Annu Rev Biochem 79: 351-379.

[13] Bitel CL, Perrone-Bizzozero NI, Frederikse PH HuB/C/D, nPTB, REST4, and miR-124 regulators of neuronal cell identity are also utilized in the lens. Mol Vis 16: 2301-2316.

[14] Kedde M, Agami R (2008) Interplay between microRNAs and RNA-binding proteins determines developmental processes. Cell Cycle 7: 899-903.

[15] Moore J, Lasko P (2009) Breaking the A chain: regulating mRNAs in development through CCR4 deadenylase. F1000 Biol Rep 1: 20.

[16] Brewer G (2002) Messenger RNA decay during aging and development. Ageing Res Rev 1: 607-625.

[17] Mignone F, Gissi C, Liuni S, Pesole G (2002) Untranslated regions of mRNAs. Genome Biol 3: REVIEWS0004.

[18] Krol J, Loedige I, Filipowicz W The widespread regulation of microRNA biogenesis, function and decay. Nat Rev Genet 11: 597-610.

[19] Misquitta CM, Chen T, Grover AK (2006) Control of protein expression through mRNA stability in calcium signalling. Cell Calcium 40: 329-346.

[20] Khabar KS (2007) Rapid transit in the immune cells: the role of mRNA turnover regulation. J Leukoc Biol 81: 1335-1344.

[21] Khabar KS, Young HA (2007) Post-transcriptional control of the interferon system. Biochimie 89: 761-769.

[22] Pascale A, Govoni S (2012) The complex world of post-transcriptional mechanisms: is their deregulation a common link for diseases? Focus on ELAV-like RNA-binding proteins. Cell Mol Life Sci 69: 501-517.

[23] Tenenbaum SA, Carson CC, Lager PJ, Keene JD (2000) Identifying mRNA subsets in messenger ribonucleoprotein complexes by using cDNA arrays. Proc Natl Acad Sci U S A 97: 14085-14090.

[24] Raghavan A, Ogilvie RL, Reilly C, Abelson ML, Raghavan S, et al. (2002) Genome-wide analysis of mRNA decay in resting and activated primary human T lymphocytes. Nucleic Acids Res 30: 5529-5538.

[25] Lam LT, Pickeral OK, Peng AC, Rosenwald A, Hurt EM, et al. (2001) Genomic-scale measurement of mRNA turnover and the mechanisms of action of the anti-cancer drug flavopiridol. Genome Biol 2: RESEARCH0041.

[26] Frevel MA, Bakheet T, Silva AM, Hissong JG, Khabar KS, et al. (2003) p38 Mitogen-activated protein kinase-dependent and -independent signaling of mRNA stability of AU-rich element-containing transcripts. Mol Cell Biol 23: 425-436.

[27] Yang E, van Nimwegen E, Zavolan M, Rajewsky N, Schroeder M, et al. (2003) Decay rates of human mRNAs: correlation with functional characteristics and sequence attributes. Genome Res 13: 1863-1872.

[28] Vlasova-St Louis I, Bohjanen PR (2011) Coordinate regulation of mRNA decay networks by GU-rich elements and CELF1. Curr Opin Genet Dev 21: 444-451.

[29] Vlasova IA, McNabb J, Raghavan A, Reilly C, Williams DA, et al. (2005) Coordinate stabilization of growth-regulatory transcripts in T cell malignancies. Genomics 86: 159-171.

[30] Vlasova IA, Tahoe NM, Fan D, Larsson O, Rattenbacher B, et al. (2008) Conserved GU-rich elements mediate mRNA decay by binding to CUG-binding protein 1. Mol Cell 29: 263-270.

[31] Paillard L, Omilli F, Legagneux V, Bassez T, Maniey D, et al. (1998) EDEN and EDEN-BP, a cis element and an associated factor that mediate sequence-specific mRNA deadenylation in Xenopus embryos. EMBO J 17: 278-287.

[32] Takahashi N, Sasagawa N, Suzuki K, Ishiura S (2000) The CUG-binding protein binds specifically to UG dinucleotide repeats in a yeast three-hybrid system. Biochem Biophys Res Commun 277: 518-523.

[33] Osborne HB, Gautier-Courteille C, Graindorge A, Barreau C, Audic Y, et al. (2005) Post-transcriptional regulation in Xenopus embryos: role and targets of EDEN-BP. Biochem Soc Trans 33: 1541-1543.

[34] Tripsianes K, Sattler M (2010) Repeat recognition. Structure 18: 1228-1229.

[35] Choi DK, Ito T, Tsukahara F, Hirai M, Sakaki Y (1999) Developmentally-regulated expression of mNapor encoding an apoptosis-induced ELAV-type RNA binding protein. Gene 237: 135-142.

[36] Good PJ, Chen Q, Warner SJ, Herring DC (2000) A family of human RNA-binding proteins related to the Drosophila Bruno translational regulator. J Biol Chem 275: 28583-28592.

[37] Li D, Bachinski LL, Roberts R (2001) Genomic organization and isoform-specific tissue expression of human NAPOR (CUGBP2) as a candidate gene for familial arrhythmogenic right ventricular dysplasia. Genomics 74: 396-401.

[38] Kress C, Gautier-Courteille C, Osborne HB, Babinet C, Paillard L (2007) Inactivation of CUG-BP1/CELF1 causes growth, viability, and spermatogenesis defects in mice. Mol Cell Biol 27: 1146-1157.

[39] Choi DK, Yoo KW, Hong SK, Rhee M, Sakaki Y, et al. (2003) Isolation and expression of Napor/CUG-BP2 in embryo development. Biochem Biophys Res Commun 305: 448-454.

[40] Yang Y, Mahaffey CL, Berube N, Maddatu TP, Cox GA, et al. (2007) Complex seizure disorder caused by Brunol4 deficiency in mice. PLoS Genet 3: e124.

[41] Wu J, Li C, Zhao S, Mao B (2010) Differential expression of the Brunol/CELF family genes during Xenopus laevis early development. Int J Dev Biol 54: 209-214.

[42] Morgan GT (2007) Localized co-transcriptional recruitment of the multifunctional RNA-binding protein CELF1 by lampbrush chromosome transcription units. Chromosome Res 15: 985-1000.

[43] Ladd AN, Stenberg MG, Swanson MS, Cooper TA (2005) Dynamic balance between activation and repression regulates pre-mRNA alternative splicing during heart development. Dev Dyn 233: 783-793.

[44] Kim-Ha J, Kerr K, Macdonald PM (1995) Translational regulation of oskar mRNA by bruno, an ovarian RNA-binding protein, is essential. Cell 81: 403-412.

[45] Milne CA, Hodgkin J (1999) ETR-1, a homologue of a protein linked to myotonic dystrophy, is essential for muscle development in Caenorhabditis elegans. Curr Biol 9: 1243-1246.

[46] Delaunay J, Le Mee G, Ezzeddine N, Labesse G, Terzian C, et al. (2004) The Drosophila Bruno paralogue Bru-3 specifically binds the EDEN translational repression element. Nucleic Acids Res 32: 3070-3082.

[47] Hashimoto Y, Suzuki H, Kageyama Y, Yasuda K, Inoue K (2006) Bruno-like protein is localized to zebrafish germ plasm during the early cleavage stages. Gene Expr Patterns 6: 201-205.

[48] Brimacombe KR, Ladd AN (2007) Cloning and embryonic expression patterns of the chicken CELF family. Dev Dyn 236: 2216-2224.

[49] Moore J, Han H, Lasko P (2009) Bruno negatively regulates germ cell-less expression in a BRE-independent manner. Mech Dev 126: 503-516.

[50] Paillard L, Osborne HB (2003) East of EDEN was a poly(A) tail. Biol Cell 95: 211-219.

[51] Paillard L, Legagneux V, Beverley Osborne H (2003) A functional deadenylation assay identifies human CUG-BP as a deadenylation factor. Biol Cell 95: 107-113.

[52] Moraes KC, Wilusz CJ, Wilusz J (2006) CUG-BP binds to RNA substrates and recruits PARN deadenylase. Rna 12: 1084-1091.

[53] Michalowski S, Miller JW, Urbinati CR, Paliouras M, Swanson MS, et al. (1999) Visualization of double-stranded RNAs from the myotonic dystrophy protein kinase gene and interactions with CUG-binding protein. Nucleic Acids Res 27: 3534-3542.

[54] Ward AJ, Rimer M, Killian JM, Dowling JJ, Cooper TA (2010) CUGBP1 overexpression in mouse skeletal muscle reproduces features of myotonic dystrophy type 1. Hum Mol Genet 19: 3614-3622.

[55] Lee JE, Lee JY, Wilusz J, Tian B, Wilusz CJ (2010) Systematic analysis of cis-elements in unstable mRNAs demonstrates that CUGBP1 is a key regulator of mRNA decay in muscle cells. PLoS One 5: e11201.
[56] Singh G, Charlet BN, Han J, Cooper TA (2004) ETR-3 and CELF4 protein domains required for RNA binding and splicing activity in vivo. Nucleic Acids Res 32: 1232-1241.
[57] Barreau C, Paillard L, Mereau A, Osborne HB (2006) Mammalian CELF/Bruno-like RNA-binding proteins: molecular characteristics and biological functions. Biochimie 88: 515-525.
[58] Timchenko LT, Timchenko NA, Caskey CT, Roberts R (1996) Novel proteins with binding specificity for DNA CTG repeats and RNA CUG repeats: implications for myotonic dystrophy. Hum Mol Genet 5: 115-121.
[59] Timchenko LT, Miller JW, Timchenko NA, DeVore DR, Datar KV, et al. (1996) Identification of a (CUG)n triplet repeat RNA-binding protein and its expression in myotonic dystrophy. Nucleic Acids Res 24: 4407-4414.
[60] Marquis J, Paillard L, Audic Y, Cosson B, Danos O, et al. (2006) CUG-BP1/CELF1 requires UGU-rich sequences for high-affinity binding. Biochem J 400: 291-301.
[61] Goraczniak R, Gunderson SI (2008) The regulatory element in the 3'-untranslated region of human papillomavirus 16 inhibits expression by binding CUG-binding protein 1. J Biol Chem 283: 2286-2296.
[62] Mori D, Sasagawa N, Kino Y, Ishiura S (2008) Quantitative analysis of CUG-BP1 binding to RNA repeats. J Biochem 143: 377-383.
[63] Suzuki H, Jin Y, Otani H, Yasuda K, Inoue K (2002) Regulation of alternative splicing of alpha-actinin transcript by Bruno-like proteins. Genes Cells 7: 133-141.
[64] Bonnet-Corven S, Audic Y, Omilli F, Osborne HB (2002) An analysis of the sequence requirements of EDEN-BP for specific RNA binding. Nucleic Acids Res 30: 4667-4674.
[65] Salisbury E, Sakai K, Schoser B, Huichalaf C, Schneider-Gold C, et al. (2008) Ectopic expression of cyclin D3 corrects differentiation of DM1 myoblasts through activation of RNA CUG-binding protein, CUGBP1. Exp Cell Res 314: 2266-2278.
[66] Cosson B, Gautier-Courteille C, Maniey D, Ait-Ahmed O, Lesimple M, et al. (2006) Oligomerization of EDEN-BP is required for specific mRNA deadenylation and binding. Biol Cell 98: 653-665.
[67] Wu C, Alwine JC (2004) Secondary structure as a functional feature in the downstream region of mammalian polyadenylation signals. Mol Cell Biol 24: 2789-2796.
[68] Mooers BH, Logue JS, Berglund JA (2005) The structural basis of myotonic dystrophy from the crystal structure of CUG repeats. Proc Natl Acad Sci U S A 102: 16626-16631.
[69] Ladd AN, Charlet N, Cooper TA (2001) The CELF family of RNA binding proteins is implicated in cell-specific and developmentally regulated alternative splicing. Mol Cell Biol 21: 1285-1296.
[70] Han J, Cooper TA (2005) Identification of CELF splicing activation and repression domains in vivo. Nucleic Acids Res 33: 2769-2780.

[71] Tsuda K, Kuwasako K, Takahashi M, Someya T, Inoue M, et al. (2009) Structural basis for the sequence-specific RNA-recognition mechanism of human CUG-BP1 RRM3. Nucleic Acids Res 37: 5151-5166.

[72] Edwards J, Malaurie E, Kondrashov A, Long J, de Moor CH, et al. (2011) Sequence determinants for the tandem recognition of UGU and CUG rich RNA elements by the two N--terminal RRMs of CELF1. Nucleic Acids Res 39: 8638-8650.

[73] Teplova M, Song J, Gaw HY, Teplov A, Patel DJ Structural insights into RNA recognition by the alternate-splicing regulator CUG-binding protein 1. Structure 18: 1364-1377.

[74] Roberts R, Timchenko NA, Miller JW, Reddy S, Caskey CT, et al. (1997) Altered phosphorylation and intracellular distribution of a (CUG)n triplet repeat RNA-binding protein in patients with myotonic dystrophy and in myotonin protein kinase knockout mice. Proc Natl Acad Sci U S A 94: 13221-13226.

[75] Kuyumcu-Martinez NM, Wang GS, Cooper TA (2007) Increased steady-state levels of CUGBP1 in myotonic dystrophy 1 are due to PKC-mediated hyperphosphorylation. Mol Cell 28: 68-78.

[76] Timchenko NA, Wang GL, Timchenko LT (2005) RNA CUG-binding protein 1 increases translation of 20-kDa isoform of CCAAT/enhancer-binding protein beta by interacting with the alpha and beta subunits of eukaryotic initiation translation factor 2. J Biol Chem 280: 20549-20557.

[77] Beisang D, Rattenbacher B, Vlasova-St Louis IA, Bohjanen PR (2012) Regulation of CUG-binding protein 1 (CUGBP1) binding to target transcripts upon T cell activation. J Biol Chem 287: 950-960.

[78] Orengo JP, Chambon P, Metzger D, Mosier DR, Snipes GJ, et al. (2008) Expanded CTG repeats within the DMPK 3' UTR causes severe skeletal muscle wasting in an inducible mouse model for myotonic dystrophy. Proc Natl Acad Sci U S A 105: 2646-2651.

[79] Wang GS, Kuyumcu-Martinez MN, Sarma S, Mathur N, Wehrens XH, et al. (2009) PKC inhibition ameliorates the cardiac phenotype in a mouse model of myotonic dystrophy type 1. J Clin Invest 119: 3797-3806.

[80] Schoser B, Timchenko L (2010) Myotonic dystrophies 1 and 2: complex diseases with complex mechanisms. Curr Genomics 11: 77-90.

[81] Huichalaf C, Sakai K, Jin B, Jones K, Wang GL, et al. (2010) Expansion of CUG RNA repeats causes stress and inhibition of translation in myotonic dystrophy 1 (DM1) cells. FASEB J 24: 3706-3719.

[82] Rattenbacher B, Beisang D, Wiesner DL, Jeschke JC, von Hohenberg M, et al. (2010) Analysis of CUGBP1 targets identifies GU-repeat sequences that mediate rapid mRNA decay. Mol Cell Biol 30: 3970-3980.

[83] Rattenbacher B, Beisang D, Wiesner DL, Jeschke JC, von Hohenberg M, et al. Analysis of CUGBP1 targets identifies GU-repeat sequences that mediate rapid mRNA decay. Mol Cell Biol 30: 3970-3980.

[84] Halees AS, Hitti E, Al-Saif M, Mahmoud L, Vlasova-St Louis IA, et al. (2011) Global assessment of GU-rich regulatory content and function in the human transcriptome. RNA Biol 8: 681-691.

[85] Graindorge A, Le Tonqueze O, Thuret R, Pollet N, Osborne HB, et al. (2008) Identification of CUG-BP1/EDEN-BP target mRNAs in Xenopus tropicalis. Nucleic Acids Res 36: 1861-1870.

[86] Le Tonqueze O, Gschloessl B, Namanda-Vanderbeken A, Legagneux V, Paillard L, et al. Chromosome wide analysis of CUGBP1 binding sites identifies the tetraspanin CD9 mRNA as a target for CUGBP1-mediated down-regulation. Biochem Biophys Res Commun 394: 884-889.

[87] Daughters RS, Tuttle DL, Gao W, Ikeda Y, Moseley ML, et al. (2009) RNA gain-of-function in spinocerebellar ataxia type 8. PLoS Genet 5: e1000600.

[88] Masuda A, Andersen HS, Doktor TK, Okamoto T, Ito M, et al. (2012) CUGBP1 and MBNL1 preferentially bind to 3' UTRs and facilitate mRNA decay. Sci Rep 2: 209.

[89] Pan Q, Shai O, Lee LJ, Frey BJ, Blencowe BJ (2008) Deep surveying of alternative splicing complexity in the human transcriptome by high-throughput sequencing. Nat Genet 40: 1413-1415.

[90] Wang ET, Sandberg R, Luo S, Khrebtukova I, Zhang L, et al. (2008) Alternative isoform regulation in human tissue transcriptomes. Nature 456: 470-476.

[91] Ladd AN, Cooper TA (2002) Finding signals that regulate alternative splicing in the post-genomic era. Genome Biol 3: reviews0008.

[92] Voelker RB, Berglund JA (2007) A comprehensive computational characterization of conserved mammalian intronic sequences reveals conserved motifs associated with constitutive and alternative splicing. Genome Res 17: 1023-1033.

[93] Dembowski JA, Grabowski PJ (2009) The CUGBP2 splicing factor regulates an ensemble of branchpoints from perimeter binding sites with implications for autoregulation. PLoS Genet 5: e1000595.

[94] Anant S, Henderson JO, Mukhopadhyay D, Navaratnam N, Kennedy S, et al. (2001) Novel role for RNA-binding protein CUGBP2 in mammalian RNA editing. CUGBP2 modulates C to U editing of apolipoprotein B mRNA by interacting with apobec-1 and ACF, the apobec-1 complementation factor. J Biol Chem 276: 47338-47351.

[95] Chen Z, Eggerman TL, Patterson AP (2007) ApoB mRNA editing is mediated by a coordinated modulation of multiple apoB mRNA editing enzyme components. Am J Physiol Gastrointest Liver Physiol 292: G53-65.

[96] Ladd AN, Taffet G, Hartley C, Kearney DL, Cooper TA (2005) Cardiac tissue-specific repression of CELF activity disrupts alternative splicing and causes cardiomyopathy. Mol Cell Biol 25: 6267-6278.

[97] Ho TH, Bundman D, Armstrong DL, Cooper TA (2005) Transgenic mice expressing CUG-BP1 reproduce splicing mis-regulation observed in myotonic dystrophy. Hum Mol Genet 14: 1539-1547.

[98] Philips AV, Timchenko LT, Cooper TA (1998) Disruption of splicing regulated by a CUG-binding protein in myotonic dystrophy. Science 280: 737-741.

[99] Savkur RS, Philips AV, Cooper TA (2001) Aberrant regulation of insulin receptor alternative splicing is associated with insulin resistance in myotonic dystrophy. Nat Genet 29: 40-47.

[100] Charlet BN, Savkur RS, Singh G, Philips AV, Grice EA, et al. (2002) Loss of the muscle-specific chloride channel in type 1 myotonic dystrophy due to misregulated alternative splicing. Mol Cell 10: 45-53.

[101] Mankodi A, Takahashi MP, Jiang H, Beck CL, Bowers WJ, et al. (2002) Expanded CUG repeats trigger aberrant splicing of ClC-1 chloride channel pre-mRNA and hyperexcitability of skeletal muscle in myotonic dystrophy. Mol Cell 10: 35-44.

[102] Ladd AN, Cooper TA (2004) Multiple domains control the subcellular localization and activity of ETR-3, a regulator of nuclear and cytoplasmic RNA processing events. J Cell Sci 117: 3519-3529.

[103] Gromak N, Matlin AJ, Cooper TA, Smith CW (2003) Antagonistic regulation of alpha-actinin alternative splicing by CELF proteins and polypyrimidine tract binding protein. RNA 9: 443-456.

[104] Charlet BN, Logan P, Singh G, Cooper TA (2002) Dynamic antagonism between ETR-3 and PTB regulates cell type-specific alternative splicing. Mol Cell 9: 649-658.

[105] Kino Y, Washizu C, Oma Y, Onishi H, Nezu Y, et al. (2009) MBNL and CELF proteins regulate alternative splicing of the skeletal muscle chloride channel CLCN1. Nucleic Acids Res 37: 6477-6490.

[106] Dujardin G, Buratti E, Charlet-Berguerand N, Martins de Araujo M, Mbopda A, et al. (2010) CELF proteins regulate CFTR pre-mRNA splicing: essential role of the divergent domain of ETR-3. Nucleic Acids Res 38: 7273-7285.

[107] Barron VA, Zhu H, Hinman MN, Ladd AN, Lou H (2010) The neurofibromatosis type I pre-mRNA is a novel target of CELF protein-mediated splicing regulation. Nucleic Acids Res 38: 253-264.

[108] Koebis M, Ohsawa N, Kino Y, Sasagawa N, Nishino I, et al. (2011) Alternative splicing of myomesin 1 gene is aberrantly regulated in myotonic dystrophy type 1. Genes Cells 16: 961-972.

[109] Terenzi F, Brimacombe KR, Penn MS, Ladd AN (2009) CELF-mediated alternative splicing is required for cardiac function during early, but not later, postnatal life. J Mol Cell Cardiol 46: 395-404.

[110] Berger DS, Moyer M, Kliment GM, van Lunteren E, Ladd AN (2011) Expression of a dominant negative CELF protein in vivo leads to altered muscle organization, fiber size, and subtype. PLoS One 6: e19274.

[111] Kalsotra A, Xiao X, Ward AJ, Castle JC, Johnson JM, et al. (2008) A postnatal switch of CELF and MBNL proteins reprograms alternative splicing in the developing heart. Proc Natl Acad Sci U S A 105: 20333-20338.

[112] Dasgupta T, Ladd AN (2012) The importance of CELF control: molecular and biological roles of the CUG-BP, Elav-like family of RNA-binding proteins. Wiley Interdiscip Rev RNA 3: 104-121.

[113] Orengo JP, Ward AJ, Cooper TA (2011) Alternative splicing dysregulation secondary to skeletal muscle regeneration. Ann Neurol 69: 681-690.

[114] Berger DS, Ladd AN (2012) Repression of nuclear CELF activity can rescue CELF-regulated alternative splicing defects in skeletal muscle models of myotonic dystrophy. PLoS Curr 4: RRN1305.

[115] Audic Y, Omilli F, Osborne HB (1998) Embryo deadenylation element-dependent deadenylation is enhanced by a cis element containing AUU repeats. Mol Cell Biol 18: 6879-6884.

[116] Richter JD, Lasko P (2011) Translational control in oocyte development. Cold Spring Harb Perspect Biol 3: a002758.

[117] Jackson RJ, Standart N (1990) Do the poly(A) tail and 3' untranslated region control mRNA translation? Cell 62: 15-24.

[118] Paillard L, Legagneux V, Maniey D, Osborne HB (2002) c-Jun ARE targets mRNA deadenylation by an EDEN-BP (embryo deadenylation element-binding protein)-dependent pathway. J Biol Chem 277: 3232-3235.

[119] Ezzeddine N, Paillard L, Capri M, Maniey D, Bassez T, et al. (2002) EDEN-dependent translational repression of maternal mRNAs is conserved between Xenopus and Drosophila. Proc Natl Acad Sci U S A 99: 257-262.

[120] Wilusz CJ, Wormington M, Peltz SW (2001) The cap-to-tail guide to mRNA turnover. Nat Rev Mol Cell Biol 2: 237-246.

[121] Chen CY, Shyu AB (2011) Mechanisms of deadenylation-dependent decay. Wiley Interdiscip Rev RNA 2: 167-183.

[122] Kim JH, Richter JD (2006) Opposing polymerase-deadenylase activities regulate cytoplasmic polyadenylation. Mol Cell 24: 173-183.

[123] Novoa I, Gallego J, Ferreira PG, Mendez R (2010) Mitotic cell-cycle progression is regulated by CPEB1 and CPEB4-dependent translational control. Nat Cell Biol 12: 447-456.

[124] Horb LD, Horb ME (2010) BrunoL1 regulates endoderm proliferation through translational enhancement of cyclin A2 mRNA. Dev Biol 345: 156-169.

[125] Nakamura A, Sato K, Hanyu-Nakamura K (2004) Drosophila cup is an eIF4E binding protein that associates with Bruno and regulates oskar mRNA translation in oogenesis. Dev Cell 6: 69-78.

[126] Barreau C, Watrin T, Beverley Osborne H, Paillard L (2006) Protein expression is increased by a class III AU-rich element and tethered CUG-BP1. Biochem Biophys Res Commun 347: 723-730.

[127] Timchenko NA, Iakova P, Cai ZJ, Smith JR, Timchenko LT (2001) Molecular basis for impaired muscle differentiation in myotonic dystrophy. Mol Cell Biol 21: 6927-6938.

[128] Timchenko NA, Patel R, Iakova P, Cai ZJ, Quan L, et al. (2004) Overexpression of CUG triplet repeat-binding protein, CUGBP1, in mice inhibits myogenesis. J Biol Chem 279: 13129-13139.

[129] Fox JT, Stover PJ (2009) Mechanism of the internal ribosome entry site-mediated translation of serine hydroxymethyltransferase 1. J Biol Chem 284: 31085-31096.

[130] Woeller CF, Fox JT, Perry C, Stover PJ (2007) A ferritin-responsive internal ribosome entry site regulates folate metabolism. J Biol Chem 282: 29927-29935.

[131] Zheng Y, Miskimins WK (2011) CUG-binding protein represses translation of p27Kip1 mRNA through its internal ribosomal entry site. RNA Biol 8: 365-371.

[132] Timchenko NA, Welm AL, Lu X, Timchenko LT (1999) CUG repeat binding protein (CUGBP1) interacts with the 5' region of C/EBPbeta mRNA and regulates translation of C/EBPbeta isoforms. Nucleic Acids Res 27: 4517-4525.

[133] Bae EJ, Kim SG (2005) Enhanced CCAAT/enhancer-binding protein beta-liver-enriched inhibitory protein production by Oltipraz, which accompanies CUG repeat-binding protein-1 (CUGBP1) RNA-binding protein activation, leads to inhibition of preadipocyte differentiation. Mol Pharmacol 68: 660-669.

[134] Karagiannides I, Thomou T, Tchkonia T, Pirtskhalava T, Kypreos KE, et al. (2006) Increased CUG triplet repeat-binding protein-1 predisposes to impaired adipogenesis with aging. J Biol Chem 281: 23025-23033.

[135] Jin J, Wang GL, Timchenko L, Timchenko NA (2009) GSK3beta and aging liver. Aging (Albany NY) 1: 582-585.

[136] Timchenko LT, Salisbury E, Wang GL, Nguyen H, Albrecht JH, et al. (2006) Age-specific CUGBP1-eIF2 complex increases translation of CCAAT/enhancer-binding protein beta in old liver. J Biol Chem 281: 32806-32819.

[137] Jones K, Timchenko L, Timchenko NA (2012) The role of CUGBP1 in age-dependent changes of liver functions. Ageing Res Rev.

[138] Iakova P, Wang GL, Timchenko L, Michalak M, Pereira-Smith OM, et al. (2004) Competition of CUGBP1 and calreticulin for the regulation of p21 translation determines cell fate. Embo J 23: 406-417.

[139] Lian XJ, Gallouzi IE (2009) Oxidative Stress Increases the Number of Stress Granules in Senescent Cells and Triggers a Rapid Decrease in p21waf1/cip1 Translation. J Biol Chem 284: 8877-8887.

[140] Fujimura K, Kano F, Murata M (2008) Dual localization of the RNA binding protein CUGBP-1 to stress granule and perinucleolar compartment. Exp Cell Res 314: 543-553.

[141] Vlasova IA, Bohjanen PR (2008) Posttranscriptional regulation of gene networks by GU-rich elements and CELF proteins. RNA Biol 5: 201-207.

[142] Le Tonqueze O, Gschloessl B, Namanda-Vanderbeken A, Legagneux V, Paillard L, et al. (2010) Chromosome wide analysis of CUGBP1 binding sites identifies the tetraspanin CD9 mRNA as a target for CUGBP1-mediated down-regulation. Biochem Biophys Res Commun 394: 884-889.

[143] Zhang L, Lee JE, Wilusz J, Wilusz CJ (2008) The RNA-binding protein CUGBP1 regulates stability of tumor necrosis factor mRNA in muscle cells: implications for Myotonic Dystrophy. J Biol Chem.

[144] Philips AV, Cooper TA (2000) RNA processing and human disease. Cell Mol Life Sci 57: 235-249.

[145] La Spada AR, Taylor JP (2010) Repeat expansion disease: progress and puzzles in disease pathogenesis. Nat Rev Genet 11: 247-258.

[146] Arnal-Estape A, Tarragona M, Morales M, Guiu M, Nadal C, et al. (2010) HER2 silences tumor suppression in breast cancer cells by switching expression of C/EBPss isoforms. Cancer Res 70: 9927-9936.

[147] Cibois M, Gautier-Courteille C, Vallee A, Paillard L (2010) A strategy to analyze the phenotypic consequences of inhibiting the association of an RNA-binding protein with a specific RNA. RNA 16: 10-15.

[148] Wang GS, Kearney DL, De Biasi M, Taffet G, Cooper TA (2007) Elevation of RNA-binding protein CUGBP1 is an early event in an inducible heart-specific mouse model of myotonic dystrophy. J Clin Invest 117: 2802-2811.

[149] Dansithong W, Wolf CM, Sarkar P, Paul S, Chiang A, et al. (2008) Cytoplasmic CUG RNA foci are insufficient to elicit key DM1 features. PLoS One 3: e3968.

[150] Koshelev M, Sarma S, Price RE, Wehrens XH, Cooper TA (2010) Heart-specific overexpression of CUGBP1 reproduces functional and molecular abnormalities of myotonic dystrophy type 1. Hum Mol Genet 19: 1066-1075.

[151] Leroy O, Wang J, Maurage CA, Parent M, Cooper T, et al. (2006) Brain-specific change in alternative splicing of Tau exon 6 in myotonic dystrophy type 1. Biochim Biophys Acta 1762: 460-467.

[152] Sofola OA, Jin P, Qin Y, Duan R, Liu H, et al. (2007) RNA-binding proteins hnRNP A2/B1 and CUGBP1 suppress fragile X CGG premutation repeat-induced neurodegeneration in a Drosophila model of FXTAS. Neuron 55: 565-571.

[153] Hino S, Kondo S, Sekiya H, Saito A, Kanemoto S, et al. (2007) Molecular mechanisms responsible for aberrant splicing of SERCA1 in myotonic dystrophy type 1. Hum Mol Genet 16: 2834-2843.

[154] Corbeil-Girard LP, Klein AF, Sasseville AM, Lavoie H, Dicaire MJ, et al. (2005) PABPN1 overexpression leads to upregulation of genes encoding nuclear proteins that are sequestered in oculopharyngeal muscular dystrophy nuclear inclusions. Neurobiol Dis 18: 551-567.

[155] Yu Z, Wang AM, Robins DM, Lieberman AP (2009) Altered RNA splicing contributes to skeletal muscle pathology in Kennedy disease knock-in mice. Dis Model Mech 2: 500-507.

[156] Cooper TA, Wan L, Dreyfuss G (2009) RNA and disease. Cell 136: 777-793.

[157] Starr TK, Allaei R, Silverstein KA, Staggs RA, Sarver AL, et al. (2009) A transposon-based genetic screen in mice identifies genes altered in colorectal cancer. Science 323: 1747-1750.

[158] Choi WT, Folsom MR, Azim MF, Meyer C, Kowarz E, et al. (2007) C/EBPbeta suppression by interruption of CUGBP1 resulting from a complex rearrangement of MLL. Cancer Genet Cytogenet 177: 108-114.

[159] Arnal-Estape A, Tarragona M, Morales M, Guiu M, Nadal C, et al. HER2 silences tumor suppression in breast cancer cells by switching expression of C/EBPss isoforms. Cancer Res 70: 9927-9936.

[160] Guerzoni C, Ferrari-Amorotti G, Bardini M, Mariani SA, Calabretta B (2006) Effects of C/EBPalpha and C/EBPbeta in BCR/ABL-expressing cells: differences and similarities. Cell Cycle 5: 1254-1257.

[161] Guerzoni C, Bardini M, Mariani SA, Ferrari-Amorotti G, Neviani P, et al. (2006) Inducible activation of CEBPB, a gene negatively regulated by BCR/ABL, inhibits

proliferation and promotes differentiation of BCR/ABL-expressing cells. Blood 107: 4080-4089.

[162] Wang GL, Salisbury E, Shi X, Timchenko L, Medrano EE, et al. (2008) HDAC1 cooperates with C/EBPalpha in the inhibition of liver proliferation in old mice. J Biol Chem.

[163] Wang GL, Salisbury E, Shi X, Timchenko L, Medrano EE, et al. (2008) HDAC1 promotes liver proliferation in young mice via interactions with C/EBP beta. J Biol Chem.

[164] Fournier MJ, Gareau C, Mazroui R (2010) The chemotherapeutic agent bortezomib induces the formation of stress granules. Cancer Cell Int 10: 12.

[165] Gareau C, Fournier MJ, Filion C, Coudert L, Martel D, et al. (2011) p21(WAF1/CIP1) upregulation through the stress granule-associated protein CUGBP1 confers resistance to bortezomib-mediated apoptosis. PLoS One 6: e20254.

[166] Iakova P, Timchenko L, Timchenko NA (2011) Intracellular signaling and hepatocellular carcinoma. Semin Cancer Biol 21: 28-34.

[167] Xiao L, Cui YH, Rao JN, Zou T, Liu L, et al. (2011) Regulation of cyclin-dependent kinase 4 translation through CUG-binding protein 1 and microRNA-222 by polyamines. Mol Biol Cell 22: 3055-3069.

[168] Cui YH, Xiao L, Rao JN, Zou T, Liu L, et al. (2012) miR-503 represses CUG-binding protein 1 translation by recruiting CUGBP1 mRNA to processing bodies. Mol Biol Cell 23: 151-162.

[169] Kalsotra A, Wang K, Li PF, Cooper TA (2010) MicroRNAs coordinate an alternative splicing network during mouse postnatal heart development. Genes Dev 24: 653-658.